# Behavioral and Mental Health Problems in Children

# Behavioral and Mental Health Problems in Children

Editor

**Tingzhong Yang**

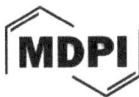

Basel • Beijing • Wuhan • Barcelona • Belgrade • Novi Sad • Cluj • Manchester

*Editor*
Tingzhong Yang
Zhejiang University
Hangzhou
China

*Editorial Office*
MDPI
St. Alban-Anlage 66
4052 Basel, Switzerland

This is a reprint of articles from the Special Issue published online in the open access journal *Children* (ISSN 2227-9067) (available at: https://www.mdpi.com/journal/children/special_issues/324PZ089H9).

For citation purposes, cite each article independently as indicated on the article page online and as indicated below:

Lastname, A.A.; Lastname, B.B. Article Title. *Journal Name* **Year**, *Volume Number*, Page Range.

**ISBN 978-3-7258-0181-7 (Hbk)**
**ISBN 978-3-7258-0182-4 (PDF)**
doi.org/10.3390/books978-3-7258-0182-4

© 2024 by the authors. Articles in this book are Open Access and distributed under the Creative Commons Attribution (CC BY) license. The book as a whole is distributed by MDPI under the terms and conditions of the Creative Commons Attribution-NonCommercial-NoDerivs (CC BY-NC-ND) license.

# Contents

**About the Editor** . . . . . . . . . . . . . . . . . . . . . . . . . . . . . . . . . . . . . . . . . . . . . . . . . . . . . . . . vii

**Preface** . . . . . . . . . . . . . . . . . . . . . . . . . . . . . . . . . . . . . . . . . . . . . . . . . . . . . . . . . . . . . . . . ix

**Tingzhong Yang and Dan Wu**
Behavioral and Mental Health Problems in Children
Reprinted from: *Children* **2023**, *10*, 1820, doi:10.3390/children10111820 . . . . . . . . . . . . . . . . . 1

**Gökçe Yağmur Efendi, Rahime Duygu Temeltürk, Işık Batuhan Çakmak and Mustafa Dinçer**
Surviving the Immediate Aftermath of a Disaster: A Preliminary Investigation of Adolescents' Acute Stress Reactions and Mental Health Needs after the 2023 Turkey Earthquakes
Reprinted from: *Children* **2023**, *10*, 1485, doi:10.3390/children10091485 . . . . . . . . . . . . . . . . 4

**Pornsiri Chatpreecha and Sasiporn Usanavasin**
Design of a Collaborative Knowledge Framework for Personalised Attention Deficit Hyperactivity Disorder (ADHD) Treatments
Reprinted from: *Children* **2023**, *10*, 1288, doi:10.3390/children10081288 . . . . . . . . . . . . . . . . 23

**Ruyu Liu, Ke Xu, Xingliang Zhang, Feng Cheng, Liangmin Gao and Junfang Xu**
HIV-Related Knowledge and Sexual Behaviors among Teenagers: Implications for Public Health Interventions
Reprinted from: *Children* **2023**, *10*, 1198, doi:10.3390/children10071198 . . . . . . . . . . . . . . . . 42

**Xiaozhao Yang and Chao Zhang**
Children's Health and Typology of Family Integration and Regulation: A Functionalist Analysis
Reprinted from: *Children* **2023**, *10*, 494, doi:10.3390/children10030494 . . . . . . . . . . . . . . . . . 53

**Chen-Ya Juan**
The Mealtime Behavior Problems of Children with Developmental Disabilities and the Teacher's Stress in Inclusive Preschools
Reprinted from: *Children* **2023**, *10*, 441, doi:10.3390/children10030441 . . . . . . . . . . . . . . . . . 63

**Ibrahim H. Acar, Sevval Nur Sezer, İlayda Uculas and Fatma Ozge Unsal**
Examining the Contributions of Parents' Daily Hassles and Parenting Approaches to Children's Behavior Problems during the COVID-19 Pandemic
Reprinted from: *Children* **2023**, *10*, 312, doi:10.3390/children10020312 . . . . . . . . . . . . . . . . . 75

**Yosi Yaffe**
Maternal and Paternal Authoritarian Parenting and Adolescents' Impostor Feelings: The Mediating Role of Parental Psychological Control and the Moderating Role of Child's Gender
Reprinted from: *Children* **2023**, *10*, 308, doi:10.3390/children10020308 . . . . . . . . . . . . . . . . . 87

**Rui Zhao, Jun Lv, Yan Gao, Yuyan Li, Huijing Shi, Junguo Zhang, et al.**
Association between Family Environment and Adolescents' Sexual Adaptability: Based on the Latent Profile Analysis of Personality Traits
Reprinted from: *Children* **2023**, *10*, 191, doi:10.3390/children10020191 . . . . . . . . . . . . . . . . . 101

**Biplab Kumar Datta, Ashwini Tiwari, Elinita Pollard and Havilah Ravula**
The Influence of Parent's Cardiovascular Morbidity on Child Mental Health: Results from the National Health Interview Survey
Reprinted from: *Children* **2023**, *10*, 138, doi:10.3390/children10010138 . . . . . . . . . . . . . . . . . 112

**Liuyue Huang, Junrun Huang, Zhichao Chen, Weiwei Jiang, Yi Zhu and Xinli Chi**
Psychometric Properties of the Chinese Version of the Brief Interpersonal Competence Questionnaire for Adolescents
Reprinted from: *Children* **2023**, *10*, 59, doi:10.3390/children10010059 . . . . . . . . . . . . . . . . . **123**

**Binyan Wang, Lihong Ye, Linshuoshuo Lv, Wei Liu, Fenfen Liu and Yingying Mao**
Psychological Resilience among Left-Behind Children in a Rural Area of Eastern China
Reprinted from: *Children* **2022**, *9*, 1899, doi:10.3390/children9121899 . . . . . . . . . . . . . . . . . **133**

**Nolwenn Dissaux, Pierre Neyme, Deok-Hee Kim-Dufor, Nathalie Lavenne-Collot, Jonathan J. Marsh, Sofian Berrouiguet, et al.**
Psychosis Caused by a Somatic Condition: How to Make the Diagnosis? A Systematic Literature Review
Reprinted from: *Children* **2023**, *10*, 1439, doi:10.3390/children10091439 . . . . . . . . . . . . . . . **147**

**Nathalie Lavenne-Collot, Nolwenn Dissaux, Nicolas Campelo, Charlotte Villalon, Guillaume Bronsard, Michel Botbol and David Cohen**
Sympathy-Empathy and the Radicalization of Young People
Reprinted from: *Children* **2022**, *9*, 1889, doi:10.3390/children9121889 . . . . . . . . . . . . . . . . . **175**

# About the Editor

**Tingzhong Yang**

Tingzhong Yang, is a Professor at and the Director of the Research Center for Digital Health Theory and Management at the National Health Big Data Institute of Zhejiang University; he is also a Distinguished Professor at the Women's Hospital of Zhejiang University School of Medicine. He was an advisor for the World Health Organization (WHO) with regard to delivering policy and programs on tobacco control to health profession students, and he served as an expert in updating the Chronic respiratory diseases (CRDs) section of the WHO Global Action Plan for the Prevention and Control of NCDs, 2013–2020. His primary academic focus is social and behavioral science in public health, and his research interests include tobacco control and mental stress. He has published more than 110 papers in peer-reviewed international journals. His research was officially reported on by the World Health Organization and was selected as one of the research highlights of the University at the celebration of the 120th anniversary of Zhejiang University . He has also published several books, including "Health Research: Social and Behavioral Theory and Methods" "Smoking Environments in China, Challenges for Tobacco Control", and "Mental Stress and Behavior Problems Among Special Groups: Social Resources, Influences on Health, and Reducing Health Inequities", as well as others. He was the Asian Editor for the American Journal of Health Behavior, and, currently, is the editor of the Global Journal of Social Sciences Studies.

# Preface

The stimulus, stress, and behavioral and mental response (SSB) model proposes that various stimuli induce stress and behavioral responses, which may, in turn, lead to health problems. In recent decades, many countries, especially some developing countries, have experienced rapid economic reform and social challenges. People in such a society, especially young parents, are under great mental stress to work and survive. Such stress can inadvertently influence their children's upbringing, potentially leading to significant behavioral and mental health concerns for their offspring. In particular, today's world is fraught with crisis and uncertainty. The Russian–Ukrainian and Israeli–Hamas wars are severe crises affecting the whole world, and they also impact global societal safety and economic stability. These situations pose a great challenge to child raising. Children are a vulnerable population who are in crisis. Approaches to address this problem need to be based on high-quality scientific research to understand the root causes and determine effective approaches to reduce behavioral and mental health problems. In order to achieve these goals, we proposed and published a new book, "Behavioral and Mental Health Problems in Children". In this book, 14 high-quality papers were published. It is truly a global collection of papers, with authors distributed across many countries, including the United States, France, China, Japan, Israel, and Thailand.

This book included two main sections. The first section aimed to provide a comprehensive understanding of the social and behavioral mechanisms leading to behavioral and mental health problems in children (BMPC). It covered some key issues related to BMPC, such as "Family integration, regulation and children's health", "The mealtime behavior problems of children", "Parents' daily hassles and parenting approaches to children's behavior problems", "Maternal and paternal authoritarian parenting and adolescents' impostor feelings", "Family environment and adolescents' sexual adaptability", "The influence of a parent's cardiovascular morbidity on a child's mental health", "Resilience among left-behind children", "Sympathy, empathy and the radicalization of young people", and "the acute stress symptoms in adolescents during the immediate post-earthquake period", as well as others. The second section aimed to develop behavioral and mental health promotion strategies and policy among children, referring to specialized policy research. The information obtained from these studies could be helpful in informing health policies, planning prevention strategies, and designing and implementing appropriate, targeted interventions, to help reduce behavioral and mental health problems in children. Many researchers have not only realized these challenges but have also put forward reasonable suggestions for policy and prevention applications. For example, Yang and Zhang posit that children with good health render it possible for a family to develop a concerted parent–child relationship, enabling families to function as unified entities. Such a finding calls for policymakers to consider the fact that children's health has consequences beyond medical and healthcare relevancy. Indeed, the health of children may be intrinsically linked to the function and vitality of familial structures and, by extension, the harmonious coexistence within a society marked by mutual solidarity and cohesion. Acar et al. underscore that interventions focusing on stress management may be effective in reducing daily parenting hassles, which may lead to a decrease in practicing negative parenting strategies and, in turn, lead to a reduction in children's behavior problems.

I believe that the new book has made a great contribution to research on BMPC, with studies that uncover social and behavioral mechanisms and put forward multidisciplinary approaches to policy application, as well as assisting in the design and implementation of effective intervention programs. The book is also beneficial for the dissemination of new knowledge and the promotion of children's mental health practices.

**Tingzhong Yang**
*Editor*

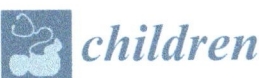 

*Editorial*

# Behavioral and Mental Health Problems in Children

Tingzhong Yang [1,2,*] and Dan Wu [3,4]

1. Women's Hospital, School of Medicine, Zhejiang University, Hangzhou 310058, China
2. Center for Tobacco Control Research, School of Medicine, Zhejiang University, Hangzhou 310058, China
3. School of Psychology, Shenzhen University, Shenzhen 518060, China; wudan.tracy@szu.edu.cn
4. Shenzhen Humanities & Social Sciences Key Research Bases of the Center for Mental Health, Shenzhen University, Shenzhen 518060, China
* Correspondence: tingzhongyang@zju.edu.cn

The stimulus, stress, and behavioral and mental response (SSB) model proposes that various stimuli induce stress and behavioral responses, which may, in turn, lead to health problems [1]. In recent decades, many countries, especially several developing countries, have experienced rapid economic development and social change. This accelerated pace of societal development and transformation invariably escalates social competition, placing considerable mental stress on the youth. Such stress can inadvertently influence their upbringing, potentially leading to significant behavioral and mental health concerns for their offspring. In particular, today's world is fraught with crisis and uncertainty. The Russian–Ukrainian and Israeli–Hamas wars are a severe crisis affecting the whole world, and they also impact global societal safety and economic stability. In recent years, the COVID-19 pandemic has not only directly led to behavioral and mental health problems in children but also greatly complicated the life and work of young parents. This poses a significant challenge to child raising and development. Children, inherently a vulnerable demographic, are at the epicenter of these crises. Many studies found that behavioral and mental problems occur in children and adolescents globally, especially in developing countries [2,3]. Given the overt nature of these issues, they may affect children's development, and the consequences can be lasting, potentially correlating with mental disorders persisting into adulthood. Children's behavioral and mental problems have become a serious social and public health problem. Governments and social health and service organizations around the world must give sufficient attention and take actionable measures to address these problems.

Numerous studies have identified several risk factors related to behavioral and mental problems of young children, including families' low socioeconomic status, family dysfunction, physical or psychological abuse, traumatic experiences, and parenting problems [4–7]. However, the majority of prior research only provides a general description of the demographic characteristics and their associations. Such studies cannot propose substantive prevention and control strategies. Additionally, the methodology and outcomes of numerous studies have failed to yield direct evidence aimed at mitigating the long-term persistence and potential exacerbation of such behavioral and mental disturbances into adulthood [8]. Approaches to address this deficiency need to be based on high-quality scientific research to understand the root causes and determine effective strategies to reduce behavioral and mental health problems. In order to achieve these goals, we proposed and published a Special Issue, "Behavioral and Mental Health Problems in Children", in the journal "*Children*". In this Special Issue, 13 papers were published, and we are pleased to find that many high-quality papers appeared in the issue. It is truly a global collection of papers, with authors distributed across many countries, including the United States, France, China, Japan, Israel, and Thailand. These studies cover some key issues related to children's behavioral and psychological problems, such as "Family integration, regulation and children's health", "The mealtime behavior problems of children", "Parents' daily

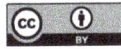

hassles and parenting approaches to children's behavior problems", "Maternal and paternal authoritarian parenting and adolescents' impostor feelings", "Family environment and adolescents' sexual adaptability", "The influence of parent's cardiovascular morbidity on child mental health", "Resilience among left-behind children", "Sympathy-empathy and the radicalization of young people", and "the acute stress symptoms in adolescents during the immediate post-earthquake period".

These papers provided a comprehensive understanding of the social and behavioral mechanisms leading to behavioral and mental health problems in children. The information obtained from these studies could be helpful in informing health policy; planning prevention strategies; and designing and implementing appropriate, targeted interventions to help reduce behavioral and mental health problems in children. Many researchers have not only realized these challenges but have also put forward reasonable suggestions for policy and prevention applications.

In this Special Issue, Yang and Zhang posit that children with good health render it possible for a family to develop a concerted parent–child relationship, enabling families to function as unified entities (contribution 1). Such a finding calls for policymakers to consider that children's health has consequences beyond medical and healthcare relevancy. Indeed, the health of children may be intrinsically linked to the function and vitality of familial structures and, by extension, the harmonious coexistence within a society marked by mutual solidarity and cohesion.

Acar et al. underscore that interventions focusing on stress management may be effective in reducing daily parenting hassles, which may lead to a decrease in practicing negative parenting strategies and, in turn, lead to a reduction in children's behavior problems (contribution 2).

Efendi and his collaborators revealed striking results in demonstrating the need for the careful evaluation of adolescents, who, despite the absence of tangible physical injuries, may exhibit signs of acute stress disorder (contribution 3). Moreover, the research emphasizes the importance of attentive consideration of the psychiatric complaints from adolescents who are willing to seek mental health assistance.

Areas for further efforts: A key issue is that some current studies are not designed from any strong theoretical model, particularly those seeking to elucidate the determinants of people's behavior. This hinders a deeper understanding of children's behavior and mental problems, signifying an avenue for scholarly enhancement. To the best of our knowledge, some papers still lack an in-depth and comprehensive overview. In terms of the social and behavioral mechanisms of behavioral and mental problems among children, these particular papers did not delve deep into the core of the matter, which is not very helpful for understanding the real world and solving problems [9]. Further studies need to provide root causes with an understanding of the social and behavioral mechanisms leading to behavioral and mental problems among children.

One objective of this issue is to disseminate knowledge of holistic, multidisciplinary approaches to policy application and to assist in the design and implementation of effective intervention programs. It must be mentioned that some research is not very targeted and is not designed according to the need to reduce behavioral and mental health problems in the current literature. Furthermore, few intervention studies aimed at resolving problems have been implemented. Further research is needed to overcome this shortcoming.

**Author Contributions:** T.Y. wrote the draft, and D.W. edited and revised the editorial. All authors have read and agreed to the published version of the manuscript.

**Funding:** This research received no external funding.

**Conflicts of Interest:** The authors declare no conflict of interest.

**List of Contributions**

1. Yang, X.; Zhang, C. Children's health and typology of family integration and regulation: A functionalist analysis. *Children* **2023**, *10*, 494. https://doi.org/10.3390/children10030494.
2. Acar, I.H.; Sezer, S.N.; Uculas, İ.; Unsal, F.O. Examining the contributions of parents' daily hassles and parenting approaches to children's behavior problems during the COVID-19 pandemic. *Children* **2023**, *10*, 312. https://doi.org/10.3390/children10020312.
3. Efendi, G.Y.; Temeltürk, R.D.; Çakmak, I.B.; Dinçer, M. Surviving the immediate aftermath of a disaster: A preliminary investigation of adolescents' acute stress reactions and mental health needs after the 2023 Turkey earthquakes. *Children* **2023**, *10*, 1485. https://doi.org/10.3390/children10091485.

**References**

1. Cottrell, R.R.; McKenzie, J.F. *Health Promotion & Education Research Methods*, 2nd ed.; Jones & Bartlett Publishers: Boston, MA, USA, 2011.
2. Kieling, C.; Baker-Henningham, H.; Belfer, M.; Conti, G.; Ertem, I.; Omigbodun, O.; Rohde, L.A.; Srinath, S.; Ulkuer, N.; Rahman, A. Child and adolescent mental health worldwide: Evidence for action. *Lancet* **2011**, *378*, 1515–1525. [CrossRef] [PubMed]
3. Polanczyk, G.V.; Salum, G.A.; Sugaya, L.S.; Caye, A.; Rohde, L.A. Annual research review: A meta-analysis of the worldwide prevalence of mental disorders in children and adolescents. *J. Child Psychol. Psychiatry* **2015**, *56*, 345–365. [CrossRef] [PubMed]
4. Van Oort, F.V.; Van Der Ende, J.; Wadsworth, M.E.; Verhulst, F.C.; Achenbach, T.M. Cross-national comparison of the link between socioeconomic status and emotional and behavioral problems in youths. *Soc. Psychiatry Psychiatr. Epidemiol.* **2011**, *46*, 167–172. [CrossRef] [PubMed]
5. Peters, R.; McMahon, R. *The Effect of Parental Dysfunction on Children*; Kluwer Academic: New York, NY, USA, 2002.
6. Norman, R.E.; Byambaa, M.; De, R.; Butchart, A.; Scott, J.; Vos, T. The long-term health consequences of child physical abuse, emotional abuse, and neglect: A systematic review and meta-analysis. *PLoS Med.* **2012**, *9*, e1001349. [CrossRef] [PubMed]
7. Perry, B.D. Stress, Trauma and Post-Traumatic Stress Disorders in Children. *Child Trauma Acad.* **2007**, *17*, 42–57. Available online: https://naturalstatecounselingcenters.com/wp-content/uploads/2020/04/PTSD_Intro_Perry_1.pdf (accessed on 14 September 2023).
8. Mulraney, M.; Coghill, D.; Bishop, C.; Mehmed, Y.; Sciberras, E.; Sawyer, M.; Efron, D.; Hiscock, H. A systematic review of the persistence of childhood mental health problems into adulthood. *Neurosci. Biobehav. Rev.* **2021**, *129*, 182–205. [CrossRef] [PubMed]
9. Yang, T. Constructing and testing for validation of social structure behavior theory and it's cross-level models. *Med. Res. Front.* **2023**, *2*, 175–182. [CrossRef]

**Disclaimer/Publisher's Note:** The statements, opinions and data contained in all publications are solely those of the individual author(s) and contributor(s) and not of MDPI and/or the editor(s). MDPI and/or the editor(s) disclaim responsibility for any injury to people or property resulting from any ideas, methods, instructions or products referred to in the content.

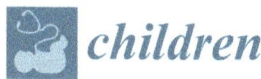 

Article

# Surviving the Immediate Aftermath of a Disaster: A Preliminary Investigation of Adolescents' Acute Stress Reactions and Mental Health Needs after the 2023 Turkey Earthquakes

Gökçe Yağmur Efendi [1,*], Rahime Duygu Temeltürk [2], Işık Batuhan Çakmak [3] and Mustafa Dinçer [1]

[1] Department of Child and Adolescent Psychiatry, Şanlıurfa Mehmet Akif İnan Training and Research Hospital, Şanlıurfa 63500, Türkiye; dincermustafamd@gmail.com
[2] Department of Child and Adolescent Psychiatry, Ankara University, Ankara 06490, Türkiye; rduygukaydok@gmail.com
[3] Department of Psychiatry, Sungurlu State Hospital, Çorum 19300, Türkiye; batuhancakmak@hotmail.com
* Correspondence: gokceefendi@gmail.com

Citation: Efendi, G.Y.; Temeltürk, R.D.; Çakmak, I.B.; Dinçer, M. Surviving the Immediate Aftermath of a Disaster: A Preliminary Investigation of Adolescents' Acute Stress Reactions and Mental Health Needs after the 2023 Turkey Earthquakes. *Children* **2023**, *10*, 1485. https://doi.org/10.3390/children10091485

Academic Editor: Tingzhong Yang

Received: 1 August 2023
Revised: 23 August 2023
Accepted: 28 August 2023
Published: 31 August 2023

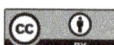

Copyright: © 2023 by the authors. Licensee MDPI, Basel, Switzerland. This article is an open access article distributed under the terms and conditions of the Creative Commons Attribution (CC BY) license (https://creativecommons.org/licenses/by/4.0/).

**Abstract:** On 6 February, southeastern Turkey and parts of Syria were struck by two powerful earthquakes, one measuring a magnitude of 7.8 and the other, nine hours later, at a magnitude of 7.5. These earthquakes have been recorded as some of the deadliest natural disasters worldwide since the 2010 Haiti earthquake, impacting around 14 million people in Turkey. For trauma survivors, the stressors associated with an event can lead to the development of acute stress disorder (ASD) or other psychiatric disorders. Trauma experiences during adolescence can impact development and affect adolescents differently than adults. Although ASD in adults has been addressed in several studies, there is much less information available about how younger populations respond to acute stress. The aim of our study was to assess the occurrence of ASD among individuals seeking help at the Şanlıurfa Mehmet Akif İnan Research and Training Hospital Child and Adolescent Outpatient Clinic following the 2023 Turkey Earthquakes and the factors associated with acute stress reactions. A child and adolescent psychiatry specialist conducted psychiatric interviews with the adolescents, and the individuals were also asked to complete 'The National Stressful Events Survey Acute Stress Disorder Short Scale' (NSESSS) to evaluate acute stress symptoms. ASD diagnoses were established according to the Diagnostic and Statistical Manual of Mental Disorders, Fifth Edition (DSM-5) criteria. Results showed that 81.6% of the participants ($n = 49$) were diagnosed with ASD, and drug treatment was initiated in 61.7% of the cases ($n = 37$). It was determined that ASD rates did not differ according to gender, and patients without physical injury had higher acute stress symptom scores ($p > 0.05$). According to the logistic regression models, paternal educational levels and adolescents' own requests for psychiatric assistance were predictors of acute stress disorder (OR 10.1, $β = 2.31$, $p = 0.006$ and OR 16.9, 95 $β = 2.83$, $p = 0.001$, respectively). Our findings revealed striking results in demonstrating the need for careful evaluation of adolescents without physical injury in terms of acute stress disorder and the need to pay close attention to the psychiatric complaints of adolescents willing to seek mental health assistance. Moreover, our study suggests that the proportion of adolescents experiencing acute stress symptoms after earthquakes might be higher than previously reported. Estimation of the incidence rate and symptoms of psychiatric distress in the short-term period following a disaster is important for establishing disaster epidemiology and implementing efficient relief efforts in the early stages. The outcomes of this study have the potential to yield novel insights into the realms of disaster mental health and emergency response policies, as well as their pragmatic implementations.

**Keywords:** acute stress disorder (ASD); earthquake; psychological needs

## 1. Introduction

In the early hours of 6 February, a powerful 7.8-magnitude earthquake struck southeastern Turkey and some parts of Syria. This was then followed by another 7.5-magnitude quake nine hours later, accompanied by over 200 aftershocks [1]. The first Pazarcık-centered earthquake was felt across a vast geography, including Turkey and Syria, as well as Lebanon, Cyprus, Iraq, Israel, Jordan, Iran, and Egypt. The two major earthquakes caused damage to an area of approximately 350,000 km$^2$, affecting approximately 14 million people in Turkey, who constituted 16% of Turkey's population [2]. These earthquakes, which occurred on the Eastern Anatolian Fault Line, caused a devastating impact, with over 50,000 people losing their lives in 11 provinces [3]. These earthquakes have also been recorded as some of the deadliest worldwide since the 2010 Haiti earthquake [4].

In the past two decades, natural disasters have resulted in millions of deaths worldwide, and hundreds of millions of people have suffered from various traumas [5]. These global disasters are characterized by their unpredictability and severity, encompassing a range of events, like earthquakes, nuclear meltdowns, pandemics, and food crises. Such catastrophic events frequently yield abrupt and overwhelming physical or psychological harm to populations, which can incite significant emotional distress and psychopathology [6]. For trauma survivors, the stressors associated with an event can lead to the development of acute stress disorder (ASD) and posttraumatic stress disorder (PTSD) or a number of other psychiatric disorders [7]. Researchers have extensively studied the psychological aftermath of natural disasters. Various studies have suggested that the percentage of individuals with psychiatric disorders could be as high as 60%, and PTSD rates might reach up to 74% following such events. However, findings have varied significantly between studies [8,9].

Childhood and adolescence are recognized as vulnerable periods for postdisaster psychological morbidity. For adolescents, experiencing trauma is especially significant, given the substantial physical and emotional growth during this phase. The stressors that adolescent encounters help shape their development and perspective and can have long-lasting impacts [10]. Traumatic events can influence the nervous and endocrine systems, even leading to structural changes in the brain due to severe stress [11]. Adolescence is also a time of social and emotional development. Trauma during this stage can result in social isolation, poor academic performance, and behavioral issues, all of which can impact both the current and future quality of life [12].

When a child or adolescent experiences a traumatic event, they may exhibit a variety of emotional responses [13,14]. While acute stress reactions in adults have been extensively studied, the understanding of how younger individuals respond to acute stress remains limited, as research has primarily concentrated on adults [15,16]. A recent meta-analysis examining acute stress disorder in children and adolescents evaluating 17 different studies reported that the evidence base is still quite limited and highly heterogeneous [17]. Recently, there has been a rise in studies focusing on acute stress symptoms among children and adolescents [18]. However, only a limited number of published investigations have explored acute stress symptoms in children and adolescents in relation to earthquake injuries [19].

ASD was introduced into the DSM-IV to describe acute stress reactions (ASRs) occurring in the initial month after exposure to a traumatic event and before the possibility of diagnosing PTSD and to identify trauma survivors in the acute phase who are at high risk for PTSD [20]. The diagnostic criteria underwent multiple changes with the introduction of the DSM-5 in 2013, and ASD was moved from the anxiety disorders category to a newly created one (i.e., trauma- and stressor-related disorders) to distinguish its characteristics further. Additionally, in contrast to DSM-IV, the diagnosis of ASD in DSM-5 no longer necessitates the presence of dissociative symptoms. While the accuracy of predicting subsequent PTSD cases is moderate, diagnosing ASD would be beneficial in acute trauma situations to identify individuals who may benefit from early interventions or ongoing monitoring [21].

In the aftermath of a disaster, it is common for the focus to be on fulfilling the community's material and physical needs. Unfortunately, this can cause the psychological needs of children to be overlooked. To ensure their wellbeing, it is crucial to incorporate child mental healthcare into public health interventions for emergencies and disasters. To address the needs of children and adolescents after a natural disaster, it is crucial to assess their mental wellbeing and psychiatric symptoms during the acute phase after a disaster. Understanding and responding to disasters is crucial, and conducting research might provide valuable insights. It is essential to establish disaster mental health systems and capabilities in advance to ensure a swift response during the initial stages of such events.

Estimation of the incidence rate and course of psychiatric distress in the short-term period following a disaster is important for establishing disaster epidemiology and implementing practical relief efforts in the early stages [22]. The aim of our study was to assess the psychological distress and the occurrence of acute stress disorder among individuals seeking help at the Şanlıurfa Mehmet Akif İnan Training and Research Hospital following the 2023 Turkey Earthquakes. Furthermore, we explored sociodemographic, clinical, and event-related factors that could potentially correlate with acute stress reactions.

The main objective of this study was to examine the acute stress symptoms in adolescents during the immediate postearthquake period following the devastating Turkey earthquakes in 2023. Additionally, building on prior research, we aimed to assess certain risk factors that might potentially make earthquake survivors more susceptible to developing ASD. These factors encompassed variables such as bodily injuries, the educational backgrounds of adolescents and their parents, and the gender of the patients. The outcomes of this study are expected to provide valuable insights for informing policy formulation, enhancing disaster readiness protocols, and advancing mental health intervention strategies within Turkey and across global contexts.

## 2. Materials and Methods

### 2.1. Data Collection

Following the earthquake on 6 February 2023, child and adolescent psychiatry clinics in hospitals across several impacted provinces faced disruptions in their services for varying durations. The hospital where this study took place was located in Şanlıurfa, one of the affected provinces. However, the hospital building remained undamaged, allowing the child and adolescent psychiatry clinic to open its doors to all patients seeking psychiatric assessment without requiring an appointment in the aftermath of the earthquake.

During the immediate aftermath of the earthquake, the principal investigator, who had not personally experienced the earthquake and was outside the city at the time of the incident, assumed responsibility for child and adolescent psychiatry outpatient services upon returning to Şanlıurfa. In contrast, the remaining child and adolescent psychiatrists at the hospital were unable to provide outpatient services for two weeks due to their direct exposure to the traumatic event. They had to deal primarily with their own vital needs and survival. While other child and adolescent psychiatrists resumed their duties after two weeks, the principal investigator continued to conduct psychiatric interviews for adolescents seeking help at the outpatient clinic. Other team members focused on providing assistance in different areas to children and adolescents affected by the earthquake, such as providing consultations for inpatients being treated for their injuries and providing families with education about the psychological effects of disasters.

Our study included children and adolescents aged 11–17 years who sought treatment between 7 February and 7 March 2023 at the Child and Adolescent Psychiatry Outpatient Clinic of Şanlıurfa Mehmet Akif İnan Training and Research Hospital. The study focused on evaluating the symptoms of patients who sought help within a month after the earthquake, as the primary goal of our study was to assess the psychiatric symptoms in children during the acute period following the traumatic experience. The reason for evaluating the symptoms of adolescents aged 11–17 in our study was to assess patients experiencing similar developmental stages.

A child and adolescent psychiatry specialist conducted psychiatric interviews with the patients, and diagnostic evaluations were based on the DSM-5 manual. Sociodemographic data forms evaluating the patients' experiences during and after the earthquake (accommodation in a place other than home, loss of housing, etc.) were completed by the parents of the patients and placed in the patient files. Adolescents aged 11–17 were also asked to fill out the DSM-5 'Severity of Acute Stress Symptoms National Stressful Events Survey Acute Stress Disorder Short Scale—Child Age 11–17' (NSESSS) form to measure the severity of acute stress symptoms of the patients and to be used in follow-ups.

Ethics approval was secured from Harran University's committee. Patient data were retrospectively collected following proper procedures. Since the Turkish Ministry of Health requested that an additional document called the 'disaster notification form' be filled out in addition to the applications of the earthquake victims, the patient files were kept in great detail. The treating physician reopened patient files to extract data for research purposes, and the data were used solely for the research, providing that results would be published in a way that did not allow patients' identification. The participants and their families were contacted and informed about the study, and their permissions were obtained. The patient files of all adolescents aged 11–17 who applied to the Child and Adolescent Psychiatry Clinic within the specified period after the earthquake were analyzed. A convenience sampling method was utilized, as all suitable cases were included over a specific time frame. There were no exclusion criteria for our study except for missing information in the patient files. Out of the 72 patients aged 11–17 who sought treatment at our outpatient clinic in the first month after the earthquake, 12 were excluded due to incomplete information in their files and forms. Missing data from the 12 excluded files were not included in the analysis.

*2.2. Measurements and Procedures*

The sociodemographic questionnaire was created by experts in the field of medicine, specifically child and adolescent psychiatrists, and included questions about demographic information and the adolescents' experience of the earthquake. Our clinic routinely employs a standard sociodemographic form to ensure comprehensive patient records. Questions about earthquake experience were added to this form after the earthquake. Demographic information obtained included data such as the age and gender of the children, whether the children continued to formal education, the educational status of the child, the education and employment status of the parents, and whether the parents were divorced. The questionnaire asked adolescents about their experiences during and after the earthquake, including whether they had lost a family member or friend, suffered injuries, or had their house destroyed. The sociodemographic form also included questions about the mental health services that adolescents required following the earthquake.

A brief ASD screening tool, the DSM-5 'Severity of Acute Stress Symptoms National Stressful Events Survey Acute Stress Disorder Short Scale—Child Age 11–17' (NSESSS), was used to screen for the presence of ASD symptoms and their severity. The NSESSS is designed to be used in the initial evaluation and treatment of children and adolescents diagnosed with acute stress disorder or individuals with acute stress disorder symptoms. This 7-item measure is designed to be completed by the child, and each item of the scale asks the child to rate the severity of their acute stress disorder during the past seven days. The total score can range from 0 to 28, with higher scores indicating greater severity of acute stress disorder. The average total score reduces the overall score to a 5-point scale, which allows the clinician to think of the severity of the child's acute stress disorder in terms of none (0), mild (1), moderate (2), severe (3), or extreme (4) [23]. A Turkish validity and reliability study of the scale was conducted by Sapmaz et al. in 2017, and it was shown that the Turkish version of the scale can be used reliably and validly, both in clinical practice and research [24].

Our hospital's Child and Adolescent Psychiatry Clinic started to provide service again on the fourth day after the earthquake. Service was provided to all patients who applied during the first month after the earthquake, including those without an appointment. First, a child and adolescent psychiatrist filled out the patients' sociodemographic forms by directing questions to the patients, and this process took approximately 10 min. Subsequently, adolescents were given an NSESSS form to fill out, which took about 5 min. Following this, the same doctor carried out psychiatric evaluations of the patients. The duration of these interviews varied but generally spanned between 40 min and an hour. On average, the evaluation of a single patient took about an hour. The information obtained was stored in the patients' electronic files on the hospital's computer system. A retrospective review of the patients' records was performed by the physician who also performed psychiatric evaluations of the patients.

*2.3. Statistical Analysis*

The sample size of the study was determined utilizing the G*Power 3.1 program [25]. A previous study examining the diagnosis and symptoms of acute stress disorder in children under 18 in Turkey after the 1999 Marmara earthquake was used as a reference. In this study, 74.5% of the children who experienced the earthquake were diagnosed with ASD [26]. With a Type-I error set at 0.05 and a targeted test power of $1 - \beta = 0.80$, the required sample size for statistical analysis was calculated as 54.

The Statistical Package for the Social Sciences (SPSS) version 23.0 program package was used for the statistical analysis of the data. Descriptive data were presented as numbers and percentages for categorical variables (e.g., sociodemographic features, psychiatric symptoms, ASD diagnosis) and means and standard deviations represented numerical data (e.g., age, scale item scores). The Shapiro–Wilk test was used to determine the normality of data distribution. NSESSS scale scores comparisons among groups (divided into groups such as according to the reasons for applying to the child psychiatry clinic and according to gender) were analyzed using the Mann–Whitney U test because of the non-normal data distribution. Chi-squared and Fisher's exact tests were used for the categorical variables, and a binary logistic regression model was conducted. All tests were two-tailed with a significance threshold of 0.05.

## 3. Results

*3.1. Sociodemographic and Clinical Characteristics of Cases*

The sociodemographic and clinical characteristics of the children are presented in Table 1. Upon examination of 16 adolescents with a family history of psychiatric illness, it was found that eight had psychiatric disorders in their mothers, four in their fathers, and four in their siblings. The most common psychiatric diagnosis was depression among parents. In contrast, psychotic disorders were the most common diagnoses in siblings.

Before the earthquake, 20 adolescents (33.3%) had consulted the Child and Adolescent Psychiatry Outpatient Clinic for support, while 40 (66.7%) had never sought psychiatric assistance. Among the 20 adolescents who had applied to child psychiatry before, 20% ($n = 4$) had attention deficit hyperactivity disorder, 20% ($n = 4$) had depressive disorder, 15% ($n = 3$) had anxiety disorder, and 15% had ($n = 3$) substance use disorder. Additionally, 15 ($n = 3$) of the patients who had previously sought psychiatric help were not formally diagnosed. It was found that 14 of the patients who had previously sought psychiatric assistance were using psychiatric drugs. The most frequently used drug combination was the combination of a selective serotonin reuptake inhibitor and an antipsychotic.

Table 1. Sociodemographic and clinical characteristics of cases.

| Sociodemographic Variables | Participants (n = 60) Mean ± SD (Min–Max)/n (%) |
|---|---|
| Gender | |
| Female | 37 (61.7) |
| Male | 23 (38.3) |
| Age (years) | 13.73 ± 1.86 (11–17) |
| Attending Formal Education | |
| Yes | 50 (83.3) |
| No | 10 (16.7) |
| Maternal Education, n (%) | |
| Literate | 17 (28.33) |
| Primary school | 24 (40) |
| Secondary school | 5 (8.33) |
| High school | 10 (16.66) |
| College degree or higher | 4 (6.66) |
| Paternal Education, n (%) | |
| Literate | 2 (3.33) |
| Primary school | 31 (51.66) |
| Secondary school | 4 (6.66) |
| High school | 16 (26.66) |
| College degree or higher | 7 (11.66) |
| Maternal Occupation, n (%) | |
| Housewife | 57 (95) |
| Laborer | 2 (3.3) |
| Civil servant | 1 (1.7) |
| Paternal Occupation, n (%) | |
| Unemployed | 6 (10) |
| Laborer | 27 (45) |
| Civil servant | 8 (13.3) |
| Tradesman | 14 (23.3) |
| Farmer | 5 (8.3) |
| Family Type, n (%) | |
| Parents married and living together | 54 (90) |
| Single-parent family | 6 (10) |
| Number of Siblings | 2.81 ± 1.45 (0–6) |
| Presence of Individuals with Psychopathology in the Family | |
| Absent | 44 (73.3) |
| Present | 16 (26.7) |

SD: Standard deviation; Min: minimum; Max: maximum.

*3.2. Earthquake-Related Experiences of the Cases*

The experiences of children and adolescents related to the earthquake are given in Table 2. Additionally, upon examining the cases who lost family members in the earthquake, it was found that three had lost one parent, six had lost both parents and siblings, two had lost grandparents, and five had lost cousins.

Out of the total number of cases, 45 (75%) reported that their most distressing experience related to the earthquake was during the event itself. The remaining 15 (25%) found the media coverage and the images they saw afterward more unsettling than the actual earthquake.

Psychiatric symptoms of the patients after the earthquake are shown in Figure 1.

Table 2. Earthquake-related experiences of the cases.

| Earthquake-Related Experiences | Participants (n = 60) n (%) |
|---|---|
| City of Residence | |
| Şanlıurfa | 43 (71.7) |
| Other cities | 17 (28.3) |
| Migration to Another City After the Earthquake | |
| Yes | 20 (33.3) |
| No | 40 (66.7) |
| Accommodation Outside the Home After the Earthquake (Ever) | |
| Yes | 54 (90) |
| No | 6 (10) |
| Accommodation Outside the Home After the Earthquake (Still at the Time of Evaluation) | |
| Yes | 22 (36.7) |
| No | 38 (63.3) |
| Damage Status of the House | |
| No damage | 20 (33.3) |
| Slightly damaged | 22 (36.7) |
| Medium–heavy damaged | 3 (5) |
| Collapsed in the earthquake | 15 (25) |
| Loss of Family Members in the Earthquake | |
| No | 44 (73.3) |
| Yes | 16 (26.7) |
| First-degree relatives | 9 (15) |
| Others | 7 (11.7) |

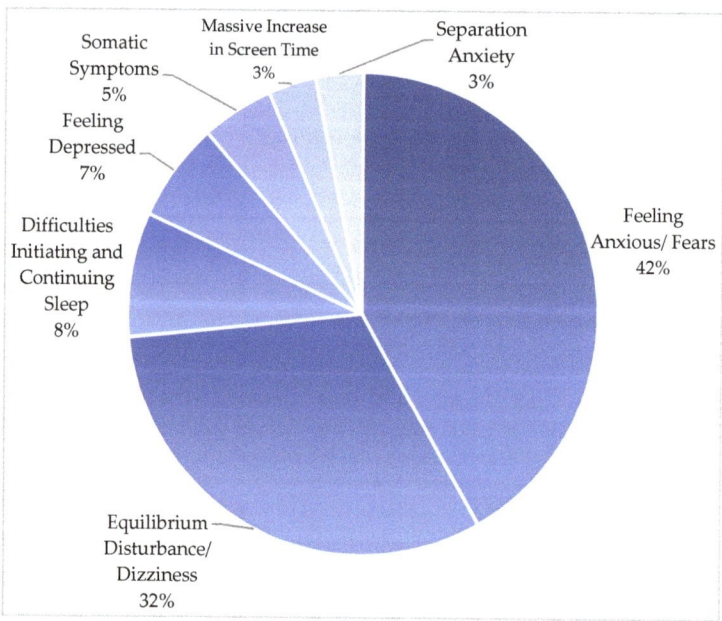

Figure 1. Psychiatric symptoms of the cases.

When the cases were examined regarding whether they had physical damage related to the earthquake, 46 (76.7%) of the cases had no bodily damage, 10 (16.66%) had a bone fracture, 2 (3.33%) had limb amputation, and 2 (3.33%) was found to have lung contusion.

### 3.3. ASD Diagnosis and Pharmacological Treatments

During evaluations at the Child and Adolescent Outpatient Clinic following the earthquake, 49 (81.6%) of the cases received an ASD diagnosis. Of the remaining 11 (18.3%) cases, all exhibited acute stress symptoms but did not meet the DSM-5 criteria for an ASD diagnosis. Among the 49 patients diagnosed with ASD, 38 (77.5%) had solely ASD without any other coexisting conditions. Additionally, nine patients (18.3%) were diagnosed with both ASD and anxiety disorder, while two patients (4%) had both ASD and depressive disorder. Following psychiatric evaluation, drug treatment was initiated in 37 out of 60 cases, constituting 61.7% of the sample. Among the commonly prescribed drug treatments, the combination of selective serotonin reuptake inhibitors (SSRIs) and atypical antipsychotics (AAs) (20%) and AAs alone (20%) were the most frequently initiated. These were followed by SSRI (6.6%) and mirtazapine (6.6%) treatment alone.

### 3.4. NSESSS Scale Scores and Their Relationships with Different Variables

Among the 7 items of the NSESSS, Item 1 evaluates 'flashbacks', the reliving of past stress as if it is recurring; Item 2 assesses intense emotional distress triggered by reminders of stress; Item 3 gauges detachment from self, body, surroundings, or memories; Item 4 examines avoidance of stress-associated thoughts, feelings, or sensations; Item 5 measures sustained hyperalertness and vigilance for danger; Item 6 rates heightened startle response due to sudden noises; and Item 7 considers extreme irritability that might result in yelling, fights, or destructive behavior.

The mean values of the scores given to the 7 items and the total scale scores for the NSESSS are shown in Table 3. According to these results, on average, the highest score was given to the sixth item on the scale, an item questioning being easily startled and frightened. The third item obtained the lowest score, and this item questioned whether the person experienced the feeling of being dissociated from their own body or environment. In addition, while 35 (58.4%) of the participants rated the sixth item as 'quite a lot/extremely', 15 (25%) gave the same answer for the third item.

Table 3. The mean values of the scores given to the items in the NSESSS.

| Scale Items | Participant ($n$ = 60) Mean ± SD |
|---|---|
| Total scale score | 1.90 ± 0.83 |
| Item 1 | 2.11 ± 1.15 |
| Item 2 | 2.30 ± 1.26 |
| Item 3 | 1.41 ± 1.25 |
| Item 4 | 1.65 ± 1.31 |
| Item 5 | 2.16 ± 1.35 |
| Item 6 | 2.53 ± 1.29 |
| Item 7 | 1.48 ± 1.08 |

SD: Standard deviation.

Participants were divided into various groups and evaluated in terms of NSESSS scores. Initially, they were separated based on their reasons for seeking help at the Child Psychiatry Clinic (self-requested counseling or family-initiated). Further analysis divided adolescents into two groups according to gender and physical injury. After assessing the normality of data distribution using the Shapiro-Wilk test, the Mann–Whitney U test was conducted due to the non-normal data distribution ($p < 0.05$). Afterward, analyses were performed by dividing the patients into two groups according to their mean NSESSS scores, as those who scored below two on the NSESSS scale (no acute stress symptoms and mild acute stress symptoms) and those who scored two and above (moderate, severe, and extreme acute stress symptoms). Gender differences between these two groups were examined categorically with the chi-squared test.

When the groups were examined according to the reasons for applying to the Child Psychiatry Clinic, the total score of the NSESSS was found to be significantly different between the groups (Mann–Whitney U test, Z = −3.29, U = 209, $p < 0.001$). Adolescents who requested psychiatric counseling on their own demand had a higher score on the scale ([Mdn (IQR) = 16 (13–19)], 95% CI = 14.24–17.26) than those who were requested to seek psychiatric counseling by their families (Mdn (IQR) = 9 (5–17), 95% CI = 7.57–13.03). No significant difference was found between the mean scores of the NSESSS between male and female patients (Mann–Whitney U test, Z = −0.38, U = 400, $p = 0.69$; Mdn (IQR) = 16 (11.5–20.5), 95% CI= 10.92–15.85 for male, Mdn (IQR) = 15 (10.5–19.5), 95% CI = 11.82–15.85 for female). We used the Mann–Whitney U test to investigate whether there were differences in the NSESSS scores between patients with and without bodily injury. Our findings revealed that patients without bodily injury had significantly higher NSESSS scores (Mann–Whitney U test, Z = −2.29, U = 191, $p = 0.02$); Mdn (IQR) = 16 (9.75–19), 95% CI = 12.86–16.35 for without, Mdn (IQR) = 11 (5–14.25), 95% CI = 7.77–13.37 for with bodily injury).

Further analyses were performed by dividing the patients into two groups according to their mean NSESSS scores, as those who scored below 2 on the NSESSS scale (no acute stress symptoms and mild acute stress symptoms) and those who scored 2 and above (moderate, severe, and extreme acute stress symptoms). A total of 27 of the adolescents (45%) had a mean NSESSS total score of less than 2, whereas 33 (55%) scored 2 or more. No statistically significant difference was observed according to gender in terms of receiving a score of less than two and a score of two or more according to the total mean score of the NSESSS (chi-squared test, $p = 0.85$).

### 3.5. Predictors of Acute Stress Disorder

A binary logistic regression was carried out to determine further sociodemographic and clinical factors that might be associated with acute stress disorder scores as evaluated by the NSESSS. After the univariate analyses, the reasons for applying to the child psychiatry clinic, paternal educational level, current use of any psychiatric medicine, and the status of attending formal education were included in the regression model ($p$ values $< 0.10$). Multicollinearity was checked using the variance inflation factor (VIF), and no problems were identified (i.e., VIF < 10). The current model, including these predictors, was significant ($p < 0.001$ and Nagelkerke $R^2$ = 0.47), and the Hosmer–Lemeshow goodness-of-fit test was insignificant [$X^2$ (8) = 11.051, $p = 0.087$], suggesting that the model fit the data well. According to the logistic regression model presented in Table 4, paternal educational levels and reasons for applying to the Child Psychiatry Clinic were predictors of acute stress disorder.

Table 4. Logistic regression model for prediction of acute stress disorder.

| | β | SE | $p$ | OR (95% CI) |
|---|---|---|---|---|
| Reason for applying to the Child Psychiatry Clinic | 2.83 | 0.88 | 0.001 | 16.94 (2.99–96.01) |
| Paternal educational level | 2.31 | 0.84 | 0.006 | 10.16 (1.94–53.27) |
| Current use of any psychiatric medicine | 1.24 | 0.84 | 0.143 | 3.45 (0.65–18.18) |
| Status of attending formal education | −1.77 | 0.95 | 0.065 | 0.17 (0.02–1.11) |

SE: standard error; OR: odds ratio.

## 4. Discussion

While there are various studies in the literature regarding the psychiatric disorders experienced by individuals after an earthquake, there is a scarcity of research focused on both the acute period following the earthquake and adolescents. Our study aimed to fill the gap in the existing literature by assessing the psychological symptoms and needs of adolescents who sought assistance at a child psychiatry clinic within the first month after experiencing an earthquake.

### 4.1. Psychiatric Symptoms of the Adolescents

In this study, we evaluated 60 earthquake-affected adolescents and identified fear/anxiety as the most prevalent psychological symptom. Among the patients, 41.6% ($n = 25$) experienced fear/anxiety, followed by equilibrium disturbances/dizziness at 31.6% ($n = 19$). In the literature, different studies dealing with postearthquake somatic and psychological symptoms have reported a remarkable increase in the patients presenting with vague, dizziness-like features, which cannot be attributed to any defined variant of vestibular disorder. Nomura et al. conducted an epidemical clinical study and labeled earthquake-associated dizziness as 'post-earthquake dizziness syndrome' following a major earthquake in Japan on 11 March 2011 [27]. In a later study conducted in Japan, 36.4% of participants reported experiencing postearthquake dizziness, and changes in living conditions and autonomic stress were found to be associated with dizziness symptoms [28]. In another study conducted with adolescents after an earthquake in China, the percentage of patients experiencing dizziness in the third month after the earthquake was found to be 41.9%, and this rate decreased to 34.8% in the sixth month. Postearthquake dizziness/equilibrium disturbance rates reported in our study are relatively lower than those reported in previous studies, and to gain a deeper understanding of this phenomenon and the progression of the symptoms, our team is closely monitoring the patients in this group through ongoing regular follow-ups.

To our knowledge, our study is one of the few studies reporting postearthquake vertigo symptoms in adolescents, and although this phenomenon has been studied and documented in adults, our research sheds new light on its occurrence in younger individuals. There is currently no established specific treatment approach for these symptoms; however, the appropriate management of such earthquake-induced psychological stress resulting in dizziness should encompass interdisciplinary assessment, appraisal of the underlying impairment, and appropriate counseling and therapeutic approaches [29].

### 4.2. The Prevalence of ASD

In this study, ASD diagnosis was assessed through clinical interviews based on DSM-5 criteria conducted by a child and adolescent psychiatrist, and a significantly higher rate than the rates of ASD reported in the literature following earthquakes was detected. In contrast to earlier findings, we found that 81.6% ($n = 49$) of cases were diagnosed with ASD. A study conducted in India reported that 48% of children aged eight years and older who visited the emergency department of a hospital after an earthquake scored above the cut-off value for stress-induced psychological disorder diagnosis on the Children Impact of Event Scale [30]. Another study evaluating acute stress symptoms in children after the 1999 earthquake in Turkey with a semistructured clinical interview reported that 74.5% of children and adolescents were diagnosed with ASD [26].

Our study found a higher percentage of patients diagnosed with acute stress disorder compared to other studies. One potential explanation for this disparity could be attributed to the severity and destructiveness of the two major earthquakes, along with the subsequent aftershocks. Gökçen et al. showed that even a moderate-intensity earthquake without any devastation might cause significant PTSD symptoms in children and adolescents; however, previous studies have indicated that individuals exposed to higher levels of trauma are likely to develop posttraumatic stress reactions [31,32]. Research indicates that previous traumatic events can be a predictor of acute stress reactions following a current traumatic experience, and it may be suggested that exposure to two major earthquakes on the same day might have exacerbated acute stress symptoms in patients by creating an additive traumatic effect [33]. Moreover, the earthquakes received extensive coverage from both national and international media. Graphic images were also shared on traditional and social media about individuals who had family members trapped under debris or who had lost their lives. Considering the fact that 25% of the patients in our study stated that what they saw in the media after the earthquake was more traumatic than the moment of the earthquake, it can be argued that, especially, the graphic images shared on social media may partly explain the high rate of ASD in our study. There are studies reporting that the interaction of media exposure with emotional reaction to media coverage in the aftermath of traumatic events might predict ongoing posttraumatic stress, and research conducted after Hurricane Sandy revealed that individuals who used social media experienced higher stress levels than those who relied solely on traditional media [34,35]. Some findings suggested that higher social media exposure was associated with an increased likelihood of experiencing acute stress symptoms, such as anxiety, fear, and sleep disturbances [36]. Although media use habits and intensities of adolescents were not examined in our study, it seems reasonable to suggest that there may be a correlation between media use and posttraumatic stress symptoms. Further research is necessary to comprehend the impact of viewing trauma-related news or images in the media on stress symptoms.

### 4.3. The Initiation of Pharmacological Treatments

Drug treatment was initiated in 61.7% of the 60 patients evaluated in our study, and the most frequently used drug groups were determined as atypical antipsychotics with a combination of SSRIs and atypical antipsychotics alone. There is a limited amount of research on the use of medication to treat ASD, as most studies on children and adolescents focus on the treatment of PTSD. In various treatment guidelines dealing with ASD treatment, pharmacological treatments are not recommended for use as an early intervention for ASD or related conditions [37]. One meta-analysis of pharmacological interventions for the prevention of PTSD found that, across 14 studies, pharmacological interventions were effective in treating ASD or preventing PTSD; however, no effect was found when only randomized, controlled trials were included [38]. While existing pharmacological trials do not provide strong evidence for specific medications to treat ASD currently, there are studies in the literature that show some benefits when initiating pharmacological treatments for individuals with ASD. These benefits might vary depending on a patient's condition. In certain cases, the use of medication is highlighted for managing acute symptoms effectively [39]. A randomized, double-blind clinical study using imipramine in pediatric burn patients suggested that imipramine may be cautiously used to reduce symptoms of ASD [40]. Another study showed that risperidone, an atypical antipsychotic, may be effective in relieving ASD symptoms in children with burns [41]. In addition, although large-scale psychopharmacology studies have not been conducted in the literature for the treatment of trauma-related disorders in children and adolescents, Cohen et al. reported that 95% of child psychiatrists had used pharmacotherapy to treat childhood and adolescent PTSD, and the medications most frequently used were selective serotonin reuptake inhibitors and $\alpha$-adrenergic agonists [42]. To the best of our knowledge, our study is the first in the literature to report the rate of drug initiation and treatments in clinical practice for adolescents diagnosed with ASD. Large-scale and longitudinal further studies are needed to evaluate factors affecting clinicians' drug choices and the efficacy of medication used off-label in children and adolescents with ASD.

There are few studies in the literature regarding the effectiveness of nonpharmacological interventions in managing the symptoms of acute stress disorder. Although psychological debriefing (PD), one of the nonpharmacological interventions for acute stress symptoms, has been frequently applied to adolescents and adults after traumatic events in the past, it was recently abandoned as it was revealed that it was not helpful [43]. There are more studies on the effectiveness of nonpsychopharmacological interventions for

PTSD symptoms in children and adolescents. Various studies have shown that cognitive behavioral therapy (CBT) and eye movement desensitization and reprocessing (EMDR) treatments can be particularly effective in the treatment of PTSD symptoms in children and adolescents [44,45]. Different global mental health organizations recommend the use of psychotherapy in the treatment of PTSD. For instance, the American Academy of Child and Adolescent Psychiatry (AACAP) recommends that trauma-focused psychotherapies should be used as the primary frontline treatment for PTSD in children and adolescents [46]. The most recent edition of the Australian guidelines for preventing and treating PTSD emphasizes the use of trauma-focused cognitive behavior therapy for children with PTSD, either alone or with a caregiver [47].

We are currently maintaining contact with the patients who participated in our study, continuing their care at our clinic. Some patients have been referred to psychologists for CBT treatment, as per recommended guidelines. Notably, the referral of the patients to psychologists commenced a month after the earthquake. This delay was due to hospital psychologists facing personal losses and being unable to return to work immediately during the initial weeks postearthquake. As our study concentrated on evaluating acute psychiatric symptoms following the earthquake, assessments of nonpharmacological treatments were not included. Findings on nonpharmacological interventions will be presented in our upcoming follow-up study.

*4.4. Evaluation of the Scores in the Acute Stress Scale*

In our study, we evaluated the responses to the NSESSS and found that the sixth item, an item asking about feeling jumpy or being easily startled upon hearing unexpected noises, had the highest average score, and 58.4% of the participants rated experiencing this sixth item as 'quite a lot/extremely'. A previous study using data from 15 studies assessing acute stress symptoms conducted with children and adolescents from 5 to 17 years of age reported that 36.3% of the participants experienced hypervigilance symptoms and about 24.7% experienced exaggerated startle responses [48]. Studies evaluating the posttraumatic stress symptoms of adolescents in the literature have mainly focused on PTSD, and symptoms regarding being easily startled and frightened have been reported frequently. A previous study examining adolescents' postdisaster experiences and psychiatric problems 13 months after the 1999 Marmara earthquake in Turkey showed that 68% of the participants experienced startling easily [49]. In addition, a study describing the posttraumatic stress disorder symptoms in adolescent survivors three months after Wenchuan Earthquake reported that 49.1% of the participants experienced symptoms of increased arousal [50]. Although studies evaluating acute stress symptoms in adolescents have reported hypervigilance symptoms at different rates, it is evident that many adolescents experience feeling jumpy or being easily startled after a traumatic experience. Zhang et al. showed that the arousal symptom cluster was one of the most influential predictors of future PTSD among trauma-exposed children and adolescents; therefore, recognizing and following up on children experiencing this cluster of symptoms might be particularly important [51]. Adolescents evaluated within the scope of our study will also be followed closely, and the relationship between this symptom cluster and PTSD will be further investigated and reported.

It was determined that the third item was the subscale that the participants in our study gave the lowest average score in the NSESSS, and only 25% of the participants rated the third item, an item questioning feelings of being detached or distant from oneself or one's physical surroundings or memories, as 'quite a lot/extremely'. In accordance with the present results of our study, previous research demonstrated that the requirement of dissociative symptoms for a diagnosis of ASD in the DSM-IV was stringent, and most patients failed to meet complete DSM-IV ASD diagnosis criteria because of lacking dissociative symptoms [52]. Furthermore, in another study, acute stress disorder minus dissociation symptoms was reported to be almost three times more sensitive in adolescents than complete DSM-IV acute stress disorder criteria in predicting later PTSD [53]. The criteria for ASD in the DSM-5 have been modified due to evidence showing that posttraumatic reactions vary greatly and that the DSM-IV's focus on dissociative symptoms was too narrow [54].

One of the remarkable results of our study is that the NSESSS scores of the adolescents who applied to the Child Psychiatry Outpatient Clinic at their own request were significantly higher than those who were brought for counseling at the request of their families. In addition, the logistic regression analyses performed determined that an adolescents' demand to apply to the psychiatry clinic predicted a clinical diagnosis of ASD. This discovery holds significant importance, as it highlights the necessity of recognizing adolescents' expressed need for psychiatric assistance and is consistent with some previously reported results from other studies. A previous study conducted to examine and identify predictors of ASD and ASD symptomatology in children hospitalized for injuries reported that parents might underestimate their children's acute distress [55]. Another study conducted by Meiser-Stedman et al. examining parent–child agreement for ASD and PTSD in children and adolescents reported that parent–child agreement for ASD was poor and child-reported ASD predicted later child-reported PTSD, while parent-reported ASD failed to predict later parent-reported PTSD. Furthermore, the same study determined that parent-reported ASD failed to predict later child-reported PTSD, suggesting that parent-only screening in the aftermath of trauma would be less than optimal [56]. In addition, a study conducted with children between ages 8 and 17 hospitalized for their injuries showed that the parent–child agreement was low for ASD diagnosis in children, and parents without ASD underestimated their child's ASD compared to the child's self-rating [57]. Considering both this study and previous studies, it can be posited that, irrespective of parental perceptions regarding the impact of traumatic events on their children, attending to adolescents' articulated desire for psychiatric support assumes paramount importance. Our study, which reported findings supporting previous research, contributes to the literature in terms of emphasizing the importance of listening to adolescents who express their need for psychiatric help.

*4.5. Physical Injury and Acute Stress*

A noteworthy finding from our study is that the NSESSS scores of adolescents who did not suffer physical injuries were notably higher than those who did. Higher mean scores on the NSESSS indicate a more intense experience of acute stress symptoms. Although many studies in the literature have shown a significant relationship between the severity of PTSD symptoms and the presence of physical injury, studies addressing the relationship between ASD and bodily injury in adolescents are scarce [58–60]. A study conducted in Turkey after the Marmara earthquakes showed that ASD and PTSD were more common in children who sustained bodily injuries, and this result was subsequently corroborated by a limited number of investigations examining the association between physical injuries and ASD symptoms in adolescents [61,62]. One possible explanation for children without physical injury having higher NSESSS scores than those with bodily injuries in our study might be that children with injuries were in contact with hospital staff while receiving medical care. This communication might have provided children with a better chance to process their trauma. Haag et al. reported that having been treated as an inpatient predicted less severe ASD in children with road traffic accidents, and injury severity was not found to be predictive of ASD severity. To explain their findings, which are similar to our results, the researchers proposed the possibility that children admitted to the hospital received more professional care, and the process of inpatient treatment helped ease the cognitive and emotional processing of the traumatic event [63]. In addition, children hospitalized for a short time due to their physical injuries were temporarily away from the images and news related to the earthquake in the external environment and the media, and it can be argued that this may be associated with lower NSESSS scores. Although more comprehensive adolescent studies addressing the relationship between physical injury and acute stress symptoms are needed, the findings of our research are important for a number of reasons. After massive natural disasters such as earthquakes, resources often focus on people with physical injuries; however, as our findings indicate, it is crucial to evaluate the psychological wellbeing of adolescents, even if they have not sustained physical injuries. Additional programs that carry child and adolescent mental health services outside of hospitals may be beneficial to reach young people after an earthquake who do not have physical injuries. After the 2023 earthquakes, mobile 'psychosocial support' tents were set up by the Ministry of Health of the Republic of Turkey in settlements in many provinces affected by the event, and our findings emphasize the importance of such interventions. Moreover, providing trauma-sensitive training to healthcare professionals can bring about added advantages, as the way children who are hospitalized for physical injuries interact with a treatment team may help alleviate any posttraumatic psychological symptoms they may be experiencing.

*4.6. Educational Status of Fathers and Acute Stress Disorder in Adolescents*

Another thought-provoking result of our study is that we showed that the fathers' education level predicted the diagnosis of ASD in adolescents. Although there are various studies in the literature reporting a relationship between fathers' education levels and PTSD symptoms in children and adolescents, to the best of our knowledge, no studies in the literature have shown a correlation between a father's education level and ASD symptoms. El-Khodary et al. reported that lower paternal education predicted a PTSD diagnosis in Palestinian children and adolescents, and they argued that parents with lower educational levels might have lower family income and more economic pressure [64]. Similarly, in a study conducted in Greenland, the low education level of the father was found to be a significant predictor of PTSD in adolescents [65]. Research has also demonstrated that, when fathers have lower levels of education, their children have a higher likelihood of experiencing various traumas [66,67]. However, to the best of our knowledge, our study is the first study in the literature to report that an increase in a father's education level predicts ASD. One factor that might explain this noteworthy result may be the relationship between the level of education and the involvement in interaction with children and the family-related processes of fathers. Marsiglio found that fathers with higher education tended to report higher levels of paternal involvement with their school-aged children, and other studies have also reported that older and more educated fathers tend to be more highly involved with their children [68–70]. Although father involvement generally affects children's mental health and development positively, it has been shown that, in some cases, it can also have adverse effects. Liu et al. reported that, at high levels of paternal inconsistency, higher father involvement was associated with higher behavioral and emotional problems in children, and when father–child relationships were poor, higher father involvement was also related to more behavioral and emotional problems [71]. Based on these previous findings, it can be suggested that fathers with higher education in our study were more involved in family relations and childcare processes. Our study did not examine the earthquake's psychological impact on fathers. However, if fathers were affected and displayed signs of acute stress, it could have impacted the acute stress symptoms of their children. This may have been more pronounced in children whose fathers had a higher education level, as they may have had more interaction with their fathers. Studies have shown that there is a link between lower levels of education among fathers and trauma-related disorders, such as PTSD, in children and adolescents [72,73]. Our study emphasizes the significance of recognizing that children of highly educated fathers may also be at risk of acute stress disorder and that they should receive thorough evaluations and attention. It would be beneficial to conduct further studies that explore the factors associated with the link between fathers' education levels and ASD in adolescents. Such studies would help shed more light on this phenomenon and enhance our understanding.

### 4.7. Limitations

The implications of this study's findings should be considered within the context of certain limitations. Our assessment was restricted to adolescents who sought care at the outpatient clinic, thereby implying that caution should be exercised when attempting to generalize the findings to the entire population. Large-scale future studies on this subject should focus on a population sample rather than a clinical sample to achieve results that can apply to the general population.

As mentioned previously, the absence of an examination of ASD symptoms in the parents could introduce an additional limitation to the study. Considering the severity and spread of the natural disaster experienced, it can be predicted that at least some parents may have psychiatric symptoms related to posttraumatic stress. Research has demonstrated that the stress symptoms and psychological resilience of parents can impact their children's posttraumatic psychiatric symptoms [74,75]. To better understand and address acute stress symptoms in adolescents following natural disasters, it would be helpful to examine the psychological reactions of parents to trauma and how these reactions may impact their children's psychiatric symptoms.

In addition, one of the study's limitations is that information about past traumas, which may affect patients' current trauma responses, was not comprehensively addressed in the patient evaluation process. Studies indicate that previous traumatic experiences may predict PTSD after subsequent traumatic events [76]. To gain a deeper understanding of how adolescents react to stress and trauma, it would be useful to conduct future studies that take into account previous traumatic experiences of adolescents. This could provide valuable insight into the topic.

Lastly, the cross-sectional design only captured data at a specific point in time, providing a snapshot of the participants' experiences without accounting for potential changes in ASD symptoms over time. Longitudinal studies would be needed to better understand the trajectory and persistence of ASD symptoms in this population following earthquake exposure. We will conduct a longitudinal evaluation of the patients in our study to understand better the long-term course of ASD symptoms in adolescents and associated factors, and we plan to report the results in a future research publication. Despite these limitations, the study provides valuable insights into the immediate effects of earthquakes on adolescent mental health, highlighting the need for further research in this area to inform targeted interventions and support strategies for this vulnerable population.

## 5. Conclusions

In conclusion, the current study contributes to the existing literature by addressing the psychological symptoms of adolescents seeking assistance at a child psychiatry clinic shortly after experiencing an earthquake. Our research adds to the existing body of knowledge by highlighting the importance of assessing teenagers for acute stress disorder who have fathers with high levels of education and no history of physical injury. This study also provides valuable insights into the psychological impact of earthquakes on adolescents and emphasizes the need for targeted interventions, such as psychosocial training of hospital staff about trauma-informed care and the utilization of mobile psychosocial support tools, in this vulnerable population. As the world is facing increasing environmental disasters, developing effective postdisaster trauma response programs and establishing trauma-related policies are critical, not only for people in developing countries but also for people worldwide. Comprehending acute stress disorder in adolescents, who constitute a significant proportion of the world population, following natural disasters is of utmost importance, yet the information on this subject is currently scarce. Longitudinal studies that examine patients from various sociodemographic and cultural backgrounds are necessary to understand this subject comprehensively, as well as treatment and follow-up studies. We believe that this study, as well as further research built upon our findings, can guide the development of comprehensive strategies and mental health policies to address the mental health needs of adolescents affected by earthquakes and other traumatic events.

**Author Contributions:** Conceptualization, G.Y.E. and M.D.; methodology, G.Y.E. and R.D.T.; validation, G.Y.E., R.D.T. and I.B.Ç.; formal analysis, G.Y.E. and R.D.T.; investigation, G.Y.E., R.D.T. and I.B.Ç.; resources, G.Y.E., R.D.T. and I.B.Ç.; data curation, G.Y.E. and M.D.; writing—original draft preparation, review and editing, G.Y.E., R.D.T. and I.B.Ç.; visualization, I.B.Ç. All authors have read and agreed to the published version of the manuscript.

**Funding:** This research received no external funding.

**Institutional Review Board Statement:** The study was conducted in accordance with the Declaration of Helsinki and approved by the Ethics Committee of Harran University (protocol code HRU/23.11.12, 19 June 2023).

**Informed Consent Statement:** Informed consent was obtained from all subjects involved in the study.

**Data Availability Statement:** Readers can access the data used in this study upon request from the corresponding author.

**Acknowledgments:** In cherished memory of those whose lives were tragically taken by the devastating earthquake, we humbly extend our heartfelt acknowledgments to all those affected. May our collective efforts pave the path toward a safer and more resilient future, honoring the memory of those we have lost.

**Conflicts of Interest:** The authors declare no conflict of interest.

# References

1. Naddaf, M. Turkey-Syria earthquake: What scientists know. *Nature* **2023**, *614*, 398–399, 505. [CrossRef] [PubMed]
2. England, A.; Smith, A.; Parrish, G.; Bernard, S. Turkey and Syria's Devastating Earthquakes in Graphics. Available online: https://www.ft.com/content/337edef6-05c9-498c-a3f0-13776082f218 (accessed on 10 April 2023).
3. 6 Şubat'taki Depremlerde Can Kaybı 50 bin 500'e Yükseldi. Available online: https://www.bbc.com/turkce/articles/c51kdv8d15jo#:~:text=%C4%B0%C3%A7i%C5%9Fleri%20Bakan%C4%B1%20S%C3%BCleyman%20Soylu%2C%206,bin%20969'unun%20enkaz%C4%B1n%C4%B1n%20kald%C4%B1r%C4%B1ld%C4%B1 (accessed on 15 June 2023).
4. The Earthquake in Turkey Is One of the Deadliest This Century. Here's Why. Available online: https://www.cbsnews.com/at-511lanta/news/the-earthquake-in-turkey-is-one-of-the-deadliest-this-century-heres-why/ (accessed on 15 June 2023).
5. Lo, H.-W.A.; Su, C.-Y.; Chou, F.H.-C. Disaster psychiatry in Taiwan: A comprehensive review. *J. Exp. Clin. Med.* **2012**, *4*, 77–81. [CrossRef]
6. Pridmore, W. 'I can see clearly now': Clarifying the role of psychiatry in global disaster. *Australas. Psychiatry* **2021**, *29*, 337–339. [CrossRef] [PubMed]
7. Sparks, S.W. Posttraumatic stress syndrome: What is it? *J. Trauma Nurs.* **2018**, *25*, 60–65. [CrossRef]
8. Sharan, P.; Chaudhary, G.; Kavathekar, S.A.; Saxena, S. Preliminary report of psychiatric disorders in survivors of a severe earthquake. *Am. J. Psychiatry* **1996**, *153*, 556–558. [CrossRef]
9. Goenjian, A. A mental health relief programme in Armenia after the 1988 earthquake: Implementation and clinical observations. *Br. J. Psychiatry* **1993**, *163*, 230–239. [CrossRef]
10. Crane, P.A.; Clements, P.T. Psychological response to disasters: Focus on adolescents. *J. Psychosoc. Nurs. Ment. Health Serv.* **2005**, *43*, 31–38. [CrossRef]
11. Spear, L.P. Neurobehavioral changes in adolescence. *Curr. Dir. Psychol. Sci.* **2000**, *9*, 111–114. [CrossRef]
12. Eckes, A.; Radunovich, H.L. Trauma and Adolescents. (FCS2280). In *IFAS Extension FCS 2280/FY1004*; University of Florida: Gainesville, FL, USA, 2007.
13. Kar, N. Psychological impact of disasters on children: Review of assessment and interventions. *World J. Psychiatry* **2009**, *5*, 5–11. [CrossRef]
14. Danese, A.; Smith, P.; Chitsabesan, P.; Dubicka, B. Child and adolescent mental health amidst emergencies and disasters. *Br. J. Psychiatry* **2020**, *216*, 159–162. [CrossRef]
15. Forbes, D.; Creamer, M.; Phelps, A.; Couineau, A.-L.; Cooper, J.A.; Bryant, R.; McFarlane, A.C.; Devilly, G.J.; Matthews, L.; Raphael, B. Treating adults with acute stress disorder and post-traumatic stress disorder in general practice: A clinical update. *Med. J. Aust.* **2007**, *187*, 120–123. [CrossRef] [PubMed]
16. Lubin, G.; Sids, C.; Vishne, T.; Shochat, T.; Ostfield, Y.; Shmushkevitz, M. Acute stress disorder and post-traumatic stress disorder among medical personnel in Judea and Samaria areas in the years 2000–2003. *Mil. Med.* **2007**, *172*, 376–378. [CrossRef] [PubMed]
17. Walker, J.R.; Teague, B.; Memarzia, J.; Meiser-Stedman, R. Acute stress disorder in children and adolescents: A systematic review and meta-analysis of prevalence following exposure to a traumatic event. *J. Affect. Disord. Rep.* **2020**, *2*, 100041. [CrossRef]
18. Cohen, M. Acute stress disorder in older, middle-aged and younger adults in reaction to the second Lebanon war. *Int. J. Geriatr. Psychiatry* **2008**, *23*, 34–40. [CrossRef]

19. Liu, K.; Liang, X.; Guo, L.; Li, Y.; Li, X.; Xin, B.; Huang, M.; Li, Y. Acute stress disorder in the paediatric surgical children and adolescents injured during the Wenchuan earthquake in China. *Stress Health* **2010**, *26*, 262–268. [CrossRef]
20. Bryant, R.A.; Friedman, M.J.; Spiegel, D.; Ursano, R.; Strain, J. A review of acute stress disorder in DSM-5. *Focus* **2011**, *9*, 335–350. [CrossRef]
21. Bryant, R.A.; Creamer, M.; O'Donnell, M.; Silove, D.; McFarlane, A.C.; Forbes, D. A comparison of the capacity of DSM-IV and DSM-5 acute stress disorder definitions to predict posttraumatic stress disorder and related disorders. *J. Clin. Psychiatry* **2014**, *76*, 3467. [CrossRef]
22. Chen, C.C.; Yeh, T.L.; Yang, Y.K.; Chen, S.J.; Lee, I.H.; Fu, L.S.; Yeh, C.Y.; Hsu, H.C.; Tsai, W.L.; Cheng, S.H.; et al. Psychiatric morbidity and post-traumatic symptoms among survivors in the early stage following the 1999 earthquake in Taiwan. *Psychiatry Res.* **2001**, *105*, 13–22. [CrossRef]
23. Kilpatrick, D.; Resnick, H.; Friedman, M. Severity of Acute Stress Symptoms—Child Age 11–17 (National Stressful Events Survey Acute Stress Disorder Short Scale [NSESSS]). 2013. Available online: https://www.psychiatry.org/File%20Library/Psychiatrists/Practice/DSM/APA_DSM5_Severity-of-Acute-Stress-Symptoms-Child-Age-11-to-17.pdf (accessed on 10 April 2023).
24. Sapmaz, S.Y.; Erkuran, H.Ö.; Ergin, D.; Celasin, N.S.; Karaarslan, D.; Öztürk, M.; Köroglu, E.; Aydemir, Ö. DSM-5 Akut Stres Belirtileri Siddet Ölçegi-Çocuk Formu Yas 11-17'nin Türkçe Güvenilirligi ve Geçerliligi/Validity and Reliability of the Turkish version of DSM-5" Severity of Acute Stress Symptoms-Child Age 11-17" Form. *Dusunen Adam* **2017**, *30*, 32. [CrossRef]
25. Buchner, A.; Erdfelder, E.; Faul, F.; Lang, A. *G\* Power 3.1 Manual*; Heinrich-Heine-Universitat Dusseldorf: Düsseldorf, Germany, 2017.
26. Abali, O.; Tüzün, ü.; Göktürk, ü.; An gürkan, K.; Alyanak, B.; Görker, I. Acute psychological reactions of children and adolescents after the marmara earthquake: A brief preliminary report. *Clin. Child Psychol. Psychiatry* **2002**, *7*, 283–287. [CrossRef]
27. Nomura, Y.; Toi, T. Post earthquake dizziness syndrome. *Equilib. Res.* **2014**, *73*, 167–173. [CrossRef]
28. Miwa, T.; Matsuyoshi, H.; Nomura, Y.; Minoda, R. Post-earthquake dizziness syndrome following the 2016 Kumamoto earthquakes, Japan. *PLoS ONE* **2021**, *16*, e0255816. [CrossRef] [PubMed]
29. Kumar, V.; Bhavana, K. Post earthquake equilibrium disturbance: A study after Nepal–India Earthquake 2015. *Indian J. Otolaryngol. Head Neck Surg.* **2019**, *71*, 1258–1265. [CrossRef] [PubMed]
30. Mondal, R.; Banerjee, I.; Sabui, T.; Saren, A.; Sarkar, S.; Hazra, A.; Majumder, D.; Dutta, S.; Pan, P. Acute stress-related psychological impact in children following devastating natural disaster, the Sikkim earthquake (2011), India. *J. Neurosci. Rural Pract.* **2013**, *4*, S19–S23. [CrossRef]
31. Lewin, T.J.; Carr, V.J.; Webster, R.A. Recovery from post-earthquake psychological morbidity: Who suffers and who recovers? *Aust. N. Z. J. Psychiatry* **1998**, *32*, 15–20. [CrossRef]
32. Gökçen, C.; Şahingöz, M.; Annagür, B.B. Does a non-destructive earthquake cause posttraumatic stress disorder? A cross-sectional study. *Eur. Child Adolesc. Psychiatry* **2013**, *22*, 295–299. [CrossRef]
33. Harvey, A.G.; Bryant, R.A. Predictors of acute stress following motor vehicle accidents. *J. Trauma. Stress* **1999**, *12*, 519–525. [CrossRef]
34. Goodwin, R.; Palgi, Y.; Hamama-Raz, Y.; Ben-Ezra, M. In the eye of the storm or the bullseye of the media: Social media use during Hurricane Sandy as a predictor of post-traumatic stress. *J. Psychiatr. Res.* **2013**, *47*, 1099–1100. [CrossRef]
35. Pfefferbaum, B.; Seale, T.W.; Brandt, E.N.; Pfefferbaum, R.L.; Doughty, D.E.; Rainwater, S.M. Media exposure in children one hundred miles from a terrorist bombing. *Ann. Clin. Psychiatry* **2003**, *15*, 1–8. [CrossRef]
36. Fraustino, J.D.; Liu, B.; Jin, Y. *Social Media Use during Disasters: A Review of the Knowledge Base and Gaps*; START: College Park, MD, USA, 2012.
37. Forbes, D.; Creamer, M.; Phelps, A.; Bryant, R.; McFarlane, A.; Devilly, G.J.; Matthews, L.; Raphael, B.; Doran, C.; Merlin, T.; et al. Australian guidelines for the treatment of adults with acute stress disorder and post-traumatic stress disorder. *Aust. N. Z. J. Psychiatry* **2007**, *41*, 637–648. [CrossRef]
38. Sijbrandij, M.; Kleiboer, A.; Bisson, J.I.; Barbui, C.; Cuijpers, P. Pharmacological prevention of post-traumatic stress disorder and acute stress disorder: A systematic review and meta-analysis. *Lancet Psychiatry* **2015**, *2*, 413–421. [CrossRef] [PubMed]
39. Howlett, J.R.; Stein, M.B. Prevention of trauma and stressor-related disorders: A review. *Neuropsychopharmacology* **2016**, *41*, 357–369. [CrossRef] [PubMed]
40. Robert, R.; Blakeney, P.E.; Villarreal, C.; Rosenberg, L.; Meyer, W.J., III. Imipramine treatment in pediatric burn patients with symptoms of acute stress disorder: A pilot study. *J. Am. Acad. Child Adolesc. Psychiatry* **1999**, *38*, 873–882. [CrossRef]
41. Meighen, K.G.; Hines, L.A.; Lagges, A.M. Risperidone treatment of preschool children with thermal burns and acute stress disorder. *J. Child Adolesc. Psychopharmacol.* **2007**, *17*, 223–232. [CrossRef] [PubMed]
42. Cohen, J.A.; Mannarino, A.P.; Rogal, S. Treatment practices for childhood posttraumatic stress disorder☆. *Child Abus. Negl.* **2001**, *25*, 123–135. [CrossRef] [PubMed]
43. Rose, S.; Bisson, J.; Churchill, R.; Wessely, S.; Cochrane Common Mental Disorders Group. Psychological debriefing for preventing post traumatic stress disorder (PTSD) Cochrane Database of Systematic Reviews. *Cochrane Database Syst. Rev.* **2010**. [CrossRef]
44. Gutermann, J.; Schreiber, F.; Matulis, S.; Schwartzkopff, L.; Deppe, J.; Steil, R. Psychological treatments for symptoms of posttraumatic stress disorder in children, adolescents, and young adults: A meta-analysis. *Clin. Child Fam. Psychol. Rev.* **2016**, *19*, 77–93. [CrossRef]

45. Lucio, R.; Nelson, T.L. Effective practices in the treatment of trauma in children and adolescents: From guidelines to organizational practices. *J. Evid. Inf. Soc. Work* **2016**, *13*, 469–478. [CrossRef]
46. Cohen, J.A.; AACAP Work Group on Quality Issues. Practice parameter for the assessment and treatment of children and adolescents with posttraumatic stress disorder. *J. Am. Acad. Child Adolesc. Psychiatry* **2010**, *49*, 414–430.
47. Phelps, A.J.; Lethbridge, R.; Brennan, S.; Bryant, R.A.; Burns, P.; Cooper, J.A.; Forbes, D.; Gardiner, J.; Gee, G.; Jones, K.; et al. Australian guidelines for the prevention and treatment of posttraumatic stress disorder: Updates in the third edition. *Aust. N. Z. J. Psychiatry* **2022**, *56*, 230–247. [CrossRef]
48. Kassam-Adams, N.; Palmieri, P.A.; Rork, K.; Delahanty, D.L.; Kenardy, J.; Kohser, K.L.; Landolt, M.A.; Le Brocque, R.; Marsac, M.L.; Meiser-Stedman, R.; et al. Acute stress symptoms in children: Results from an international data archive. *J. Am. Acad. Child Adolesc. Psychiatry* **2012**, *51*, 812–820. [CrossRef] [PubMed]
49. Dogan, A. Adolescents' posttraumatic stress reactions and behavior problems following Marmara earthquake. *Eur. J. Psychotraumatol.* **2011**, *2*, 5825. [CrossRef] [PubMed]
50. Zhang, W.; Jiang, X.; Ho, K.w.; Wu, D. The presence of post-traumatic stress disorder symptoms in adolescents three months after an 8· 0 magnitude earthquake in southwest China. *J. Clin. Nurs.* **2011**, *20*, 3057–3069. [CrossRef]
51. Zhang, J.; Sami, S.; Meiser-Stedman, R. Acute stress and PTSD among trauma-exposed children and adolescents: Computational prediction and interpretation. *J. Anxiety Disord.* **2022**, *92*, 102642. [CrossRef]
52. Meiser-Stedman, R.; Dalgleish, T.; Yule, P.S.A.W.; Bryant, B.; Ehlers, A.; Mayou, R.A.; Winston, N.K.A.A.F. Dissociative symptoms and the acute stress disorder diagnosis in children and adolescents: A replication of the Harvey and Bryant (1999) study. *J. Trauma. Stress* **2007**, *20*, 359–364. [CrossRef]
53. Dalgleish, T.; Meiser-Stedman, R.; Kassam-Adams, N.; Ehlers, A.; Winston, F.; Smith, P.; Bryant, B.; Mayou, R.A.; Yule, W. Predictive validity of acute stress disorder in children and adolescents. *Br. J. Psychiatry* **2008**, *192*, 392–393. [CrossRef] [PubMed]
54. Highlights of Changes from DSM-IV-TR to DSM-5. Available online: https://practicumsupport-psych.sites.olt.ubc.ca/files/2013/05/Summary-of-DSM-V-Changes.pdf (accessed on 10 April 2023).
55. Daviss, W.B.; Racusin, R.; Fleischer, A.; Mooney, D.; Ford, J.D.; McHUGO, G.J. Acute stress disorder symptomatology during hospitalization for pediatric injury. *J. Am. Acad. Child Adolesc. Psychiatry* **2000**, *39*, 569–575. [CrossRef]
56. Meiser-Stedman, R.; Smith, P.; Glucksman, E.; Yule, W.; Dalgleish, T. Parent and child agreement for acute stress disorder, post-traumatic stress disorder and other psychopathology in a prospective study of children and adolescents exposed to single-event trauma. *J. Abnorm. Child Psychol.* **2007**, *35*, 191–201. [CrossRef]
57. Kassam-Adams, N.; Garcia-Espana, J.F.; Miller, V.A.; Winston, F. Parent-child agreement regarding children's acute stress: The role of parent acute stress reactions. *J. Am. Acad. Child Adolesc. Psychiatry* **2006**, *45*, 1485–1493. [CrossRef]
58. Hsu, C.-C.; Chong, M.-Y.; Yang, P.; Yen, C.-F. Posttraumatic stress disorder among adolescent earthquake victims in Taiwan. *J. Am. Acad. Child Adolesc. Psychiatry* **2002**, *41*, 875–881. [CrossRef]
59. Tian, Y.; Wong, T.K.; Li, J.; Jiang, X. Posttraumatic stress disorder and its risk factors among adolescent survivors three years after an 8.0 magnitude earthquake in China. *BMC Public Health* **2014**, *14*, 1073. [CrossRef] [PubMed]
60. Farooqui, M.; Quadri, S.A.; Suriya, S.S.; Khan, M.A.; Ovais, M.; Sohail, Z.; Shoaib, S.; Tohid, H.; Hassan, M. Posttraumatic stress disorder: A serious post-earthquake complication. *Trends Psychiatry Psychother.* **2017**, *39*, 135–143. [CrossRef]
61. Demir, T.; Demir, D.E.; Alkas, L.; Copur, M.; Dogangun, B.; Kayaalp, L. Some clinical characteristics of children who survived the Marmara earthquakes. *Eur. Child Adolesc. Psychiatry* **2010**, *19*, 125–133. [CrossRef] [PubMed]
62. Berkem, M.; Bildik, T. Izmit depreminde hospitalize edilen depremzede çocuk ve ergenlerin klinik özellikleri/The clinical features of children who are hospitalized after earthquake. *Anadolu Psikiyatr. Derg.* **2001**, *2*, 133.
63. Haag, A.-C.; Zehnder, D.; Landolt, M.A. Guilt is associated with acute stress symptoms in children after road traffic accidents. *Eur. J. Psychotraumatol.* **2015**, *6*, 29074. [CrossRef] [PubMed]
64. El-Khodary, B.; Samara, M.; Askew, C. Traumatic events and PTSD among Palestinian children and adolescents: The effect of demographic and socioeconomic factors. *Front. Psychiatry* **2020**, *11*, 4. [CrossRef] [PubMed]
65. Karsberg, S.H.; Lasgaard, M.; Elklit, A. Victimisation and PTSD in a Greenlandic youth sample. *Int. J. Circumpolar Health* **2012**, *71*, 18378. [CrossRef]
66. Usta, J.; Farver, J. Child sexual abuse in Lebanon during war and peace. *Child Care Health Dev.* **2010**, *36*, 361–368. [CrossRef]
67. Liang, Y.; Zhou, Y.; Liu, Z. Traumatic experiences and posttraumatic stress disorder among Chinese rural-to-urban migrant children. *J. Affect. Disord.* **2019**, *257*, 123–129. [CrossRef]
68. Marsiglio, W. Paternal engagement activities with minor children. *J. Marriage Fam.* **1991**, *53*, 973–986. [CrossRef]
69. King, V.; Harris, K.M.; Heard, H.E. Racial and ethnic diversity in nonresident father involvement. *J. Marriage Fam.* **2004**, *66*, 1–21.
70. Lerman, R.; Sorensen, E. *Fatherhood*; Routledge: London, UK, 2014; pp. 137–158. ISBN 9780203708347.
71. Liu, Y.; Dittman, C.K.; Guo, M.; Morawska, A.; Haslam, D. Influence of father involvement, fathering practices and father-child relationships on children in mainland China. *J. Child Fam. Stud.* **2021**, *30*, 1858–1870. [CrossRef]
72. Dietrich, H.; Al Ali, R.; Tagay, S.; Hebebrand, J.; Reissner, V. Screening for posttraumatic stress disorder in young adult refugees from Syria and Iraq. *Compr. Psychiatry* **2019**, *90*, 73–81. [CrossRef] [PubMed]
73. Silwal, S.; Dybdahl, R.; Chudal, R.; Sourander, A.; Lien, L. Psychiatric symptoms experienced by adolescents in Nepal following the 2015 earthquakes. *J. Affect. Disord.* **2018**, *234*, 239–246. [CrossRef] [PubMed]

74. Thakar, D.; Coffino, B.; Lieberman, A.F. Maternal symptomatology and parent–child relationship functioning in a diverse sample of young children exposed to trauma. *J. Trauma. Stress* **2013**, *26*, 217–224. [CrossRef] [PubMed]
75. Zhai, Y.; Liu, K.; Zhang, L.; Gao, H.; Chen, Z.; Du, S.; Zhang, L.; Guo, Y. The relationship between post-traumatic symptoms, parenting style, and resilience among adolescents in Liaoning, China: A cross-sectional study. *PLoS ONE* **2015**, *10*, e0141102. [CrossRef]
76. McLaughlin, K.A.; Koenen, K.C.; Hill, E.D.; Petukhova, M.; Sampson, N.A.; Zaslavsky, A.M.; Kessler, R.C. Trauma exposure and posttraumatic stress disorder in a national sample of adolescents. *J. Am. Acad. Child Adolesc. Psychiatry* **2013**, *52*, 815–830. [CrossRef]

**Disclaimer/Publisher's Note:** The statements, opinions and data contained in all publications are solely those of the individual author(s) and contributor(s) and not of MDPI and/or the editor(s). MDPI and/or the editor(s) disclaim responsibility for any injury to people or property resulting from any ideas, methods, instructions or products referred to in the content.

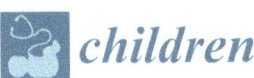 

Article

# Design of a Collaborative Knowledge Framework for Personalised Attention Deficit Hyperactivity Disorder (ADHD) Treatments

Pornsiri Chatpreecha and Sasiporn Usanavasin *

School of Information, Computer and Communication Technology, Sirindhorn International Institute of Technology, Thammasat University, Pathum Thani 12000, Thailand; pornsirichat@pim.ac.th
* Correspondence: sasiporn.us@siit.tu.ac.th

**Abstract:** Attention deficit hyperactivity disorder (ADHD) is a neurodevelopmental disorder. From the data collected by the Ministry of Public Health, Thailand, it has been reported that more than one million Thai youths (6–12 years) have been diagnosed with ADHD (2012–2018) This disorder is more likely to occur in males (12%) than females (4.2%). If ADHD goes untreated, there might be problems for individuals in the long run. This research aims to design a collaborative knowledge framework for personalised ADHD treatment recommendations. The first objective is to design a framework and develop a screening tool for doctors, parents, and teachers for observing and recording behavioural symptoms in ADHD children. This screening tool is a combination of doctor-verified criteria and the ADHD standardised screening tool (Vanderbilt). The second objective is to introduce practical algorithms for classifying ADHD types and recommending appropriate individual behavioural therapies and activities. We applied and compared four well-known machine-learning methods for classifying ADHD types. The four algorithms include Decision Tree, Naïve Bayes, neural network, and k-nearest neighbour. Based on this experiment, the Decision Tree algorithm yielded the highest average accuracy, which was 99.60%, with F1 scores equal to or greater than 97% for classifying each type of ADHD.

**Keywords:** attention deficit hyperactivity disorder; machine learning; knowledge framework; screening tool

Citation: Chatpreecha, P.; Usanavasin, S. Design of a Collaborative Knowledge Framework for Personalised Attention Deficit Hyperactivity Disorder (ADHD) Treatments. *Children* 2023, 10, 1288. https://doi.org/10.3390/children10081288

Academic Editor: Tingzhong Yang

Received: 29 June 2023
Revised: 20 July 2023
Accepted: 23 July 2023
Published: 26 July 2023

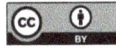

**Copyright:** © 2023 by the authors. Licensee MDPI, Basel, Switzerland. This article is an open access article distributed under the terms and conditions of the Creative Commons Attribution (CC BY) license (https:// creativecommons.org/licenses/by/ 4.0/).

## 1. Introduction

Attention deficit hyperactivity disorder (ADHD) is a complex mental health disorder that affects children aged six to twelve years [1–3]. ADHD is classified into three main subtypes: inattentive, impulsive–hyperactive, and a combination of the two. An individual with the inattentive subtype has difficulty paying attention and staying focused, while an individual with the impulsive–hyperactive type not only often feels restless and yields to impulses easily compared to other children in the equivalent development stage, but also has difficulty paying attention, similar to the inattentive subtype [1,2,4,5]. To diagnose a pupil with any of the subtypes mentioned earlier, they must show at least six of the nine given symptoms for at least six months [2,6,7].

ADHD is a severe neurodevelopmental disorder that has multiple aetiologies, but it is quite complicated to pinpoint a single factor that might be the cause. Mainly, it is caused by a combination of environmental and genetic factors. Environmental factors include lead poisoning from maternal smoking during pregnancy, a less supportive home environment, and recent studies even show that the number of hours of watching television or using other media devices might contribute to environmental factors causing ADHD [4,5,8,9]. As for the genetic factors, these may be due to parental genes, which influence or regulate the production of neurotransmitters in a child's brain during their development. The lack of neurotransmitters like dopamine (impulsiveness) or norepinephrine (attention) might result in the child being diagnosed with ADHD [3,4,10–14]. Unfortunately, at present, there is no available cure for ADHD, but if diagnosed early, help is provided as soon as symptoms surface, risks are detected, or ADHD predisposition is diagnosed. EI aims to help, to the fullest potential, promote physical, emotional, mental, social, and intellectual development. If a child is being supported from the beginning, the child is deemed to have the development of an average individual. In addition, the action reduces the cost and burden incurred [2,7,15,16].

If behavioural syndrome goes untreated, there might be problems for individuals in the long run. The patients might be at risk of other health conditions. They would also suffer from decreased social life quality, unsatisfactory academic performance, unpleasant relationships, comorbid psychiatric conditions, and much more. If not treated until adulthood, the symptoms may affect the health and lifestyle of the patients in many aspects. According to research about the persistence rate of ADHD into adulthood, the psychiatric comorbidities of adult ADHD, and the risk of serious adverse outcomes, such as criminality and mortality, ADHD should no longer be viewed only as a disorder primarily affecting the behaviour and learning of children [17,18]. ADHD should also be regarded as a significant health condition that confers an increased risk for early death due to suicide. In addition, although nearly one-third of children with ADHD will continue to fulfil norm-referenced criteria for ADHD as adults, most will also have at least one mental health problem in adulthood.

Children with ADHD experience far more obstacles compared to their average counterparts. While many children diagnosed with ADHD receive some special school services to improve their learning environment and experience, this might not always be the case [19]. Consequently, parents must observe their children's behaviour when at home, and teachers can help by monitoring and evaluating the behaviour while individuals are at school. For the assessment, teachers and parents can use the questionnaires of the DSM-5 standard [4,20], particularly the Vanderbilt ADHD Diagnostic Rating Scale (VADRS) (Thai version) [21]. Furthermore, teachers should become involved, as they know the students personally and academically. In addition, there are chances that the child's ADHD symptoms could be neglected and considered as habits by their parents. Therefore, having multiple perspectives and integrating all the results from different informants would be most optimal. With the expertise and evaluation of the assessment tests, physicians could then recommend and guide teachers and parents with methodologies and strategies which would ensure that, if followed, the children would be able to manage their symptoms [19,21,22].

The primary purpose of this research was to design a collaborative knowledge framework for personalised ADHD treatments. The main objectives included (1) a design of a collaborative framework and a screening tool for ADHD symptoms that could be used by medical professionals, parents, and teachers, and (2) the introduction of a practical algorithm for the classification of the types of ADHD with sets of recommended individual behavioural therapies and activities for different types of ADHD. To find an appropriate classification technique for the types of behavioural syndrome and address the need for such a machine learning algorithm in Thailand, we use machine learning to help with early intervention and learn student behaviour to assess the risk of having ADHD and find a solution; this will help children and those around them to heal and increase their chances of recovering. With the advancement of machine learning, we can classify symptoms more precisely and support large amounts of data, so there are advantages to using machine learning over queries alone.

We applied different machine learning algorithms, compared the results, and utilised the best algorithm in our framework. The expected outcome of our proposed framework was to provide an effective way to classify the types of behavioural syndrome and to recommend appropriate treatments and therapies based on the individual's behaviour.

For example, the prevalence of ADHD worldwide ranges between 0.1 and 8.1%. In Thailand, the prevalence is between 4.2 and 8.1% [23,24]. The prevalence of ADHD in children in Africa is 7.47% [25]. In 2016, an estimated 6.1 million U.S. children 2–17 years of age (9.4%) had received an ADHD diagnosis and 5.4 million children currently have ADHD [26]. The difference is due to the variety of population groups, ADHD study tools, and research procedures. For Thailand, only regional-level research was conducted.

This paper is organised as follows: Section 2 summarises previous studies that led to the motivation of this research. Section 3 describes the proposed approach and methods utilised in this research. Section 4 explains our experimental results, and Section 5 provides a discussion and conclusion for this work.

## 2. Related Work

Children are taken to the doctor for the early diagnosis and treatment of ADHD when behaviour resembling ADHD symptoms is observed during the evaluation. For instance, a child is much more mischievous than usual and exhibits emotional outbursts and lacks learning concentration. Hence, ADHD should be diagnosed based on an evaluation of learning, behavioural, and emotional issues. When determining the diagnosis of ADHD, it is critical to consider the following evaluations: (1) an evaluation of the patient's history and current conditions, (2) an evaluation by the parents and teachers, (3) a psychological assessment, and (4) discussion and treatment recommendations [1,2,5,15,20,27].

The development of technology related to health informatics is underway. This includes a decision support system (DSS) and patient follow-up care in the healthcare system [28]. Effective systems require cohesive and synergistic thinking, including collaborations between doctors and patients for an appropriate design [29]. Thus, it is important to have a DSS for the ADHD screening and diagnosing process for young patients with ADHD. De Silva et al. [30] proposed the development of a DSS for ADHD based on knowledge of the patterns from past screening support systems. This was able to distinguish children with ADHD from other similar children's behavioural disorders. In addition, in designing a system, there would be important aspects that would need to be considered, such as diagnostic and monitoring approaches.

The Vanderbilt ADHD Diagnostic Rating Scale (VADRS) is a well-known standardised screening approach that aids doctors in making ADHD diagnoses based on the Diagnostic and Statistical Manual of Mental Disorders, Fifth Edition (DSM-5) standard [1,2,15,19] and assessing comorbid conditions. VADRS includes 18 symptoms described in the DSM-5. VADRS separates the teachers' (VADTRS) and parents' (VADPRS) versions of the assessment forms [22,31–34]. Additionally, VADRS contains comprehensive information to make an appropriate DSM-5-based diagnosis of ADHD and screens for common commodities. Moreover, VADRS has scales that allow for measuring the comorbidities by externalising and aiding in providing appropriate treatment plans. The only setback is its lack of data validity, data supporting stability, and discriminant validity in evaluation and treatment [22,33–35].

Contemporary machine learning techniques are used in several healthcare applications [28,36–38]. They are employed to predict future diseases and offer a desirable decision from a data set. We describe and compare the advantages and disadvantages of machine learning in Table 1.

Many researchers have used machine learning algorithms to indicate diseases such as liver disease (logistic regression with 95.8% accuracy) [38], breast cancer (support vector machine with 99% accuracy) [39], and Alzheimer's disease (neural networks with 98.3% accuracy) [40]. There are previous studies that have also proposed various machine learning algorithms to predict and classify ADHD. Krishnaveni and Radhamani [41] used Naïve Bayes and the J48 classifier as machine learning techniques with questionnaires as a tool to classify ADHD. The results achieved a classification accuracy of 100%. Additionally, Deping Kuang and Lianghua He [42] utilised the deep belief network (DBN) with a magnetic resonance imaging (MRI) method to indicate ADHD, which achieved a classification accuracy of 85%. Likewise, Öztoprak et al. [43] used the Disruptive Behaviour Disorders Rating Scale Form (DBDRS), for a study that employed a Decision Tree (DT) (CART), DT

(CHAID), and neural network to yield prediction accuracies of 69.1%, 70.6%, and 61.8%, respectively. Bo Miao and Yulin Zhang Das [44] used the feature selection algorithm of three methods, for which accuracies of 77.92%, 80.52%, and 98.04% were obtained for the relief algorithm (Relief), verification accuracy (VA-Relief), and minimum redundancy maximum relevance (mRMR), respectively. Likewise, Khanna and Das [45] used the feature selection algorithm and achieved a prediction accuracy of 82.10%. Jian Peng et al. [46] used a neural network algorithm with MRI to indicate the types of ADHD, yielding 72.89% accuracy. Cordova et al. [47] incorporated data from the DSM-IV-TR and used the Random Forest algorithm to predict ADHD and the types of autism spectrum disorder (ASD) with an accuracy of 72.70%. Radhamani and Krishnaveni [48] employed a hybrid approach integrating a support vector machine (SVM) and DT algorithms. The hybrid model gave an accuracy of 100% for classification and prediction. Parashar et al. [49] used the SVM, Random Forest, and AdaBoost Classifier (applied algorithm) to predict the types of ADHD, and they obtained an accuracy of 58%, 82%, and 84%, respectively. Furthermore, Lizhen Shao et al. [50] used the SVM and MRI and obtained an accuracy of 92.68%.

Table 1. Comparison of advantages and disadvantages of machine learning models.

| No | Classification Technique | Description | Pros | Cons |
|----|--------------------------|-------------|------|------|
| 1 | Decision Tree | A Decision Tree is a supervised learning technique that can be used for both classification and regression problems, but mostly it is preferred for solving classification problems. | - Structured data/Unstructured data<br>- easy implementation | - slight variation in data can lead to a different decision tree<br>- does not work well with small data |
| 2 | Naïve Bay | The KNN algorithm classifies data by comparing information of interest to others. The algorithm returns a result based on the information that is most similar to the information of interest. | - Structured data/Unstructured data<br>- easy implementation<br>- high computation efficiency, classification rate, and accuracy. | - precision of the algorithm decreases with fewer data<br>- an extensive number record is required for accuracy |
| 3 | KNN | The Naive Bay algorithm is a data mining classifier. The technique was developed based on the principle of Probably Naïve Bayesian Classification. It is used to analyze the probability of an unprecedented event from occurred events. | - Unstructured data<br>- suitable for multimodal class<br>- If the decision-making conditions are complex, this approach can create efficient models<br>- a small dataset and the data is noise-free and labeled. | - excessive time to find the nearest neighbors in an extensive training data set<br>- performance of the algorithm depends on the number of dimensions used |
| 4 | Neural Network | This algorithm is one of the data mining techniques. It is a mathematical model for processing information with a connected computation (Connectionist). The algorithm is used to simulate the functioning of neural networks in the human brain to create a tool capable of learning pattern recognition, knowledge extraction (Knowledge Extraction), and the human brain capabilities. | - Structured data/ Unstructured data<br>- simple to use with a few parameters to adjust<br>- applicable to a wide range of problems in real life | - requires high processing time if the neural network is large<br>- difficult to know the required number of neurons and layers |

In the case of this research, the aim was to examine and apply the most suitable algorithm to predict and classify the types of ADHD by using the collected and observed data from teachers and parents in real cases. The method for the data collection is also explained in this paper. Compared to the previous work, different assessment techniques were used for screening and predicting the types of ADHD and oppositional defiant disorder (ODD). Input data were obtained by using a standardised screening tool based on the behaviour and culture of Thai children (VADRS), which was evaluated by a group of teachers. In this work, the classification results and the physicians' diagnoses were compared to validate our results. Based on the previous study, the four techniques (DT, Naïve Bay, neural network, and k-nearest neighbour (KNN)) that provided highly accurate results were examined and tested with our data set. The classification results from these four models were compared, and we selected the model that could return the most accurate result to be used in our framework. The DT is known to support non-linear data, and it could provide highly accurate results with a trained model. The results from the DT were straightforward, and the model could be improved easily based on the interpretation of the results. The Naïve Bay algorithm is a data mining classifier. It offers extensive features and data that could also be used to classify data that had multiclass characteristics. The neural network algorithm is flexible and simple to use with a few parameters to adjust. It can simulate problems and remember a series of input–output pairs that are complex and cannot be replicated in a probabilistic way. The KNN is also a straightforward technique that can be used for data classification.

In this work, we applied the mentioned four models to the input data that we had collected by using the developed screening tool in our framework. This input data were provided by a group of teachers who regularly observed the behaviour of their students in class. The input form was developed based on the VADRS. The results of each model were validated and compared with the results of the diagnoses from the doctors. Thus, we applied the model with the best results for the classification module of the types of ADHD in our framework.

### 3. Research Methodology

This section presents the proposed research methodology, research framework, and classification technique for the types of ADHD, and the recommendation system based on behavioural therapy and activities for ADHD children. Before starting the process of the research methodology, we approved the ethics via the Human Research Ethics Committee of Thammasat University (Science) (HREC-TUSc)) and the participant recruitment process in Figure 1.

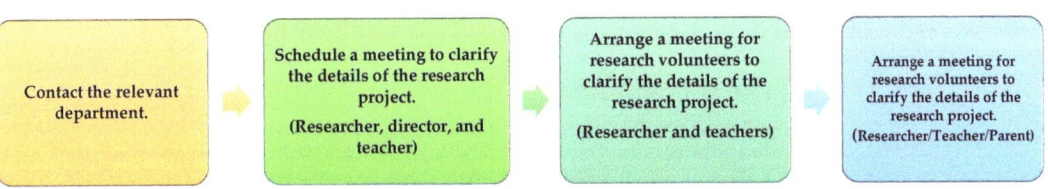

**Figure 1.** Participant recruitment process.

Figure 1 describes the selection and recruitment process of volunteers. The steps are as follows:

1. Ban Rat Niyom School (Jor Prayoon Upatham) was contacted with detailed documents about research work. The documents related to research work were presented to the school's director.
2. After receiving approval from the school's director, the researcher arranged a meeting to explain the details of the research process, activities, recruitment, and other information related to conducting research for the upcoming project.

3. Volunteer recruitment for teachers was conducted. After that, an appointment was made to meet and clarify the research implementation requirements. Documents relevant to the study and the activities to take place were presented throughout the research project.
4. The supervised teachers chose students. Then, they sent the parents the participant data sheet and consent letter. If the parents had any doubts regarding student participation, teachers could contact researchers to arrange meetings for clarification.

Participants were selected according to the following inclusion criteria.

(Inclusive criteria for teachers):

- Only homeroom teachers were selected, and they must have the following qualifications.
- The teachers must teach and supervise children of age 6–12 years old who study at the primary level (grade 1–6) at Ban Ratniyom School (Jorprayoon Upatham).
- The teachers have knowledge of and understand information about ADHD in children. They can assess and observe student behaviour in their supervising classes and are able to use a tool to screen behavioural/emotional problems, including the Strengths and Weaknesses Scale (SDQ, Teacher Student Behaviour Assessment Scale).

(Inclusive criteria for students):

- Students must be 6–12 years old and study at the primary level (grade 1–6) at Ban Rat Niyom School (Jor Prayun Upatham). They are in the class of the teachers under the criteria stated above. The participating teachers selected students for this study.

(Inclusive criteria for parents):

- Parents of the selected students, who were willing to participate, were included.

The exclusion criteria for research volunteers are as follows:

- Teachers who cannot participate in activities during the specified period of the research project were excluded.
- Teachers who could not assess and observe students' behaviours in their supervised classes according to the specified criteria and within the duration of the research project were excluded.
- There were no exclusion criteria for students and parents.

*3.1. Design and Development of the Proposed Collaborative Framework*

In this framework, there were three types of participants: teachers, parents, and doctors. The framework provided a collaborative tool for all participants to provide collaborative information based on the VADRS for preliminary assessment.

Workflow of the Collaborative Framework

The roles and responsibilities of the participants in the framework are shown in Figure 1. In this framework, the teacher evaluated the students using the VADRS, and the parents assessed their children using the same screening scale. The doctor determined and validated the results. The doctor could request to have a discussion and consultation with the teacher or parent for the appropriate treatment. The system used recorded information from the teachers and parents to perform the classification of the types of ADHD and provided recommendations for behavioural therapy for each student based on his/her type of ADHD. The treatments in the recommendation system were pre-input according to the medical recommendations based on the different types of ADHD (Figure 1).

Figure 2 shows the workflow for this research framework. The solid arrows indicate the sequence and direction of the process. The dashed line represents the data flow between the process and the database in the system. The overall process is described as follows:

- The role of the teacher was to evaluate students using the VADRS (refer to T1.1 in the framework) and view the screening of the result (T1.2). The teacher could also view the recommended behavioural therapy for each type of ADHD from the system (T1.3). The teacher could consult with the doctor if he/she had any questions about

how to apply the therapy or activity based on the recommendations from the system. After the teacher applied some therapies and/or treatment activities to the student, the teacher could update the information about the student's behaviour in the system for further assessment (T1.4). The updated data would also be used for updating the classification model for improvement.
- The parents could evaluate their child using the same VADRS (P2.1) and view the screening result from the system (P2.2). The parents could update the child's behaviour in the system for further assessment (P2.3) and view the recommended behavioural therapy for each type of ADHD from the system (P2.4).
- The doctors viewed and confirmed the results of the classification of ADHD that was returned by the system (D3.1) and recommended behavioural therapies based on the different types of ADHD (D3.2). They could view and record the discussions (D3.3) and give the teachers consultation from the system (D3.4) with follow-ups (D3.5).
- Our system consisted of three processes comprising the classification process (SA4.1), the update process for data and consultation discussion (SB4.1), and the update process for the activities and recommendations for behavioural therapy (SB4.2).

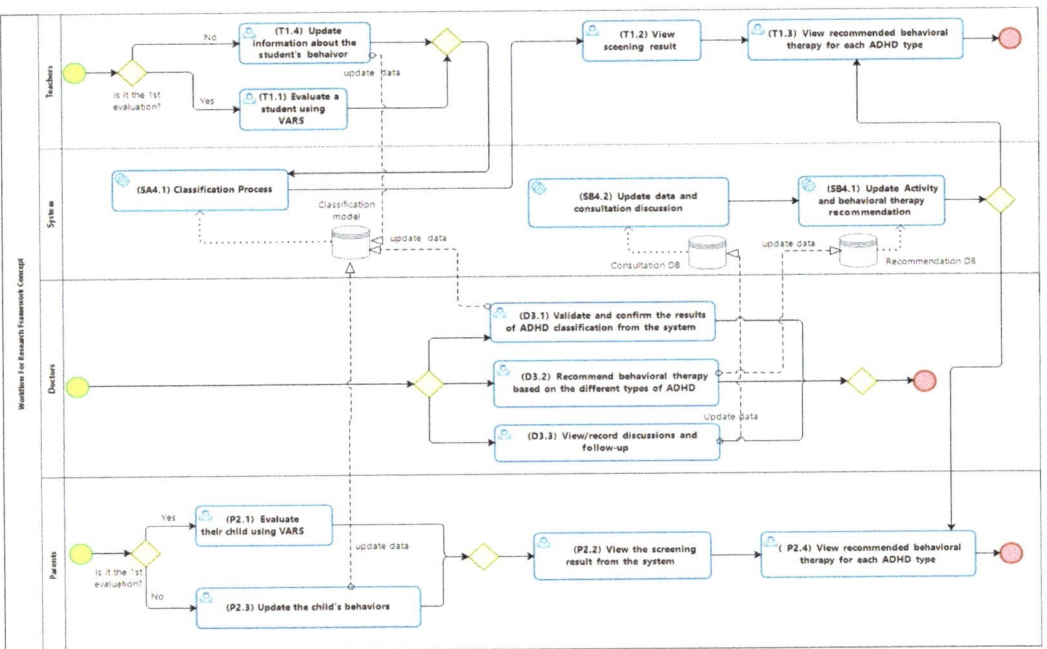

**Figure 2.** Workflow of the proposed framework.

This section provides a detailed explanation of SA4.1, SB4.1, and SB4.2 in Figure 2, respectively.

### 3.2. The Classification Process (SA4.1)

The classification was proposed based on the use of the VADRS and machine learning techniques. The results from this classification process were compared with the results evaluated by doctors who were consultants in child and adolescent psychiatry and developmental behavioural paediatrics. The following processes were performed to implement the classification process used in this framework:

(a) Data collection and analysis process

The main data set used in this work was collected from the data provided by the teachers and parents. The system automatically generated a set of questionnaires based on the VADRS and allowed the teachers and parents to evaluate their children via the system. After the system received the data from the teachers and parents, it generated the data set files that were used for the classification process. In this work, we obtained data for 420 cases.

(b) Model generation process

After the data set files were created from the previous step, these data set files were pre-processed to remove any duplicates, missing data, and inconsistencies. We exploited 52 attributes of the VADRS for learning and generating a model. To do so, the data set was imported and divided into two parts with a ratio of 80% for training the model and 20% for testing the model. The development of the model by training the data process utilised the feature extraction approach. The SelectPercentile module from the sci-kit-learn tool decreased the number of attributes and selected only the important features (selection) or converted features (transformation) to reduce the dimensions. After the data were declined dimensionally, they were processed for classification. The performance of the model was tested with the data set by specifying the percentage of the properties to be chosen rather than the number of properties to be determined. The top N% percentile was chosen to acquire the procedure of the whole 10 properties. This could be summarised as follows:

1. Set SelectPercentile = N%.
2. No. of the remaining attributes $\leq$ N%.
3. Update the set of attributes based on the SelectPercentile.
4. Return the attribute selection result.

Based on the above procedure, we could reduce the matrix dimension by using the SelectPercentile of 40% for optimisation. A low percentage led to fewer attributes that were utilised to create the model, thus making it unable to extract the data accurately. Still, a high percentage resulted in the model structure having a high complexity. The value of 40 gave the best result from the experiments, with eight remaining attributes being significant for the results of the experiment. Next, we applied various machine learning algorithms and tested each algorithm separately to determine the performance of each model. These algorithms were the DT, Naïve Bayes, neural network, and KNN.

(c) Prediction process

This sub-process was to query the model from the database system. After selecting the model algorithm, the system prediction was saved to the database, and the predicted model algorithm was yielded.

(d) Verification of the result of the predicted model

To verify the results from our classification models, the models' results were reviewed and validated by the doctors. These doctors specialised in child and adolescent psychiatry and developmental behavioural paediatrics. By comparing the accuracy and performance of all the models, the most appropriate classifier was discovered and selected for classifying the types of ADHD in our framework.

*3.3. The Activity and Behavioural Therapy Recommendation Process (SB4.1)*

This section explains how the system recommended activities and behavioural therapy for ADHD children based on the different types of ADHD. In this process, the system recommended the appropriate activity and behavioural therapy based on the classified type of ADHD the child shows. The information is summarised as follows [13,51–53].

Table 2 shows recommending activities for ADHD children by type as defined below (Recommend by the doctor).

1. Mix-type is a symptom of the hyperactivity–impulsivity and inattention type of ADHD. The activities for this type focus on organisation and discipline activities (AOCD) and medication activities (AMOD).
2. Hyperactivity is a symptom of a hyperactivity–impulsivity type of ADHD. The activities for this type include organisation and discipline activities (AOCD).
3. Inattention is a symptom of a lack of concentration. The activities for the children involve increasing concentration (AIC).
4. ODD is oppositional defiant disorder ADHD. The activities focus on those that can control behaviour (ACB).

Table 2. Recommended activities and behavioural therapy for different types of ADHD.

| No | ADHD Type | Activities | Description | Example for Activities |
|---|---|---|---|---|
| 1 | Mix-type | AOCD and AMOD | Organization and Discipline Activities and Medication Activities | Play toys or games that require concentration. Training the child to play with one toy at a time will help the child to concentrate on playing longer and Listen—play good music for concentration. |
| 2 | hyperactivity | AOCD | Activities Organization/Discipline Activities | Activities that require calmness, such as building blocks of wood or making towers of coins, Feed the eggs with a spoon. |
| 3 | inattention | AMOD | Activities Medication Activities | Activities that use distance, such as throwing a ball into the basket, threading the needle, stringing the beads, or stringing the garland, |
| 4 | ODD | ACB | Activities Control Behavioral | Create a daily schedule of activities, such as doing homework before play. |
| 5 | Non-ADHD | NO-Activities | Non-ADHD | General activities that increase concentration, such as reading stories. |

To implement this process, the following sub-processes were performed.

(a) Data collection and algorithm design

In this sub-process, three tasks were performed.

(i) Questionnaires, interviews, focus group discussions, and social media were employed to collect the data sources from the parents, teachers, and doctors. This information was determined and used for designing the recommendation process and the algorithm used in the framework.
(ii) We studied and evaluated the classification algorithms for the classification of the types of ADHD based on the VADRS [4,20].
(iii) We designed an algorithm to provide the appropriate recommendations for behavioural therapy and treatment activities based on the different types of ADHD. The verified information on the behavioural therapy and treatment activities was provided by the doctors, and it was pre-input into the system for the recommendation process.

(b) Review the recommended information and algorithm

The recommended information and algorithm were reviewed and validated by the doctors.

- Update data and consultation discussion (SB4.2)

The teachers and parents could have consultations with the doctors for more detailed recommendations and discussions about the recommended therapies and activities. After the discussions, which were conducted manually, the doctors updated the information in the system, so the teachers and parents could view the doctor's recommendation and discussion details via the system.

## 4. Experiments and Results

*4.1. Analysis of the Classification Results*

The classification results and the results from the behavioural therapy-based recommendation system for ADHD children from the experiments are presented in this section.

To evaluate the classification models, a confusion matrix was widely used for the performance measurement. The confusion matrix was a table of size $n$ by $n$ that was given for the $n$ classes. If the incident was positive and classified as such, it was considered a true positive (TP). It was considered a false negative (FN) if it was labelled as negative. If the incident was negative and characterised as such, it was considered a true negative (TN). If it was classed as positive, it was considered a false positive (FP) [50–54].

True positive and true negative are performance matrices for classification performance for machine learning models. In a classification problem with five classes, the concepts of true positive and true negative can be a bit different compared to binary classification. TP represents the true positives, indicating the instances correctly classified for each class. FN (false negative) represents the instances that belong to a particular class but are incorrectly classified as one of the other four classes. Each cell in the matrix that is not a TP represents an FN for that specific class. There are no TN (true negative) values explicitly defined in this case since they are related to correctly classifying instances as not belonging to the specific class in consideration. Based on the experimental results, we chose a classification model that provided the best performance and used this model for our screening tool to classify ADHD types. After the system identifies the ADHD type, the system recommends appropriate treatments and activities based on the ADHD type.

For a confusion matrix for a two-class classification problem, the numbers along the diagonal, from upper-left to lower-right, reflect the correct decisions, whereas the numbers outside of this diagonal represent errors. The TP and TN values estimate a classifier's overall accuracy. Other aggregated performance indicators were calculated using recall (sensitivity), specificity, and the F-measure. As defined below, the performance measurements were calculated.

$$\text{Classifier Accuracy} = \frac{TP + TN}{TP + TN + FP + FN} \tag{1}$$

$$\text{True Positive Rate (TPR)} = \frac{TP}{TP + FN} \tag{2}$$

$$\text{True Negative Rate (TNR)} = \frac{TN}{TN + FP} \tag{3}$$

$$\text{Recall (RC)} = \frac{TP}{TP + FN} \tag{4}$$

$$\text{Precision (PR)} = \frac{TP}{TP + FP} \tag{5}$$

$$F1 - \text{score (F1)} = \frac{2 * (\text{Precision} + \text{Recall})}{(\text{Precision} + \text{Recall})} \tag{6}$$

$$\text{Average Accuracy} = \frac{\sum_{i=1}^{l} \frac{TP_i + TN_i}{TP_i + FN_i + FP_i + TN_i}}{l} \tag{7}$$

The classifier accuracy (Equation (1)) is a measurement used to assess which model would be the most appropriate at recognising the correlations and patterns between the variables in the data set based on the inputs (or training data). A good classification model should have high accuracy. Equation (2) shows the TPR or sensitivity, which refers to the probability of a positive test, conditioned on truly being positive.

Equation (3) shows the TNR or specificity, which refers to the probability of a negative test, conditioned on truly being negative. Contrary to the other equations, a more favourable result for this equation was closer to 0. A result of 0 referred to a 0% chance of a model predicting a case incorrectly.

Equation (4) shows recall (RC). It is also known as sensitivity or TPR, which is the measure of our model correctly identifying the TPs.

Equation (5) shows precision (PR), which is the ratio between the TPs and all the positives.

Equation (6) shows the F1 score (F1), which is a metric that takes into account both precision and recall precision.

Equation (7) shows the average accuracy, which is the average effectiveness per class of the classifier.

Table 3 shows the summary of the cross-validation of the four classifiers. It also compares the outcomes between the system results and the validated results from the doctor. For this experiment, there were 336 records of training data (80%), 84 records of test data (20%), and 420 cases of doctor-confirmed outcomes.

Table 3. Statistical data analysis of the ADHD classes.

| No | Type of ADHD | Data | Number of Data | % | All Data |
|---|---|---|---|---|---|
| 0 | Mix -Type | train | 188 | 80 | 235 |
|   |   | test | 47 | 20 |   |
| 1 | Non-ADHD | train | 28 | 80 | 35 |
|   |   | test | 7 | 20 |   |
| 2 | ODD | train | 12 | 80 | 15 |
|   |   | test | 3 | 20 |   |
| 3 | hyperactivity | train | 32 | 80 | 40 |
|   |   | test | 8 | 20 |   |
| 4 | inattention | train | 76 | 80 | 95 |
|   |   | test | 19 | 20 |   |

In Table 4, the results of the four classifiers were tabulated for comparison. Based on the results (Table 5), the DT and neural network models provided the highest accuracy. The DT method and neural network algorithm provided an accuracy of 99.57%, while the KNN algorithm achieved up to 98.72%. The Naïve Bay algorithm yielded an accuracy of 94.47%.

The average accuracy of the classification was 99.60% for the DT and neural network models. The KNN algorithm provided an average accuracy of 98.40%, whereas the Naïve Bayes yielded 94.00%. Furthermore, as shown in Table 3, the DT and neural network models produced the same values of the TPR, TNR, PR, RC, AC, and F1 for all types of ADHD. Both models had values greater than 97% for the TPR, RC, and F1. The PR of 95% and the TNR of 2% indicated the low probability of TN testing.

The classification results of the KNN algorithm showed 100% TPR for all cases except for 94% for the mix-type. A TNR of 0% was also yielded for cases except for inattention, for which the model could predict the case incorrectly with a 5% chance. For PR, only inattention yielded results of 86%, while it had a 100% ratio for the TPs and all the positives for the other types of ADHD. RC showed 100% for all cases, except for 94% for the mix-type. For AC and F1, only the mix-type and inattention did not have a result of 100%.

Table 4. Comparison of the results of the four classifiers.

| No | Type of ADHD | Test | Decision Tree | | | | | KNN | | | | | Naive Bayes | | | | | Neural Network | | | | |
|---|---|---|---|---|---|---|---|---|---|---|---|---|---|---|---|---|---|---|---|---|---|---|
| | | | Cor | % | Inc | % | Cor | % | Inc | % | Cor | % | Inc | % | Cor | % | Inc | % |
| 0 | Mix-type | 47 | 46 | 97.87 | 1 | 2.13 | 44 | 93.62 | 3 | 6.38 | 34 | 72.34 | 13 | 27.66 | 46 | 97.87 | 1.00 | 2.13 |
| 1 | Non-ADHD | 7 | 7 | 100.00 | 0 | 0.00 | 7 | 100.00 | 0 | 0.00 | 7 | 100.00 | 0 | 0.00 | 7 | 100.00 | 0.00 | 0.00 |
| 2 | ODD | 3 | 3 | 100.00 | 0 | 0.00 | 3 | 100.00 | 0 | 0.00 | 3 | 100.00 | 0 | 0.00 | 3 | 100.00 | 0.00 | 0.00 |
| 3 | hyperactivity | 8 | 8 | 100.00 | 0 | 0.00 | 8 | 100.00 | 0 | 0.00 | 8 | 100.00 | 0 | 0.00 | 8 | 100.00 | 0.00 | 0.00 |
| 4 | inattention | 19 | 19 | 100.00 | 0 | 0.00 | 19 | 100.00 | 0 | 0.00 | 19 | 100.00 | 0 | 0.00 | 19 | 100.00 | 0.00 | 0.00 |
| | Total (case) | 84 | | 99.57 | | 0.43 | | 98.72 | | 1.28 | | 94.47 | | 5.53 | | 99.57 | | 0.43 |
| | % Total Cases | | | 99.57 | | | | 98.72 | | | | 94.47 | | | | 99.57 | | |

Note: Cor = no. of correct results and Inc = no. of incorrect results.

Table 5. Performance comparison of the four classifiers.

| No | Type of ADHD | Decision Tree | | | | | | KNN | | | | | | Naive Bayes | | | | | | Neural Network | | | | | |
|---|---|---|---|---|---|---|---|---|---|---|---|---|---|---|---|---|---|---|---|---|---|---|---|---|---|
| | | TPR | TNR | PR | RC | AC | F1 | TPR | TNR | PR | RC | AC | F1 | TPR | TNR | PR | RC | AC | F1 | TPR | TNR | PR | RC | AC | F1 |
| 0 | Mix-type | 0.98 | 0 | 1 | 0.98 | 0.99 | 0.99 | 0.94 | 0 | 1 | 0.94 | 0.96 | 0.97 | 0.72 | 0 | 1 | 0.72 | 0.85 | 0.84 | 0.98 | 0 | 1 | 0.98 | 0.99 | 0.99 |
| 1 | Non-ADHD | 1 | 0 | 1 | 1 | 1 | 1 | 1 | 0 | 1 | 1 | 1 | 1 | 1 | 0 | 1 | 1 | 1 | 1 | 1 | 0 | 1 | 1 | 1 | 1 |
| 2 | ODD | 1 | 0 | 1 | 1 | 1 | 1 | 1 | 0 | 1 | 1 | 1 | 1 | 1 | 0 | 1 | 1 | 1 | 1 | 1 | 0 | 1 | 1 | 1 | 1 |
| 3 | hyperactivity | 1 | 0 | 1 | 1 | 1 | 1 | 1 | 0 | 1 | 1 | 1 | 1 | 1 | 0 | 1 | 1 | 1 | 1 | 1 | 0 | 1 | 1 | 1 | 1 |
| 4 | inattention | 1 | 0.02 | 0.95 | 1 | 0.99 | 0.97 | 1 | 0.05 | 0.86 | 1 | 0.96 | 0.93 | 1 | 0.2 | 0.59 | 1 | 0.85 | 0.75 | 1 | 0.02 | 0.95 | 1 | 0.99 | 0.97 |
| | Average Accuracy | | | 0.996 | | | | | | 0.984 | | | | | | 0.94 | | | | | | 0.996 | | | |

Note: TPR = rate of true positives; TNR = true negative rate; PR = precision; RC = recall; AC = accuracy; and F1 = F1 score.

*4.2. Analysis of the Recommendation Process*

This section explains how the system recommends activities and behavioural therapy for ADHD children based on the different types of ADHD. In this process, we used the DT algorithm for finding the appropriate recommendations for each type of ADHD.

From our experiments, the average classification accuracy offered by the Decision Tree and neural network models is equivalent to and better than other models. However, the main reason that we chose Decision Tree is because we found that it also provides better computation time compared to the neural network model. Table 6 shows an example of computation time offered by the Decision Tree and neural network from our experiments.

**Table 6.** Comparison of model time between the Decision Tree and neural network models.

| No. | Computation Time | |
|---|---|---|
| | Decision Tree Model | Neural Network |
| 1 | 0.031229 | 1.040929 |
| 2 | 0.055537 | 1.110908 |
| 3 | 0.061133 | 1.175104 |
| 4 | 0.051996 | 2.634261 |
| 5 | 0.074594 | 1.068259 |
| 6 | 0.052359 | 1.24145 |
| 7 | 0.050016 | 1.313238 |
| 8 | 0.047997 | 1.392138 |
| 9 | 0.073211 | 1.600991 |
| 10 | 0.078132 | 2.092879 |
| 11 | 0.058697 | 1.389741 |
| 12 | 0.057674 | 1.334164 |
| 13 | 0.062324 | 1.848112 |
| 14 | 0.082012 | 1.639582 |
| 15 | 0.091128 | 1.899683 |
| 16 | 0.070998 | 1.397739 |
| 17 | 0.044996 | 1.257645 |
| 18 | 0.058901 | 1.204572 |
| 19 | 0.045997 | 1.127632 |
| 20 | 0.056571 | 1.180286 |
| 21 | 0.049337 | 1.2724 |
| 22 | 0.063612 | 1.046959 |
| 23 | 0.064478 | 1.25124 |
| 24 | 0.063231 | 1.501523 |
| 25 | 0.063992 | 3.656594 |
| 26 | 0.083996 | 1.15601 |
| 27 | 0.058533 | 1.216549 |
| 28 | 0.050994 | 1.071333 |
| 29 | 0.048935 | 1.203264 |
| 30 | 0.048 | 1.352984 |
| 31 | 0.047018 | 1.296979 |
| 32 | 0.081719 | 1.195881 |
| 33 | 0.045019 | 1.038161 |
| 34 | 0.052759 | 1.117537 |
| 35 | 0.048993 | 1.120578 |
| 36 | 0.063812 | 1.11737 |
| 37 | 0.053889 | 1.229534 |
| 38 | 0.054619 | 1.55222 |
| 39 | 0.050994 | 1.119644 |
| 40 | 0.060458 | 1.255233 |
| 41 | 0.051103 | 1.493202 |
| 42 | 0.050003 | 1.005049 |
| 43 | 0.05909 | 1.304165 |
| 44 | 0.052995 | 1.251586 |
| 45 | 0.061735 | 1.457659 |

Table 6. *Cont.*

| No. | Computation Time | |
|---|---|---|
| | Decision Tree Model | Neural Network |
| 46 | 0.050007 | 1.086125 |
| 47 | 0.052067 | 1.379029 |
| 48 | 0.051687 | 1.133587 |
| 49 | 0.050996 | 1.049925 |
| 50 | 0.044999 | 1.177412 |
| 51 | 0.064901 | 1.06846 |
| 52 | 0.056602 | 0.970769 |
| 53 | 0.051998 | 1.345009 |
| 54 | 0.046708 | 1.189245 |
| 55 | 0.047584 | 1.125525 |
| 56 | 0.089003 | 1.555476 |
| 57 | 0.0625 | 2.134213 |
| 58 | 0.086094 | 2.15842 |
| 59 | 0.068346 | 1.812286 |
| 60 | 0.059886 | 1.31289 |
| 61 | 0.0644 | 1.274483 |
| 62 | 0.053056 | 1.663544 |
| 63 | 0.077142 | 1.632083 |
| 64 | 0.084134 | 2.141111 |
| 65 | 0.074552 | 1.464199 |
| 66 | 0.057663 | 1.094026 |
| 67 | 0.048291 | 1.640016 |
| 68 | 0.044992 | 1.486279 |
| 69 | 0.049449 | 1.069333 |
| 70 | 0.046227 | 1.450437 |
| 71 | 0.063584 | 1.509127 |
| 72 | 0.075065 | 1.465219 |
| 73 | 0.047998 | 1.345517 |
| 74 | 0.047002 | 1.229406 |
| 75 | 0.056996 | 1.622626 |
| 76 | 0.048608 | 1.10312 |
| 77 | 0.046375 | 1.286845 |
| 78 | 0.047895 | 1.19502 |
| 79 | 0.054994 | 1.117199 |
| 80 | 0.074998 | 1.395097 |
| 81 | 0.05399 | 1.271263 |
| 82 | 0.053778 | 1.882056 |
| 83 | 0.065562 | 1.208384 |
| 84 | 0.055619 | 1.22781 |
| 85 | 0.047999 | 1.047544 |
| 86 | 0.048203 | 1.251664 |
| 87 | 0.04885 | 1.160577 |
| 88 | 0.050631 | 0.874186 |
| 89 | 0.055177 | 1.260275 |
| 90 | 0.049021 | 1.201123 |
| 91 | 0.044018 | 1.254685 |
| 92 | 0.046995 | 1.244649 |
| 93 | 0.047016 | 1.05943 |
| 94 | 0.052024 | 0.944234 |
| 95 | 0.042279 | 1.299954 |
| 96 | 0.059698 | 1.503714 |
| 97 | 0.047133 | 1.13383 |
| 98 | 0.060916 | 1.063454 |
| 99 | 0.047019 | 0.98657 |
| 100 | 0.05708 | 1.087645 |
| Average computation time | 0.057146 | 1.348791 |

## The Decision Tree Graph

As the average accuracy of the classification was 99.60% for the DT and the neural network models, the DT algorithm was selected because the value of the F1 was greater than 97%, while PR was 95%. Its FPR of 0.02 indicated a low probability of a wrong prediction. From several experiments of the data sets, we found that the DT algorithm gave predictive accuracy close to the results of each experiment (Table 7).

**Table 7.** Performance metric of the DT classifier (for the recommended activities).

| No | Type of ADHD | Decision Tree | | | | | |
|---|---|---|---|---|---|---|---|
| | | TPR | TNR | PR | RC | AC | F1 |
| 0 | Mix-type (AOCD + AMOD + ACB) | 0.98 | 0 | 1 | 0.98 | 0.99 | 0.99 |
| 1 | hyperactivity (AOCD) | 1 | 0 | 1 | 1 | 1 | 1 |
| 2 | inattention (AIC) | 1 | 0 | 1 | 1 | 1 | 1 |
| 3 | ODD (ACB) | 1 | 0 | 1 | 1 | 1 | 1 |
| 4 | Non-ADHD (No) | 1 | 0.02 | 0.95 | 1 | 0.99 | 0.97 |
| | Accuracy average | | | 0.996 | | | |

The description for the parameter in the tree graph (Figure 3) is as follows:

(1). The samples parameter is the number of data items compatible with that node, so as the decision moved down the depth of the tree, the number of samples of a node in each layer tended to decrease over time.

(2). Gini indicates the "purity" of a node. Where Gini = 0, this infers that all the data items in the node belong to the same class. In comparison, Gini = 0.5 indicates that the data items in the node belong to two similar types, which represent the values, such as the value of R1 = [136, 0, 12 0, 0] in the child node to the right of the root node. This infers the 148 entries of 15 at this node condition. If the answer was false (child node left R1) and the value was [0, 0, 12, 0, 0], there would be 12 entries in the ODD classification. However, if the answer was true and the value was [136, 0, 0, 0, 0] (child node right R1), there would be 136 entries in the mix-type classification. This assumes that the data meeting this node's condition is in the ODD and mix-type classifications.

(3). Value is used to indicate the class of the predicted activities by the types of ADHD. The activities of the five classes were mix-type (index [0]), non-ADHD (index [1]), ODD (index [2]), hyperactivity (index [3]), and inattention (index [4]).

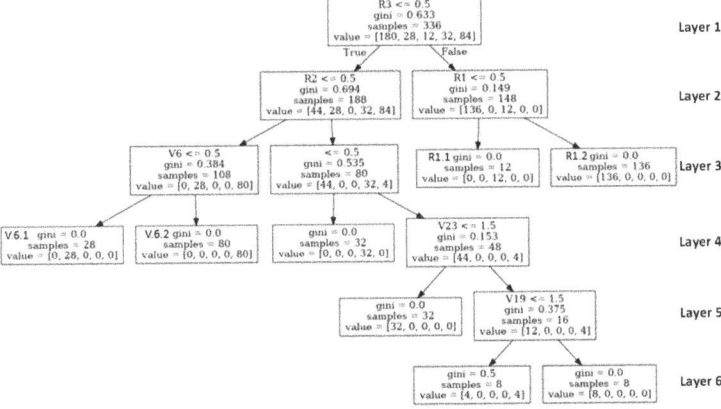

**Figure 3.** The Decision Tree graph.

We tested the DT algorithm for processing the recommendations of the activities for ADHD children. The results are shown in Table 5. The PR and TNR were 0.95 and 0.02, respectively, and the average accuracy was 0.996. This result was reviewed and validated by doctors, and the accuracy was acceptable.

## 5. Discussion and Conclusions

In this research, we aimed to overcome the mentioned problems by proposing a methodology and framework that teachers or parents could use to evaluate and screen their children's behaviour and determine if they were consistent with the types of ADHD. The framework provided recommendations for the appropriate treatments for different types of ADHD children. The expected outcome of our proposed framework was to provide an effective way to screen and classify the types of ADHD and recommend appropriate treatments and therapy based on individual behaviour.

The average classification accuracy of 99.60% was achieved by the DT and neural network algorithms. On the other hand, the KNN approach had an average classification accuracy of 98.40%, whereas the Naïve Bay technique had an average classification accuracy of 94.00%. Although the DT and neural network algorithms returned similar accuracy, in this work, we chose the DT algorithm as the main model for the classification of the types of ADHD and recommendations of the activities because the tree structure could be easily explained to all the participants for analysis, change, and future improvement. In addition, the performance, when adding a new data set to the training model, required a shorter time compared to the time required to fine-tune the neural network.

The limitation of our research is data collection. During our data collection process, the COVID-19 pandemic was seriously occurring in Thailand and all schools were closed, so it was very difficult to collect data from all participants in the study. This resulted in the small amount of data we used in this work. Also, due to the pandemic situation, we could not directly interview each student to obtain the child's opinion, which we believe can be valuable and useful for further analysis. Therefore, in our future work, we plan to improve our research by gathering more data from various groups of children such as children in big cities, children in rural areas, etc. Moreover, we will improve our tools, which would better support communications among participants (teachers, doctors, parents) to share information and follow up cases. In Thailand, the employment of machine learning technology in the children's health care system is limited. This is especially true for ADHD. Moreover, when a child is found with a condition or a tendency to have ADHD, the child relies on many elements to support the treatment, including access to disease information, medical treatment, specialised doctors related to psychiatry, travelling method to the hospital, and unforeseen expenses incurred by the family.

For future work to improve our framework, we would like to generate and expand the data collection and conduct further experiments to design and build more efficient algorithms of the sub-activities based on different types of ADHD. Although the current work could achieve high accuracy for classifying the types of ADHD, some cases would still need to be improved (e.g., classifying an inattention type and mix-type). We also plan to train the model for different scenarios and try to enhance the model's accuracy and UX/UI design based on feedback from the users (e.g., teachers and doctors).

**Author Contributions:** Conceptualisation, P.C. and S.U.; methodology, P.C. and S.U.; software, P.C.; validation, P.C. and S.U.; formal analysis, P.C. and S.U.; investigation, P.C.; resources, P.C.; data curation, P.C. and S.U.; writing—original draft preparation, P.C. and S.U.; writing—review and editing, P.C. and S.U.; visualisation, P.C.; supervision, S.U. All authors have read and agreed to the published version of the manuscript.

**Funding:** This research received no external funding.

**Institutional Review Board Statement:** The study was conducted in accordance with the Declaration of Helsinki and approved by the Ethics Committee of Thammasat University (Science) (protocol code 032/2526 and date of approval 27 July 2022).

**Informed Consent Statement:** Not applicable.

**Data Availability Statement:** Data sharing is not applicable.

**Acknowledgments:** The authors would like to thank the reviewers for their thoughtful comments and efforts towards improving this manuscript; Sija Leela and Thanyaporn Mekrungcharas, Division of Developmental and Behavioural Paediatrics, Department of Paediatrics Queen Sirikit National Institute of Child Health, Bangkok, Thailand, for their valuable advice, suggestions, and consulting on the research; Vilawan Chirdkiatgumchai, Division of Developmental and Behavioural Paediatrics Department of Paediatrics Ramathibodi Hospital, Mahidol University Bangkok, Thailand, and Mark Wolraich supporting the screening tool, the Vanderbilt Assessment Scale—Teacher Informant (Thai Version); the Research Fund of the Sirindhorn International Institute of Technology (SIIT) Thammasat University.

**Conflicts of Interest:** The authors declare no conflict of interest.

# References

1. Al-Ghannami, S.S.; Al-Adawi, S.; Ghebremeskel, K.; Cramer, M.T.; Hussein, I.S.; Min, Y.; Jeyaseelan, L.; Al-Sibani, N.; Al-Shammakhi, S.M.; Al-Mamari, F.; et al. Attention Deficit Hyperactivity Disorder and Parental Factors in School Children Aged Nine to Ten Years in Muscat, Oman. *Oman Med. J.* **2018**, *33*, 193–199. [CrossRef] [PubMed]
2. Posner, J.; Polanczyk, G.V.; Sonuga-Barke, E. Attention-deficit hyperactivity disorder. *Lancet* **2020**, *395*, 450–462. [CrossRef]
3. Rohde, L.; Buitelaar, J.K.; Gerlach, M.; Faraone, S.V.; Coghill, D. The world federation of ADHD guide. *Porto Alegre Artmed* **2019**, 66–70.
4. Swanson, J.M.; Wigal, T.; Lakes, K. DSM-V and the future diagnosis of attention-deficit/hyperactivity disorder. *Curr. Psychiatry Rep.* **2009**, *11*, 399–406. [CrossRef] [PubMed]
5. American Psychiatric Association. *Diagnostic and Statistical Manual of Mental Disorders: DSM-5*; American Psychiatric Association: Washington, DC, USA, 2013.
6. Sonne, T.; Marshall, P.; Obel, C.; Thomsen, P.H.; Grønbæk, K. An assistive technology design framework for ADHD. In Proceedings of the 28th Australian Conference on Computer-Human Interaction–OzCHI'16, Launceston, Australia, 29 November–2 December 2016.
7. Dreyer, B.P. The Diagnosis and Management of Attention-Deficit/Hyperactivity Disorder in Preschool Children: The State of Our Knowledge and Practice. *Curr. Probl. Pediatr. Adolesc. Health Care* **2006**, *36*, 6–30. [CrossRef]
8. Gallo, E.F.; Posner, J. Moving towards causality in attention-deficit hyperactivity disorder: Overview of neural and genetic mechanisms. *Lancet Psychiatry* **2016**, *3*, 555–567. [CrossRef]
9. Sibley, M.H.; Pelham Jr, W.E.; Molina, B.S.; Gnagy, E.M.; Waschbusch, D.A.; Garefino, A.C.; Kuriyan, A.B.; Babinski, D.E.; Karch, K.M. Diagnosing ADHD in adolescence. *J. Consult. Clin. Psychol.* **2012**, *80*, 139. [CrossRef]
10. Jain, R.A. *To Study the Attention Deficit Hyperactivity Disorder (ADHD) and to Evaluate the Cognitive, Hyperactive and Impulsive Behavior against 6-OHDA Hbr Lesioned Sprague Dawley Neonates Using Hyperaxe, Curcumin & Quercetin*; CL Baid Metha College of Pharmacy: Chennai, India, 2017.
11. Kalaman, C.R.; Ibrahim, N.; Shaker, V.; Cham, C.Q.; Ho, M.C.; Visvalingam, U.; Shahabuddin, F.A.; Rahman, F.N.A.; Halim, M.R.T.A.; Kaur, M.; et al. Parental Factors Associated with Child or Adolescent Medication Adherence: A Systematic Review. *Healthcare* **2023**, *11*, 501. [CrossRef]
12. Mick, E.; Biederman, J.; Faraone, S.V.; Sayer, J.; Kleinman, S. Case-Control Study of Attention-Deficit Hyperactivity Disorder and Maternal Smoking, Alcohol Use, and Drug Use During Pregnancy. *J. Am. Acad. Child Adolesc. Psychiatry* **2002**, *41*, 378–385. [CrossRef] [PubMed]
13. Perrin, J.M.; Stein, M.T.; Amler, R.W.; Blondis, T.A.; Feldman, H.; Meyer, B.; Shaywitz, B.; Wolraich, M. Clinical practice guideline: Treatment of the school-aged child with attention-deficit/hyperactivity disorder. *Pediatrics* **2001**, *108*, 1033–1044.
14. Wender, P.H.; Tomb, D.A. Attention-Deficit Hyperactivity Disorder in Adults: An Overview. *Atten.-Deficit Hyperact. Disord. (ADHD) Adults* **2010**, *176*, 258447. [CrossRef]
15. Alamuti, E. Mohammadi, M.R. Comparison of Child and Parent Cognitive Behaviour Therapy on Reduction of Attention Deficit Hyperactivity Disorder Symptoms in Children. *J. Child Adolesc. Behav.* **2016**, *4*, 285. [CrossRef]
16. Chu, S. Occupational Therapy for Children with Attention Deficit Hyperactivity Disorder: A Survey on the Level of Involvement and Training Needs of Therapists. *Br. J. Occup. Ther.* **2003**, *66*, 209–218. [CrossRef]
17. Barbaresi, W.J.; Colligan, R.C.; Weaver, A.L.; Voigt, R.G.; Killian, J.M.; Katusic, S.K.; Chawla, A.; Sprinz, P.G.; Welch, J.; Heeney, M.; et al. Mortality, ADHD, and Psychosocial Adversity in Adults With Childhood ADHD: A Prospective Study. *Pediatrics* **2013**, *131*, 637–644. [CrossRef] [PubMed]
18. Fogler, J.M.; Weaver, A.L.; Katusic, S.; Voigt, R.G.; Barbaresi, W.J. Recalled Experiences of Bullying and Victimization in a Longitudinal, Population-Based Birth Cohort: The Influence of ADHD and Co-Occurring Psychiatric Disorder. *J. Atten. Disord.* **2020**, *26*, 15–24. [CrossRef] [PubMed]

19. Singh, I. A Framework for Understanding Trends in ADHD Diagnoses and Stimulant Drug Treatment: Schools and Schooling as a Case Study. *Biosocieties* **2006**, *1*, 439–452. [CrossRef]
20. Lahey, B.B.; Pelham, W.E.; Loney, J.; Lee, S.S.; Willcutt, E. Instability of the DSM-IV Subtypes of ADHD From Preschool through Elementary School. *Arch. Gen. Psychiatry* **2005**, *62*, 896–902. [CrossRef]
21. Paholpak, S.; Arunpongpaisal, S.; Krisanaprakornkit, T.; Khiewyoo, J. Validity and reliability study of the Thai version of WHO schedules for clinical assessment in neuropsychiatry: Sections on psychotic disorders. *J. Med. Assoc. Thail.* **2008**, *91*, 408.
22. Minor, E.C.; Porter, A.C.; Murphy, J.; Goldring, E.B.; Cravens, X.; Elliott, S.N. A known group analysis validity study of the Vanderbilt Assessment of Leadership in Education in US elementary and secondary schools. *Educ. Assess. Eval. Acc.* **2014**, *26*, 29–48. [CrossRef]
23. Health, M.O.P. Thai Children are more likely to Have ADHD than One Year ago. 2008. Available online: https://www.dmh.go.th/newsdmh/ (accessed on 27 March 2023).
24. Choopun, K.; Boonlue, N. Attention Deficit Hyperactivity Disorder in Primary School Chiang Mai, Thailand. *Int. J. Child Dev. Ment. Health* **2022**, *10*.
25. Ayano, G.; Yohannes, K.; Abraha, M. Epidemiology of attention-deficit/hyperactivity disorder (ADHD) in children and adolescents in Africa: A systematic review and meta-analysis. *Ann. Gen. Psychiatry* **2020**, *19*, 21. [CrossRef]
26. Danielson, M.L.; Bitsko, R.H.; Ghandour, R.M.; Holbrook, J.R.; Kogan, M.D.; Blumberg, S.J. Prevalence of Parent-Reported ADHD Diagnosis and Associated Treatment Among U.S. Children and Adolescents, 2016. *J. Clin. Child Adolesc. Psychol.* **2018**, *47*, 199–212. [CrossRef]
27. Hoang, H.H.; Tran, A.T.N.; Nguyen, V.H.; Nguyen, T.T.B.; Le, D.D.; Jatho, A.; Onchonga, D.; Van Duong, T.; Nguyen, M.T.; Tran, B.T. Attention Deficit Hyperactivity Disorder (ADHD) and Associated Factors Among First-Year Elementary School Students. *J. Multidiscip. Health* **2021**, *14*, 997–1005. [CrossRef] [PubMed]
28. Rissanen, M. Translational health technology and system schemes: Enhancing the dynamics of health informatics. *Health Inf. Sci. Syst.* **2020**, *8*, 39. [CrossRef] [PubMed]
29. Albahar, F.; Abu-Farha, R.K.; Alshogran, O.Y.; Alhamad, H.; Curtis, C.E.; Marriott, J.F. Healthcare Professionals' Perceptions, Barriers, and Facilitators towards Adopting Computerised Clinical Decision Support Systems in Antimicrobial Stewardship in Jordanian Hospitals. *Healthcare* **2023**, *11*, 836. [CrossRef]
30. De Silva, S.; Dayarathna, S.; Ariyarathne, G.; Meedeniya, D.; Jayarathna, S.; Michalek, A.M.P. Computational Decision Support System for ADHD Identification. *Int. J. Autom. Comput.* **2020**, *18*, 233–255. [CrossRef]
31. Bard, D.E.; Wolraich, M.L.; Neas, B.; Doffing, M.; Beck, L. The Psychometric Properties of the Vanderbilt Attention-Deficit Hyperactivity Disorder Diagnostic Parent Rating Scale in a Community Population. *J. Dev. Behav. Pediatr.* **2013**, *34*, 72–82. [CrossRef]
32. Becker, S.P.M.; Langberg, J.M.; Vaughn, A.J.; Epstein, J.N. Clinical Utility of the Vanderbilt ADHD Diagnostic Parent Rating Scale Comorbidity Screening Scales. *J. Dev. Behav. Pediatr.* **2012**, *33*, 221–228. [CrossRef] [PubMed]
33. Kądziela-Olech, H. The measurement of the symptoms of ADHD in the NICHQ Vanderbilt Assessment Scale for Parent (VADPRS) and for Teacher (VADTRS). *Psychiatr. I Psychol. Klin.* **2014**, *14*, 277–283. [CrossRef]
34. Murphy, J.F.; Goldring, E.B.; Cravens, X.C.; Elliott, S.N.; Porter, A.C. The Vanderbilt assessment of leadership in education: Measuring learning-centered leadership. *J. East China Norm. Univ.* **2007**, *29*, 1–10.
35. Porter, A.C.; Polikoff, M.S.; Goldring, E.B.; Murphy, J.; Elliott, S.N.; May, H. Investigating the Validity and Reliability of the Vanderbilt Assessment of Leadership in Education. *Elem. Sch. J.* **2010**, *111*, 282–313. [CrossRef]
36. Saputra, D.C.E.; Sunat, K.; Ratnaningsih, T. A New Artificial Intelligence Approach Using Extreme Learning Machine as the Potentially Effective Model to Predict and Analyze the Diagnosis of Anemia. *Healthcare* **2023**, *11*, 697. [CrossRef] [PubMed]
37. Ferdous, M.; Debnath, J.; Chakraborty, N.R. Machine Learning Algorithms in Healthcare: A Literature Survey. In Proceedings of the 2020 11th International Conference on Computing, Communication and Networking Technologies (ICCCNT), Kharagpur, India, 1–3 July 2020. [CrossRef]
38. Shobana, G.; Umamaheswari, K. Prediction of Liver Disease using Gradient Boost Machine Learning Techniques with Feature Scaling. In Proceedings of the 2021 5th International Conference on Computing Methodologies and Communication (ICCMC), Erode, India, 8–10 April 2021; IEEE: Piscataway Township, NJ, USA; pp. 1223–1229. [CrossRef]
39. Zahoor, S.; Shoaib, U.; Lali, I.U. Breast Cancer Mammograms Classification Using Deep Neural Network and Entropy-Controlled Whale Optimization Algorithm. *Diagnostics* **2022**, *12*, 557. [CrossRef] [PubMed]
40. Dashtipour, K.; Taylor, W.; Ansari, S.; Zahid, A.; Gogate, M.; Ahmad, J.; Assaleh, K.; Arshad, K.; Imran, M.A.; Abbasi, Q. Detecting Alzheimer's disease using machine learning methods. In Proceedings of the Body Area Networks. Smart IoT and Big Data for Intelligent Health Management: 16th EAI International Conference, BODYNETS 2021, Virtual Event, 25–26 October 2021; Springer: Berlin/Heidelberg, Germany, 2022; pp. 89–100.
41. Krishnaveni, K.; Radhamani, E. Diagnosis and evaluation of ADHD using Naïve Bayes and J48 classifiers. In Proceedings of the 2016 3rd International Conference on Computing for Sustainable Global Development (INDIACom), New Delhi, India, 16–18 March 2016; IEEE: Piscataway Township, NJ, USA; pp. 1809–1814.
42. Kuang, D.; He, L. Classification on ADHD with Deep Learning. In Proceedings of the 2014 International Conference on Cloud Computing and Big Data, Wuhan, China, 12–14 November 2014.

43. Oztoprak, H.; Toycan, M.; Alp, Y.K.; Arikan, O.; Dogutepe, E.; Karakas, S. Machine-based learning system: Classification of ADHD and non-ADHD participants. In Proceedings of the 2017 25th Signal Processing and Communications Applications Conference (SIU), Antalya, Turkey, 15–18 May 2017; IEEE: Piscataway Township, NJ, USA; pp. 1–4. [CrossRef]
44. Miao, B.; Zhang, Y. A feature selection method for classification of ADHD. In Proceedings of the 2017 4th International Conference on Information, Cybernetics and Computational Social Systems (ICCSS), Dalian, China, 24–26 July 2017; IEEE: Piscataway Township, NJ, USA; pp. 21–25. [CrossRef]
45. Khanna, S.; Das, W. A Novel Application for the Efficient and Accessible Diagnosis of ADHD Using Machine Learning. In Proceedings of the 2020 IEEE/ITU International Conference on Artificial Intelligence for Good (AI4G), Geneva, Switzerland, 21–25 September 2020; IEEE: Piscataway Township, NJ, USA; pp. 51–54. [CrossRef]
46. Peng, J.; Debnath, M.; Biswas, A.K. Efficacy of novel Summation-based Synergetic Artificial Neural Network in ADHD diagnosis. *Mach. Learn. Appl.* **2021**, *6*, 100120. [CrossRef]
47. Cordova, M.; Shada, K.; Demeter, D.V.; Doyle, O.; Miranda-Dominguez, O.; Perrone, A.; Schifsky, E.; Graham, A.; Fombonne, E.; Langhorst, B.; et al. Heterogeneity of executive function revealed by a functional random forest approach across ADHD and ASD. *NeuroImage Clin.* **2020**, *26*, 102245. [CrossRef]
48. Radhamani, E.; Krishnaveni, K. Diagnosis and Evaluation of ADHD using MLP and SVM Classifiers. *Indian J. Sci. Technol.* **2016**, *9*, 93853. [CrossRef]
49. Parashar, A.; Kalra, N.; Singh, J.; Goyal, R.K. Machine Learning Based Framework for Classification of Children with ADHD and Healthy Controls. *Intell. Autom. Soft Comput.* **2021**, *28*, 669–682. [CrossRef]
50. Shao, L.; Xu, Y.; Fu, D. Classification of ADHD with bi-objective optimization. *J. Biomed. Informatics* **2018**, *84*, 164–170. [CrossRef]
51. Felt, B.T.; Biermann, B.; Christner, J.G.; Kochhar, P.; Van Harrison, R. Diagnosis and management of ADHD in children. *Am. Fam. Physician* **2014**, *90*, 456–464.
52. Pfiffner, L.J.; Mikami, A.Y.; Huang-Pollock, C.; Easterlin, B.; Zalecki, C.; McBurnett, K. A randomized, controlled trial of integrated home-school behavioral treatment for ADHD, predominantly inattentive type. *J. Am. Acad. Child Adolesc. Psychiatry* **2007**, *46*, 1041–1050. [CrossRef]
53. McVoy, M.; Findling, R.L. *Clinical Manual of Child and Adolescent Psychopharmacology*; American Psychiatric Pub: Washington, DC, USA, 2017.
54. Sokolova, M.; Lapalme, G. A systematic analysis of performance measures for classification tasks. *Inf. Process. Manag.* **2009**, *45*, 427–437. [CrossRef]

**Disclaimer/Publisher's Note:** The statements, opinions and data contained in all publications are solely those of the individual author(s) and contributor(s) and not of MDPI and/or the editor(s). MDPI and/or the editor(s) disclaim responsibility for any injury to people or property resulting from any ideas, methods, instructions or products referred to in the content.

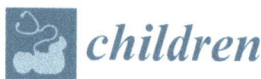 

Article

# HIV-Related Knowledge and Sexual Behaviors among Teenagers: Implications for Public Health Interventions

Ruyu Liu [1], Ke Xu [2], Xingliang Zhang [2], Feng Cheng [3,4], Liangmin Gao [5] and Junfang Xu [1,6,*]

1. Center for Health Policy Studies, School of Public Health, Zhejiang University School of Medicine, Hangzhou 310058, China
2. Hangzhou Center for Disease Control and Prevention, Hangzhou 310021, China
3. Vanke School of Public Health, Tsinghua University, Beijing 100084, China
4. Institute for Healthy China, Tsinghua University, Beijing 100084, China
5. Institute for International and Area Studies, Tsinghua University, Beijing 100084, China
6. Department of Pharmacy, Second Affiliated Hospital, Zhejiang University School of Medicine, Hangzhou 310000, China
* Correspondence: xujf2019@zju.edu.cn

**Abstract: Background:** Teenagers are at a turning point in people's physical and psychological maturity and are also in a critical period in reproductive and sexual health. It is reported that the initial age at first sexual behavior is younger than decades ago, which implies that the risky sexual behavior among teenagers may be on the rise. However, it is unclear about the changes of sexual knowledge and behaviors in recent years. **Methods:** Based on the national sentinel surveillance survey in 2011–2021 among students in Hangzhou, we selected out teenagers aged 10–19 years as our study sample. Demographic characteristics (gender, age, marital status, etc.), knowledge of HIV and sexual behaviors were collected. The sexual knowledge score and sexual behaviors were analyzed, and their influencing factors were explored. **Results:** In total, 1355 teenagers were incorporated in this study; the awareness rates of sexual knowledge in 2011, 2013, 2014 and 2021 were 74.9%, 71.8%, 89.3% and 95.8%, respectively, which showed an overall upward trend. The results of binary logistic regression showed that the survey year, whether students had received and participated in HIV-related publicity services and whether they had sexual behaviors, had a significant influence on whether the awareness rate ≥ 75%. The survey year and whether the awareness rate ≥ 75% had a significant influence on whether students had sexual behaviors. **Conclusions:** Both the average scores and awareness rates of teenagers' sexual knowledge showed an overall upward trend from 2011 to 2021. Teenagers' initial sexual behavior was at a low age, and the proportion of teenagers who had fixed, temporary and commercial heterosexual sex was still relatively high despite no significant increasing. Therefore, we should further strengthen health education on the risks of sexual behaviors from schools, families and health-related institutions to ensure teenagers receive HIV-related publicity services.

**Keywords:** sexual knowledge; sexual behaviors; teenager; public health interventions; implications

**Citation:** Liu, R.; Xu, K.; Zhang, X.; Cheng, F.; Gao, L.; Xu, J. HIV-Related Knowledge and Sexual Behaviors among Teenagers: Implications for Public Health Interventions. *Children* **2023**, *10*, 1198. https://doi.org/10.3390/children10071198

Academic Editor: Jane D. Champion

Received: 23 May 2023
Revised: 27 June 2023
Accepted: 30 June 2023
Published: 11 July 2023

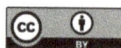

**Copyright:** © 2023 by the authors. Licensee MDPI, Basel, Switzerland. This article is an open access article distributed under the terms and conditions of the Creative Commons Attribution (CC BY) license (https:// creativecommons.org/licenses/by/ 4.0/).

## 1. Background

Teenagers are at a turning point in people's physical and psychological maturity and are also in a critical period in reproductive and sexual health [1]. With socio-economic development and cultural and ideological changes, currently teenagers in adolescence may be becoming open to sexuality, which may increase the probability of having sexual behaviors, which may cause sexual violence, premature unwanted pregnancies and unsafe abortion [2–4]. For example, a history of sexual abuse during adolescence has consistently been found to be significantly associated with increased health risks and health risk behaviors in both men and women [5]. Additionally, a cross-sectional analysis about primarily students aged 13–15 years from Namibia, Swaziland, Uganda, Zambia and Zim-babwe [6] found that 23% reported having experienced sexual violence, i.e., being physically forced to have sexual intercourse at some point in their lives. These experiences were moderately-to-strongly associated with multiple adverse health behaviors, such as multiple sexual partners, poor mental health, suicidal ideation and a history of a sexually transmitted infection. For premature unwanted pregnancies, it has major effects on mother and child health, particularly in underdeveloped nations where health care is not as advanced. One of the main causes of mortality for females between the ages of 15 and 19 is pregnancy and delivery problems [7]. It also brings up a number of human rights issues. For example, a pregnant teenage girl who is forced to miss school is not only deprived of her right to education but is also prevented from her right to health at the same time because she is not allowed to access any kind of contraception or knowledge on reproductive health [7]. Additionally, now many teenagers are not physically or mentally prepared for pregnancy or delivery, which increases the risk of problems and even life-threatening health effects [8]. Moreover, risky sexual behaviors are also the main transmission route of sexually transmitted diseases, including HIV. One study has estimated that one in four sexually active teenager females has a sexually transmitted disease such as HIV, trichomoniasis or HPV [9]. Young people aged 15 to 24 are less likely to be proactive about their HIV status than older adults, which means that they may become infected with or transmit HIV [10].

The Office of AIDS Prevention Education Project for Chinese Youth released a white paper on the exploration and practice of the AIDS Prevention Education Project for Chinese Youth, which showed that nearly 3000 HIV new cases of young students aged 15–24 were reported nationwide in 2020, with sexual transmission accounting for 98.6% [11]. Similarly, UNAIDS [12] indicated that 36.7 million [32.3–41.9 million] adults aged 15 years or older and 1.7 million [1.3–2.1 million] children aged 0–14 years were living with HIV in 2021. Despite remarkable achievements in the prevention and treatment of HIV, global progress has been uneven. More than half of the world's new infections were among women and teenagers, and nearly 2 million teenagers aged 10–19 years were living with HIV worldwide [13]. Relevant studies have also shown that somatic pubertal development [14], curiosity about sex [15], a relative lack of knowledge about sexual health [16] and accessing explicit sexual content indiscriminately on the internet [17] could increase the risk of having unsafe and unprotected sexual behaviors among teenagers.

On 29 February 2012, China's 12th Five-Year Plan of Action for Preventing HIV was promulgated [18], requiring all general secondary schools, secondary vocational schools and general higher education schools to carry out special education activities on HIV knowledge every school year, especially for teenagers. The 13th Five-Year Plan of Action for Preventing HIV in China, dated 5 February 2017, set the work target of over 90% awareness rate of prevention and treatment among key populations including young students [19]. It can be seen that China attaches great importance to the prevention and control of sexually transmitted diseases among teenagers. However, it is unclear about the changes of sexual behaviors and HIV-related knowledge among teenagers, which could provide evidence for the future public health interventions to reduce the risk of sexual health among teenagers.

## 2. Methods

### 2.1. Participants and Data Collection

The data were collected from national HIV sentinel surveillance in Hangzhou conducted between 2011 and 2021 except the year 2012. HIV sentinel surveillance of young students was located in universities and secondary vocational colleges, and phased cluster sampling was used to collect the data during the monitoring period. Personnel specifically engaged in health behaviors monitoring are selected as the leading surveyors, and they receive strict training from the Hangzhou Center for Disease Control and Prevention, which undertakes national HIV surveillance. Everyone is also allowed to exit at any time during the filling process. Additionally, the World Health Organization identified adolescence as 10–19 years old [20], so we screened 10–19 years old from the youth sentinel and finally obtained our survey population. Among all the data, we screened out the 1355 teenagers, aged 15 years at the youngest and 18 years at the oldest. However, the psychological support for the respondents, especially the underage persons, was not assessed during the HIV sentinel surveillance investigation. The following information were collected: social demographic characteristics (gender, age, marital status, ethnicity, grade, etc.), HIV-related knowledge and sexual behaviors (drug usage, fixed heterosexual sexual behavior, temporary heterosexual sexual behavior, commercial heterosexual sexual behavior, homosexual sexual behavior, condom usage, etc.).

*2.2. Measurement*

HIV-related knowledge was measured using the 8-item HIV Knowledge Questionnaire, which has been widely applied in HIV-related surveys in China and has been proved to have good validity [21,22]. One point was given for the correct answer, and 0 points were given for the wrong answer or not knowing. Therefore, the maximum score is 8, and the minimum score is 0. Additionally, a high knowledge score indicates a good understanding of HIV transmission and prevention. The awareness rate of sexual knowledge was calculated according to the requirements of "China AIDS Prevention and Control Supervision and Evaluation Framework (Trial)" [23], which indicated that if they answer 6 or more questions correctly ($\geq 75\%$), they would be considered as having knowledge awareness. In our study, sexual behaviors did not include touching but engaged in a coital relationship. Risky sexual behaviors included fixed heterosexual sex, temporary heterosexual sex, commercial heterosexual sex and homosexual sex. Fixed heterosexual sex refers to sexual behaviors with spouses or ongoing partners. Temporary heterosexual sex refers to sexual behaviors with strangers or acquaintances for once. Commercial sexual behaviors represented paying for sexual behaviors, which included commercial heterosexual behaviors and commercial homosexual behaviors. Homosexual behaviors refer to sexual behaviors with the partner who has the same gender as him or her. Unprotected sexual behaviors mean that someone did not use condom in every sexual behavior. Participation in HIV publicity services refers to the voluntary provision of relevant services as opposed to receiving publicity services. Questions asked to measure the respondents' level of knowledge have been included in the annex.

*2.3. Statistical Analysis*

Frequency, percentage and mean $\pm$ SD were used to describe social demographic characteristics, HIV related knowledge and sexual behaviors of teenagers. Univariate analysis and binary logistic regression analysis were used to explore the factors influencing the HIV-related knowledge score and sexual behaviors. The independent variables included the survey year, gender, ethnicity, grade and whether they had received and participated in HIV-related publicity services within one year to date of the corresponding survey years. All data analyses were based on statistical software SPSS 23.0 software (IBM, Armonk, NY, USA). Variables with $p < 0.05$ were considered statistically significant.

## 3. Results

*3.1. Basic Characteristics of Teenagers*

A total of 1355 teenagers under 19 years old were incorporated in our study, with 891 (65.8%) males and 464 (34.2%) females. In terms of age, the largest number of teenagers was 17 years old (688, 50.8%), followed by 18 years old (526, 38.8%). For marital status, most (1351, 99.9%) were unmarried. Moreover, there were 511 (37.9%) teenagers in grade 1 and 797 (59.0%) in grade 2. Some 694 (52.7%) and 278 (22.9%), respectively, had received and participated in HIV-related publicity services within one year to date of the corresponding survey years (Table 1).

**Table 1.** Basic characteristics of teenagers.

| Items | | Frequency | Percentage (%) |
|---|---|---|---|
| Gender | | | |
| | Male | 891 | 65.8 |
| | Female | 464 | 34.2 |
| Age(year) | | | |
| | 15 | 3 | 0.2 |
| | 16 | 138 | 10.2 |
| | 17 | 688 | 50.8 |
| | 18 | 526 | 38.8 |
| Marital Status * | | | |
| | Unmarried | 1351 | 99.9 |
| | Married | 1 | 0.1 |
| | Cohabiting | 1 | 0.1 |
| Ethnicity * | | | |
| | Han | 1315 | 97.3 |
| | Other | 37 | 2.7 |
| Grade * | | | |
| | Grad 1 | 511 | 37.9 |
| | Grade 2 | 797 | 59.0 |
| | Grade 3 and above | 42 | 3.1 |
| Whether they had received HIV-related publicity services * | | | |
| | Yes | 694 | 52.7 |
| | No | 623 | 47.3 |
| Whether they had participated in HIV-related publicity services * | | | |
| | Yes | 278 | 22.9 |
| | No | 937 | 77.1 |
| Total | | 1355 | 100 |

Note: * indicates that 2, 3, 5, 38, and 140 people were missing for marital status, ethnicity, grade, whether they had received HIV-related publicity services and whether they had participated in HIV-related publicity services, respectively.

### 3.2. Teenagers' HIV-Related Knowledge Scores and Awareness Rates

The average scores of teenagers' HIV related knowledge in 2011, 2013, 2014 and 2021 were 6.25, 6.09, 6.68 and 7.22, respectively, and the awareness rates of sexual knowledge were 74.9%, 71.8%, 89.3% and 95.8%, respectively (Figure 1).

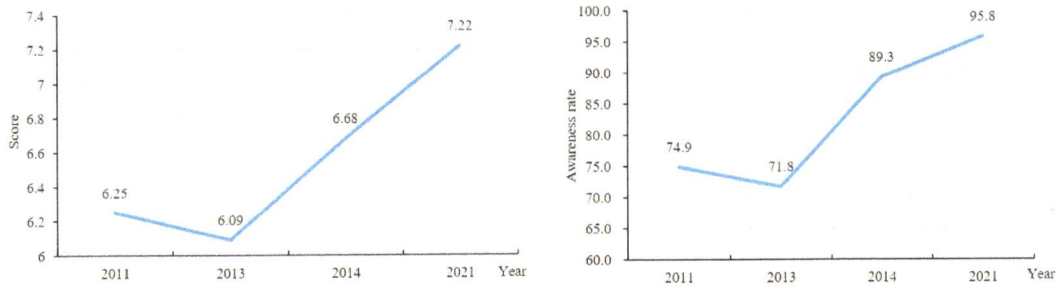

**Figure 1.** Teenagers' HIV-related knowledge scores and awareness rates.

### 3.3. Sexual Behaviors of Teenagers

Among teenagers, 5 (0.4%) of them used drugs, and 83 (6.2%) had sexual behaviors before, and 1265 had (93.8%) not. The average age of their initial sexual behaviors was 16.23 ± 1.29. Among those who had experienced sex, 65 (82.3%) had their initial sexual behavior with their romantic partners, and 2 (2.5%), 9 (11.4%) and 3 (3.8%) engaged in sexual behavior with commercial sexual partners, temporary sexual partners and homosexual partners, respectively. Totals of 39 (2.9%), 45 (3.3%) and 9 (0.7%) had fixed, temporary and commercial heterosexual sex within one year to date of the corresponding survey years, respectively. For males, 1 (0.1%) had homosexual sex within one year to date of the corresponding survey years. In addition, 30 (53.6%) of the teenagers who had sexual behaviors within one year to date of the corresponding survey years had unprotected sex (Table 2).

Table 2. Sexual behaviors of teenagers.

| Items | | Frequency | Percentage (%) |
|---|---|---|---|
| Drug using [a] | | | |
| | Yes | 5 | 0.4 |
| | No | 1295 | 99.6 |
| Whether they had sexual behaviors before [b] ($n$ = 1355) | | | |
| | Yes | 83 | 6.2 |
| | No | 1265 | 93.8 |
| Age of initial sexual behaviors (M ± SD) | 16.23 ± 1.29 | | |
| The object of initial sexual behaviors [c] ($n$ = 83) | | | |
| | Romantic partner | 65 | 82.3 |
| | Commercial sexual partner | 2 | 2.5 |
| | Temporary sexual partner | 9 | 11.4 |
| | Homosexual partner | 3 | 3.8 |
| Fixed heterosexual sex [d] ($n$ = 1355) | | | |
| | Yes | 39 | 2.9 |
| | No | 1305 | 97.1 |
| Temporary heterosexual sex [e] ($n$ = 1355) | | | |
| | Yes | 45 | 3.3 |
| | No | 1299 | 96.7 |
| Commercial heterosexual sex [f] ($n$ = 1355) | | | |
| | Yes | 9 | 0.7 |
| | No | 1335 | 99.3 |
| Homosexual sex [g] ($n$ = 891) | | | |
| | Yes | 1 | 0.1 |
| | No | 881 | 99.9 |
| Unprotected sex [h] | | | |
| | Yes | 30 | 53.6 |
| | No | 26 | 46.4 |

Note: [a], [b], [c], [d], [e], [f], [g], [h] indicates that 55, 7, 4, 11, 11, 11, 9, 4 were missing for drug using, whether they had sexual behaviors before, the object of initial sexual behaviors, fixed heterosexual sex, temporary heterosexual sex, commercial heterosexual sex, homosexual sex and unprotected sex, respectively.

From 2011 to 2021, percentages of those who had sexual behaviors within one year to date of the corresponding survey years were 5.25%, 5.08%, 7.14% and 2.35%, respectively. Among them, percentages of having fixed heterosexual sex were 3.4%, 3.7%, 3.6% and 1.3%, respectively, and having temporary heterosexual sex decreased from 3.6% in 2011 to 1.8% in 2021 (Figure 2).

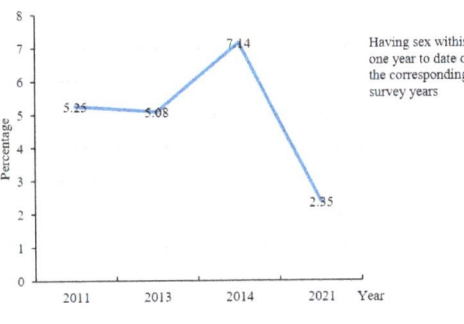 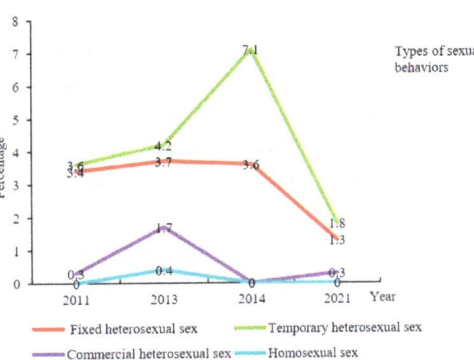

**Figure 2.** Teenagers' risky sexual behaviors.

### 3.4. Influencing Factors of HIV-Related Knowledge and Sexual Behaviors

The results of binary logistic regression showed that the survey year ($p < 0.001$, OR = 3.314), whether they had received HIV-related publicity services ($p < 0.001$, OR = 1.933), whether they had participated in HIV-related publicity services ($p = 0.019$, OR = 1.818) and whether they had sexual behaviors ($p = 0.005$, OR = 0.416) had a significant influence on the HIV-related knowledge scores. With the progress of the survey year, teenagers' HIV knowledge scores showed an upward trend. Teenagers who had received or participated in HIV-related publicity services scored higher on HIV knowledge than those who had not (Table 3).

**Table 3.** Influencing factors of sexual knowledge scores.

| Variable | | Univariate Analysis | | Multivariate Analysis | |
|---|---|---|---|---|---|
| | | Crude OR | $p$ Value | Adjusted OR | $p$ Value |
| Year | | | <0.001 | | <0.001 |
| | 2011 (ref) | | | | |
| | 2013 | 0.850 | 0.285 | 0.838 | 0.349 |
| | 2014 | 2.790 | 0.097 | 1.913 | 0.314 |
| | 2021 | 7.680 | <0.001 | 3.314 | <0.001 |
| Gender | | | | | |
| | Male (ref) | | | | |
| | Female | 1.491 | 0.008 | 1.146 | 0.428 |
| Ethnicity | | | | | |
| | Han (ref) | | | | |
| | Other | 1.279 | 0.585 | 1.100 | 0.855 |
| Grade | | | <0.001 | | 0.100 |
| | Grade 1 (ref) | | | | |
| | Grade 2 | 1.655 | <0.001 | 1.065 | 0.741 |
| | Grade ≥ 3 | 0.510 | 0.044 | 0.491 | 0.043 |
| Whether they had received HIV-related publicity services | | | | | |
| | No (ref) | | | | |
| | Yes | 2.733 | <0.001 | 1.933 | <0.001 |
| Whether they had participated in HIV-related publicity services | | | | | |
| | No (ref) | | | | |
| | Yes | 3.009 | <0.001 | 1.818 | 0.019 |
| Whether they had sexual behaviors | | | | | |
| | No (ref) | | | | |
| | Yes | 0.471 | 0.008 | 0.416 | 0.005 |

The results of binary logistic regression showed that the survey year ($p = 0.004$, OR = 0.174) and whether the awareness rate was ≥75% ($p = 0.007$, OR = 0.426) had a significant influence on whether they had sexual behaviors. With the progress of the survey year or the awareness rate ≥ 75%, the probability of risky sexual behaviors among teenagers would be downward (Table 4).

Table 4. Influencing factors of sexual behaviors.

| Variable | | Univariate Analysis | | Multivariate Analysis | |
|---|---|---|---|---|---|
| | | Crude OR | p Value | Adjusted OR | p Value |
| Year | | | 0.144 | | 0.033 |
| | 2011 (ref) | | | | |
| | 2013 | 0.966 | 0.910 | 0.628 | 0.206 |
| | 2014 | 1.387 | 0.665 | 1.473 | 0.627 |
| | 2021 | 0.434 | 0.030 | 0.174 | 0.004 |
| Gender | | | | | |
| | Male (ref) | | | | |
| | Female | 0.571 | 0.072 | 0.783 | 0.488 |
| Ethnicity | | | | | |
| | Han (ref) | | | | |
| | Other | 1.238 | 0.772 | 0.761 | 0.793 |
| Grade | | | 0.646 | | 0.378 |
| | Grade 1 (ref) | | | | |
| | Grade 2 | 0.916 | 0.753 | 1.639 | 0.167 |
| | Grade ≥ 3 | 1.632 | 0.441 | 1.382 | 0.622 |
| Whether they had received HIV-related publicity services | | | | | |
| | No (ref) | | | | |
| | Yes | 1.032 | 0.907 | 0.979 | 0.953 |
| Whether they had participated in HIV-related publicity services | | | | | |
| | No (ref) | | | | |
| | Yes | 1.948 | 0.024 | 2.909 | 0.005 |
| Awareness rate ≥ 75% | | | | | |
| | No (ref) | | | | |
| | Yes | 0.471 | 0.008 | 0.426 | 0.007 |

## 4. Discussion

In our study, the average scores and awareness rates of teenagers' sexual knowledge both showed an overall upward trend from 2011 to 2021, like the results of previous research [24]. It may be that China attaches great importance to AIDS prevention and intervention and has achieved some success in the promoting of publicity and education on AIDS prevention and treatment [25]. Additionally, it is also possible that as the Internet grows, teenagers go online more frequently, and they will actively search the Internet for sexual-related knowledge and education, resulting in increasing accessibility of HIV knowledge to teenagers [26–28]. Meanwhile, in our study, the awareness rate reached 95.8% in 2021, which is the goal of the 13th Five-Year Plan of Action for Curbing and Preventing AIDS in China, that is, to reach more than 90% among key populations including teenagers. However, one study by Sun Lixiang et al. [21] on the characteristics of AIDS prevalence and results of sentinel surveillance among young students in Liaoning province found that some teenagers still had a low awareness rate of HIV knowledge, indicating that there were some misunderstandings in the population's understanding or mastery of the characteristics of AIDS.

We consider 16.23 ± 1.29 as the average age of sexual initiation in our study to be an age at which teenagers are still considered minors in China and, according to Yan Zhang et al. [29], may expose them to increased risk of unplanned pregnancy, mental health problems or infection of sexually transmitted diseases. Additionally, there were 60 people who had sex within one year to date of the corresponding survey years, among which 30 people had unprotected sex, accounting for 53.6%, indicating that the current situation of condom use among teenagers is not optimistic, and the awareness of self-protection in the process of having sex is still insufficient, which is consistent with the findings of Liu et al. [30] Therefore, providing health education on the risk of sexual behaviors including unprotected sexual behaviors is still important. Meanwhile, carrying out intervention activities of condom promotion use [31], such as setting up condom self-service free distribution machines in schools, may help reduce the spread of sexually transmitted diseases among teenagers. Moreover, currently, teenagers' access to prevention and treatment of sexually transmitted diseases mainly comes from some health education curriculums and less through parents and other means [32], and age-appropriate online sex education has become a more acceptable form of sex education for college students [26], indicating that there is still much room for improvement in the development of education from family members and schools. Studies have shown that teenagers without parental family members are 1.93 times more likely to engage in risky sexual behaviors than those who are living with parental family members [33], possibly because parental involvement restrains them from committing risky sexual behaviors. Thus, parents of teenagers also need to learn about relevant sexual knowledge and master parent–child communication skills to improve family sex education [34]. In addition, some studies also showed that new media could expand efficiency and coverage [35], which also allows participants to communicate and interact with each other and provides timely and convenient information feedback and thus may be more attractive to teenagers [19,36].

However, for risky sexual behaviors, the proportion of teenagers who had fixed, temporary and commercial heterosexual sex was still relatively high despite no significant increasing. Among these, temporary heterosexual sex among teenagers accounted for the highest proportion among all types of sexual behaviors. This was probably because our research population was about teenagers, not about men who had sex with men, thus the probability of homosexual sex was relatively low. Moreover, our research also found that commercial heterosexual sex also existed in the teenage population.

Teenagers who had received ($p < 0.001$, OR = 1.933) or participated in ($p = 0.019$, OR = 1.818) HIV-related publicity services within one year to date of the corresponding survey years had a higher awareness rate of sexual knowledge than those who had not, which could be that they had more exposure to HIV-related education and were more aware and familiar with AIDS. Meanwhile, risky sexual behaviors among teenagers were significantly lower in 2021 ($p = 0.004$, OR = 0.174) compared to 2011, which is different from the study of Sun Lixiang et al. [21]. This difference may be due to differences in the population of the sentinel sites included in the study. Our study included people under 19 years of age with the minimum age of 15 years (0.2%) and the maximum of 18 years (38.8%), while the Sun Lixiang's study included people aged 15–29 years with an average age of $20.7 \pm 1.6$. It is also speculated that this may be due to the increase in knowledge of HIV among teenagers causing the corresponding decrease in risky sexual behaviors. Thirdly, indeed, social distancing has proven to be an active factor in controlling the spread of infectious diseases [37,38]. According to the study of Guanjian Li et al. [39], due to the COVID-19 pandemic and related containment measures, 22% of participants reported a decrease in sexual desire; 41% experienced a decrease in sexual intercourse frequency. Therefore, we have reason to believe that in the context of the outbreak of COVID-19 in 2020, maintaining social distance, avoiding mobility and reporting of geographic location carried out to prevent COVID-19 transmission [38–40] may also lead to lower interpersonal sexual interactions among teenagers, resulting in a decrease in the proportion of risky sexual behaviors.

## 5. Conclusions

We found that both the average scores and awareness rates of teenagers' sexual knowledge showed an overall upward trend from 2011 to 2021; teenagers' initial sexual behavior was at a low age, and the proportion of teenagers who had fixed, temporary and commercial heterosexual sex was still relatively high despite no significant increasing. Therefore, it is important to further strengthen health education on the risks of sexual behaviors, guide the establishment of correct relationship concepts (for example, gender relationship education should not become empty moral education or traditional "chastity" education, but rather the dissemination of scientific knowledge and social values, so that young people can gain knowledge of sexual physiology and psychology in line with their age), eliminate anxiety, ambiguity and other bad emotions in sexual development, correctly understand and deal with the morality and law of gender relations, enhance a sense of the responsibility of their own sexual behaviors, carry out intervention activities of condom promotion use, such as setting up condom self-service free distribution machines in schools, and encourage teenagers to receive HIV-related publicity services. Parents of teenagers should also be encouraged to learn about relevant sexual knowledge and master parent–child communication skills to improve family sex education. All these require the organization and publicity of policies of the health-related institutions at all levels in order to build a coordinated and synchronized whole.

## 6. Limitations

There are some limitations of this study. For example, we did not assess whether the gender of the participants was transgender of cisgender although being transgender is very rare in China. Secondly, the data collected did not cover all regions of China, and the findings may not be representative of China as a whole. In addition, by using a nationally standardized sentinel questionnaire, we were unable to explore the influences of factors not included in the questionnaire. Although the overall number of questions was the same, some questions regarding AIDS knowledge in 2021 differed from those in 2011, 2013 and 2014. Therefore, readers should be cautious when comparing the knowledge level in 2021 with other years.

**Author Contributions:** Conceptualization, J.X.; Formal analysis, R.L.; Project administration, J.X.; Writing—original draft, R.L.; Writing—review and editing, K.X., X.Z., F.C., L.G. and J.X. All authors have read and agreed to the published version of the manuscript.

**Funding:** This work was supported by China Medical Board (Project No. 20-391), Fundamental Research Funds for the Central Universities, Zhejiang Province Medical and Health General Project (Project No. 2020KY777), Special Research Program of Pharmacoeconomics and Health Technology Assessment Committee of Zhejiang Pharmaceutical Association and Sanming Project of Medicine in Shenzhen (Project NO. SZSM202111001).

**Institutional Review Board Statement:** The study protocol and consent procedure were approved by Medical Ethics Committee of School of Public Health Zhejiang University (ZGL202203-5).

**Informed Consent Statement:** Informed consent was obtained from all subjects involved in the study.

**Data Availability Statement:** All of the main data have been included in the results. Additional materials with details may be obtained from the corresponding author.

**Conflicts of Interest:** The authors declare no conflict of interest.

## References

1. Blum, R.W.; Mmari, K.N. *Risk and Protective Factors Affecting Adolescent Reproductive Health in Developing Countries: An Analysis of Adolescent Sexual and Reproductive Health Literature from Around the World: Summary*; World Health Organization: Geneva, Switzerland, 2004; p. 13.
2. Nie, Y.; Zheng, R.; Luo, X.; Xu, Y. Investigation and analysis of sexual development situation and knowledge, attitude and behavior about sexual and reproductive health of 15415 adolescents in China. *Chin. J. Woman Child Health* **2022**, *33*, 68–74. (In Chinese)
3. Centers for Disease Control and Prevention. Sexual Risk Behaviors: HIV, STD, & Teen Pregnancy Prevention. Available online: www.cdc.gov/healthyyouth/yrbs/pdf/us_overview.2016 (accessed on 20 January 2023).
4. Alamrew, Z.; Bedimo, M.; Azage, M. Risky sexual practices and associated factors for HIV/AIDS infection among private college students in Bahir Dar City, Northwest Ethiopia. *Int. Sch. Res. Not.* **2013**, *2013*, 763051. [CrossRef]
5. Maniglio, R. The impact of child sexual abuse on health: A systematic review of reviews. *Clin. Psychol. Rev.* **2009**, *29*, 647–657. [CrossRef] [PubMed]
6. Brown, D.W.; Riley, L.; Butchart, A.; Meddings, D.R.; Kann, L.; Harvey, A.P. Exposure to physical and sexual violence and adverse health behaviours in African children: Results from the Global School-based Student Health Survey. *Bull. World Health Organ.* **2009**, *87*, 447–455. [CrossRef]

7. Chakole, S.; Akre, S.; Sharma, K.; Wasnik, P.; Wanjari, M.B.; Wasnik Sr, P. Unwanted Teenage Pregnancy and Its Complications: A Narrative Review. *Cureus* **2022**, *14*, e32662. [CrossRef]
8. Ghose, S.; John, L.B. Adolescent pregnancy: An overview. *Int. J. Reprod. Contracept. Obstet. Gynecol.* **2017**, *6*, 4197. [CrossRef]
9. Forhan, S.E.; Gottlieb, S.L.; Sternberg, M.R.; Xu, F.; Datta, S.D.; McQuillan, G.M.; Berman, S.M.; Markowitz, L.E. Prevalence of sexually transmitted infections among female adolescents aged 14 to 19 in the United States. *Pediatrics* **2009**, *124*, 1505–1512. [CrossRef]
10. Zhao, J.; Chen, P.; Li, N. College students are the fresh troops to prevent AIDS. *Chin. J. Sch. Health* **2006**, *27*, 988–989. (In Chinese)
11. China National Emergency Broadcasting. More than 1.05 Million People Are Infected with AIDS in China. These Two Groups Deserve Attention. Available online: http://www.cneb.gov.cn/2021/12/01/ARTI1638321459504521.shtml (accessed on 20 January 2023). (In Chinese)
12. UNAIDS Global HIV & AIDS Statistics—Fact Sheet. Available online: https://www.unaids.org/en/resources/fact-sheet (accessed on 20 January 2023).
13. United Nations Children's Fund. *For Every Child, End AIDS: Seventh Stocktaking Report*; United Nations Children's Fund: New York, NY, USA, 2016.
14. Baams, L.; Dubas, J.S.; Overbeek, G.; van Aken, M.A. Transitions in body and behavior: A meta-analytic study on the relationship between pubertal development and adolescent sexual behavior. *J. Adolesc. Health* **2015**, *56*, 586–598. [CrossRef]
15. Yu, X.; Pan, Y.; Wang, J.; Ji, H.; Yang, Y.; Yang, S. A Comparative Study on Pubertal Development and Sexual Behaviors among Middle School Students in Beijing and Tianjin. *Chin. J. Sch. Health* **2002**, *23*, 292–293. (In Chinese)
16. Chen, Y.; Xu, J.; Cheng, L. The status of premarital sexual behavior of Chinese adolescents and the methods to reduce unwanted pregnancy. *Chin. J. Fam. Plan.* **2005**, *13*, 572–574. (In Chinese)
17. Young, S.D.; Rice, E. Online social networking technologies, HIV knowledge, and sexual risk and testing behaviors among homeless youth. *AIDS Behav.* **2011**, *15*, 253–260. [CrossRef] [PubMed]
18. General Office of the State Council. The General Office of the State Council on the Issuance of the "12th Five-Year Plan of Action" to Curb and Prevent AIDS in China. Available online: http://www.gov.cn/zwgk/2012-02/29/content_2079097.htm (accessed on 20 January 2023). (In Chinese)
19. General Office of the State Council. The General Office of the State Council on the Issuance of the "13th Five-Year Plan of Action" to Curb and Prevent AIDS in China. Available online: http://www.gov.cn/zhengce/content/2017-02/05/content_5165514.htm (accessed on 20 January 2023). (In Chinese)
20. Xu, J.; Qian, X. Review and trend analysis of adolescent reproductive health policy in China. *Chin. J. Health Policy* **2013**, *6*, 49–55. (In Chinese)
21. Sun, L.; Zhou, D.; Zhao, Y.; Pan, S.; Wang, L. Characteristics of AIDS prevalence and results of sentinel surveillance among young students in Liaoning province, 2016–2019. *J. Trop. Med.* **2022**, *22*, 1149–1152. (In Chinese)
22. Liu, J.; Yang, H.; Pan, X.; Gu, C.; Qian, J.; Guo, X.; Luo, Z. Results of AIDS sentinel surveillance of young students in Songjiang district of Shanghai. *Chin. J. AIDS STD* **2019**, *25*, 1067–1070+1084. (In Chinese)
23. China Center for Disease Control and Prevention. *China AIDS Prevention and Control Supervision and Evaluation Framework (Trial)*; People's Medical Publishing House: Beijing, China, 2007. (In Chinese)
24. Luo, Y.; Zhao, G.; Jin, J.; Zhang, X. Analysis of AIDS epidemic situation and knowledge, belief and practice among young students in Hangzhou from 2016 to 2019. *Prev. Med.* **2020**, *32*, 1034–1037. (In Chinese)
25. Zhang, J. Knowledge, attitude and behavior about AIDS prevention among college students in Shanghai. *Chin. J. Public Health* **2015**, *31*, 1352–1353. (In Chinese)
26. Lv, J. *Research on Current Status and Influencing Factors of University Students' Sexual Knowledge, Sexual Attitudes and Sexual Behavior*; Zhejiang University: Hangzhou, China, 2021. (In Chinese)
27. Lu, A. *Knowledge of AIDS and Use of Media: An Empirical Study Based on Young Students*; Southwest Jiaotong University: Chengdu, China, 2016. (In Chinese)
28. Wang, W. *Influence of Network Media on HIV/AIDS Related Knowledge, Attitude and Behavior of College Students Study—Take Undergraduate in Nanjing as an Example*; Nanjing University of Posts and Telecommunications: Nanjing, China, 2020. (In Chinese)
29. Zhang, Y.; Han, L.; Gao, L.; Zhang, Y.; Shen, J. Investigation on the Status and Relative Factors of Unsafe Sex among College Students in Beijing. *Chin. J. Fam. Plan.* **2019**, *27*, 1585–1588+1594. (In Chinese)
30. Liu, J.; Luo, Y.; Chen, H.; Chen, F. Investigation on knowledge, behavior and infection of AIDS among male college students. *Chin. J. Public Health* **2013**, *29*, 582–583. (In Chinese)
31. Duan, A.; Feng, Y.; Zhao, F.; Liu, B. Evaluation on integrated trinity model for STD/HIV crisis intervention. *Chin. J. Public Health* **2013**, *29*, 763–766. (In Chinese)
32. Huang, X.; He, J.; Tian, C. Knowledge, attitude and behavior about AIDS prevention among college students. *Chin. J. Public Health* **2015**, *31*, 249–251. (In Chinese)
33. Srahbzu, M.; Tirfeneh, E. Risky Sexual Behavior and Associated Factors among Adolescents Aged 15–19 Years at Governmental High Schools in Aksum Town, Tigray, Ethiopia, 2019: An Institution-Based, Cross-Sectional Study. *BioMed. Res. Int.* **2020**, *2020*, 3719845. [CrossRef] [PubMed]
34. Ye, H.; Yang, M.; Jiang, J. Research and analysis on current situation and attitude toward commercial sex in different populations. *Chin. J. Hum. Sex.* **2017**, *26*, 139–144. (In Chinese)

35. Wadham, E.; Green, C.; Debattista, J.; Somerset, S.; Sav, A. New digital media interventions for sexual health promotion among young people: A systematic review. *Sex. Health* **2019**, *16*, 101–123. [CrossRef] [PubMed]
36. Gao, Y.; Wang, H.; Q, Q.; Xue, F. Status of aids knowledge, attitude and behavior of college students and health education for them in Inner Mongolia. *Chin. Gen. Pract.* **2011**, *14*, 782–784. (In Chinese)
37. Pennanen-Iire, C.; Prereira-Lourenço, M.; Padoa, A.; Ribeirinho, A.; Samico, A.; Gressler, M.; Jatoi, N.-C.; Mehrad, M.; Girard, A. Sexual health implications of COVID-19 pandemic. *Sex. Med. Rev.* **2021**, *9*, 3–14. [CrossRef]
38. Sun, S.; Zhang, Y. Social Distance Keeping Behavior of the Population in the Context of Respiratory Infectious Disease Epidemics. *Adv. Psychol. Sci.* **2022**, *30*, 1612–1625. (In Chinese) [CrossRef]
39. Li, G.; Tang, D.; Song, B.; Wang, C.; Qunshan, S.; Xu, C.; Geng, H.; Wu, H.; He, X.; Cao, Y. Impact of the COVID-19 Pandemic on Partner Relationships and Sexual and Reproductive Health: Cross-Sectional, Online Survey Study. *J. Med. Internet Res.* **2020**, *22*, e20961. [CrossRef]
40. The Joint Prevention and Control Mechanism of the State Council for COVID-19. Notice on Further Optimization of the COVID-19 Prevention and Control Measures to Do a Good Job of Prevention and Control with Scientific Precision. Available online: https://www.gov.cn/xinwen/2022-11/11/content_5726122.htm (accessed on 15 June 2023). (In Chinese)

**Disclaimer/Publisher's Note:** The statements, opinions and data contained in all publications are solely those of the individual author(s) and contributor(s) and not of MDPI and/or the editor(s). MDPI and/or the editor(s) disclaim responsibility for any injury to people or property resulting from any ideas, methods, instructions or products referred to in the content.

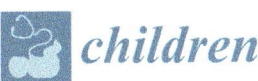

Article

# Children's Health and Typology of Family Integration and Regulation: A Functionalist Analysis

Xiaozhao Yang and Chao Zhang *

School of Journalism and Communication, Sun Yat-sen University, Guangzhou 510275, China
* Correspondence: zhangchao5@mail.sysu.edu.cn; Tel.: +86-02039332651

**Abstract:** Rationale: Children's health is conventionally studied as an ultimate consequence resulting from various social and biological processes that jointly channel the risk factors and pathogens toward an individual health outcome. What is currently neglected is the rich tradition of a functionalist analysis of children's health as a necessary function in the family institution. Children's health may be associated with how children are integrated into the family's core functioning and how parents regulate children's behaviors. Methods: The current study used a cross-sectional sample of 891 parents from 2018 southern Jiangsu and surveyed information about children's health and family activities. Employing a latent class analysis, we established four types of families based on children's integration and parental regulation: loose, free, pressed, and concerted. Results: The regression results showed that a child's health is associated with the concerted family type (OR = 3.6, $p < 0.05$), indicating the necessary functionality of health in heavily regulated and mobilized families. Conclusion: This study broadens the perspective on children's health by ushering back functionalism and placing health in its social implications.

**Keywords:** self-reported health; child–parent relationship; functionalism; family regulation

## 1. Introduction

### 1.1. Children in the Family Institution

The boundary between childhood and adulthood has become increasingly ambiguous and the social roles assigned to each are increasingly opaque [1]. If anything, the conventional relationship between adults and their children has melted in the air as a myriad of formative socio-demographic conditions for traditional adulthood have permanently changed, including the delayed entrance into the labor force, delayed or entirely extinct marital union, earlier romantic relationship, digitized social interaction, and the rise of a precarious gig economy, among others.

Functionalism is a paradigm that views each of the components in an organic institution, such as family or religion, operating latently or explicitly to sustain the survival of the institution. Functionalism posits that all constituents of a society—institutions, roles, norms, etc.—serve their purpose for the long-term survival of the society [2]. From a functionalist perspective, the family institution survives on the basis of its own functioning components, including the health of family members. Instead of a "product" of the family, the functionalist perspective argues that children are necessary components contributing to the functioning and survival of the family institution by reproducing the existing relations and resources in the family [3–5]. Children's health, rather than as an outcome, is regarded as an integral component for facilitating the function of the family. A child is integrated into the family by participating as an agent in family activities, including leisure activities, emotional correspondence, and labor activities [6,7].

Recently, the children's agency in the family institution has received rising attention in academia [4,8–11]. Some scholars have classified parental style into four general types: neglectful, permissive, authoritarian, and authoritative [12–15]. Certain parenting

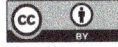

styles contribute to different child development outcomes, such as delinquency, academic performance, and mental health [16–19].

*1.2. Children's Health and the Family Institution*

A child who may not perform the normative social role due to irresistible non-personal causes unwillingly disrupts the integration between him/her and other members, and undermines the function of his/her family in society [20]. The most common among these types of irresistible causes is disease and disability [21–23]. Talcott Parsons was the first to formulate the patient's role as an integrated and necessary part of a functional society [24]. Scholars later introduced the intersectional perspective based on identities—racial, gender, ageism—to studying how health shapes our normative role in an institution such as family [25–28].

In the world of the family institution, unhealthy children may not be expected to partake in certain social activities and may be exempted from family obligations that the family would otherwise prescribe [29]. Most contemporary studies on social activities, manifested in various forms pertaining to their respective conceptional traditions, such as social capital theory, social support, and routine activity theory, seek to establish a directional causal relationship between health and social integration [30–32]. Children with health problems may be discouraged from participating in family decision and collective activities by their caregivers [33]. People suffering from disease or general infirmity are expected by the social norm to proactively seek to improve their current infirmary condition and resume their previous social functions. When they fail to achieve this, sanctions and stigma befall their existing functions in the social relation nexus and they tend to be excluded from further participating in other social activities [22,24].

*1.3. Gaps in the Literature*

While a considerable portion of the literature on child and health has noticed the importance of the family environment, very few studies have considered child health as a condition for social integration in the family. The current study builds on a sample of 891 parents of young children and investigates how social integration is an embedded function of health. Specifically, we proposed to examine the focal research question on the functional role of health in children's familial and extra-family social integration: does health provide function for family solidarity in terms of child–parent integration and parent–child regulation; is health functional for participating in social activities outside of a child's family? We illustrate this framework with Figure 1. Here, parents and children mutually regulate and integrate into each other, while the health of the children is associated with the extent to which such regulation and integration can fully realize.

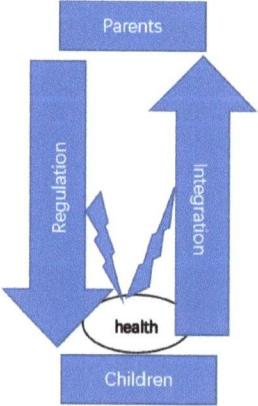

**Figure 1.** Conceptual Diagram for the Functions of Children's Health in Family Relations.

## 2. Methodology

### 2.1. Sample

The individual-level family data of this study come from a field survey from December 2018 to January 2019. The empirical survey was carried out among the parents of senior primary students from four urban ordinary primary schools in two coastal cities in eastern China. Based on the population of the city and assuming simple random sampling, the desired minimum sample size of was determined according to the formula: $n = \frac{1.96^2 * 0.5 * 0.5}{1 + 1.96^2 * 0.25} N = 384$. The investigators reached to the administrators and teachers at four primary schools. The administrators in each class unit then distributed the survey invitation to students, who, in turn, would invite their parents to respond to a self-administered survey. Parents reserve the right to voluntarily participate or withdraw at any point of the survey. Eligibility: pupils who did not attend the school at the day or could not inform their parents of the survey did not contribute to the data collection. Although the survey did not initiate a pilot test, its questionnaires comprised standardized format for most questions. The measurement includes household size, parent–child relationship, family integration, family regulation, child's social participation, child's healthy and demographic variables, etc. Finally, 900 samples were collected, and the invalid samples were listwise removed. The total number of valid samples was 891, which constituted the basic database for this study. The equivalent to the Institutional Review Board that approved the study design was an ethics committee of Soochow University.

### 2.2. Measurement

Health status of the child was self-reported by parents to the question "your child's health condition is: very bad, somewhat bad, okay, somewhat good, very good". We concatenated categories from somewhat good to very good into healthy status, and the remaining three were combined into unhealthy status.

Family integration was measured by summating three questions. For questions "when your family decide the child's extra-curriculum activities", "when your family makes major financial decisions", "when your family makes familial decisions", each question yields 1 point if the parent chose "mainly decided by the child" or "will incorporate child's decision". The score of family integration ranges from 0 to 3.

Family regulation was measured by summated average of parental involvement in the child's behaviors in the following categories: making friends at school, making friends outside school, dressing, using the Internet, watching TV. Regulation score also ranges from 0 to 3 after we divided the raw score into equidistant four categories.

Control variables included household size, gender, parent's education, parent's subjective class, parent's spousal relation, the child's willingness to participate in extra-curriculum activities, and the child's actual participation in extra-curriculum activities.

### 2.3. Analytical Strategy

To categorize population into conceptually distinct typologies based on the two dimensions of family structure—integration and regulation—we used latent class analysis that a posteriori creates group labels based on the observed data. Because the group labels are created based on the best fit from maximum likelihood function, we selected the best model based on fit indices such as BIC and log-likelihood change [34]. The estimation of the probability of belonging to each class y expresses the joint probability of the K-class-specific probability, conditioning on a set of variables; that is:

$$P(y|x) = \prod_{k=1}^{k} P(y_k|x) \pi_k$$

With the probability of each latent class for individual calculated, we used the cut-off threshold of 0.5 to assign class membership. Logistic regression was then applied to children's health status with the latent classes of family integration and family regulation as the key independent variables. Analyses were conducted with Stata 16.

## 3. Results

In Table 1, descriptive statistics of the sample composed of 891 respondents demonstrate the characteristics of key study variables and the demographic information. The sample is equally divided between male and female children, with 47.6% being females. The vast majority (90.8%) of the children are reported to be healthy or very healthy by their parents, leaving one tenth of the children in the categories below and including "okay". The average household size in this study is 2.45, which is within the typical range of household size that was formed under the one-child policy. The average highest parent education is 4.7, corresponding approximately to the vocational school. The parents' subjective class on average is unsurprisingly 3.09, corresponding to "at the average level". The mean relational conflict between spouses is 1.49, which is between "very harmonious" and "relatively harmonious". Out of four levels, children's integration into the family averages at 1.49, and their level of being regulated by parents averages at 1.66. The average level of social participation among children is 2.29, and their willingness to participate averages at 2.13.

Table 1. Sample descriptive statistics.

|  | Mean (s.d.) | N (%) |
| --- | --- | --- |
| Gender (female) |  | 424 (47.6%) |
| Healthy |  | 809 (90.8%) |
| Parental status |  |  |
| -father |  | 178 (20%) |
| -mother |  | 713 (80%) |
| Household size | 2.45 (0.91) |  |
| Parent education | 4.7 (1.43) |  |
| Parent subjective class | 3.09 (0.59) |  |
| Parent relation | 1.49 (0.71) |  |
| Family integration | 0.85 (0.83) |  |
| Family regulation | 1.66 (1.14) |  |
| Child's social participation | 2.29 (0.55) |  |
| Child's participation willingness | 2.13 (0.57) |  |

The children's integration into family decisions, management, and arbitrations conceptually refers to a down-to-top pipeline of forming solidarity within the family domain, and the level of regulation imposed on children's decisions and arbitrations represents a top-to-down channel of enforcing family solidarity from parents as the administrators of the organization. Each dimension of family solidarity as a functional representation of an organization is measured and quantified into four levels. The interactive juxtaposition of these two dimensions—integration and regulation—produces several idealtypical classes of intra-family relational types. In the left panel of Table 2, the entire sample can be divided into four groups along the levels of regulation and integration, with values smaller than and equal to 1 as the cut-off for low and high levels. Then, we arrive at the right panel of Table 2 as a conceptual construction of family solidarity types: the "loose" type has low levels in both regulation and integration; the "free" type has children highly integrated into the family but receiving little regulation; the "pressed" type is highly regulated and weakly integrated; the "concerted" type is high in both regulation and integration.

Table 2. Number of people by levels of regulation and integration in the family sphere.

|  |  | Regulation→ | | | |
|---|---|---|---|---|---|
|  |  | 0 | 1 | 2 | 3 |
| Integration→ | 0 | 75 | 97 | 73 | 104 |
|  | 1 | 76 | 92 | 78 | 109 |
|  | 2 | 28 | 32 | 30 | 63 |
|  | 3 | 6 | 7 | 3 | 18 |
|  |  | low | | High | |
|  | low | "Loose" 340 | | "Pressed" 364 | |
|  | high | "Free" 73 | | "Concerted" 114 | |

The grouping in Table 2 springs from conceptual construction. Now, we examine the empirical fitness and validity of such constructs with a latent class analysis. Using integration and regulation as manifest indicators regressing on a categorical latent construct, Table 3 shows that the four-group construction retains the highest fitness and parsimony. Such a four-group latent class outcome is described in Table 4. Class 1 is low in both regulation and integration, corresponding to the "loose" ideal type in Table 2. Class 2 is low in terms of regulation but high in integration, representing the "free" ideal type. Class 3 is high in regulation but low in integration, representing the "pressed" type, while class 4 is high in both regulation and integration.

Table 3. Model fit evaluation information.

|  | Log-Likelihood | BIC |
|---|---|---|
| 1 group | −2483 | 4994 |
| 2 groups | −2339 | 4726 |
| 3 groups | −2327 | 4722 |
| 4 groups | −2282 | 4652 |
| 5 groups | −2271 | 4653 |

Table 4. Four-class model by latent class analysis.

| N = 891 | Class 1 (Loose) | Class 2 (Free) | Class 3 (Pressed) | Class 4 (Concerted) |
|---|---|---|---|---|
| Intercept | 1 | −1.49 (0.15) | 0.04 (0.08) | −1.06 (0.12) |
| Regulation | 0.58 (0.03) | 0.55 (0.07) | 2.58 (0.03) | 2.72 (0.05) |
| Integration | 0.50 (0.03) | 2.08 (0.08) | 0.52 (0.03) | 2.10 (0.06) |
| Probability | 0.38 (0.02) | 0.09 (0.11) | 0.40 (0.02) | 0.13 (0.01) |

The probability of each individual belonging in each latent class indicates the certainty of assigning individuals to each construct. Figure 2 demonstrate that our latent classes are highly deterministic and the certainty of assignment group membership is almost absolute. The bimodal shapes of probability distributions indicate that each respondent is either a member of one latent class or not a member, with little ambiguity and overlap. When 0.5 is used as the cut-off of the posterior probabilities, the sizes of latent classes are exactly the same as that of the idealtypical classes in Table 2, confirming the empirical validity of the conceptual construction of family types.

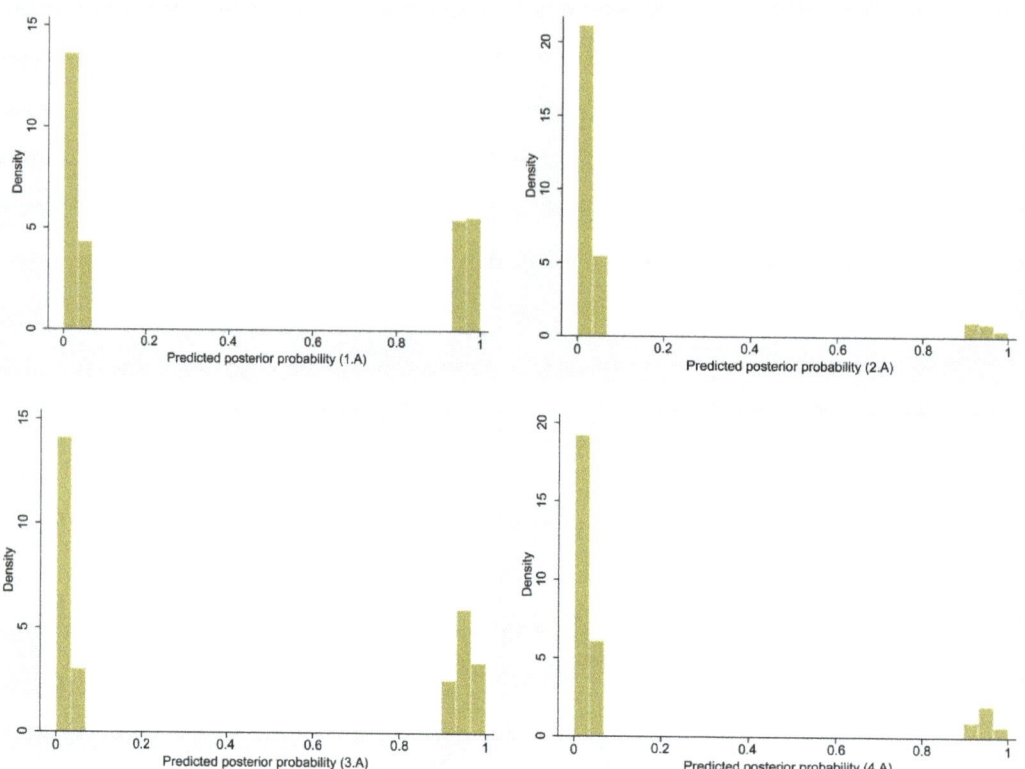

**Figure 2.** Bimodal distributions of the estimated probability of belonging to each latent class, from class 1 to class 4 (from 1.A to 4.A). N1 ($p > 0.5$) = 340, N2 ($p > 0.5$) = 73, N3 ($p > 0.5$) = 364, N4 ($p > 0.5$) = 114.

Table 5 contains logistic models regressing on health by the step-wise inclusion of independent variables. Model 1 shows that child health is positively associated with more social participation (OR = 1.94, $p < 0.01$), where a healthy child is 1.94 times more likely to have one greater level of social participation compared to an unhealthy child. Compared to the "loose" family type, the concerted family is associated with child health by 3.6 times the odds ratio. Children in the concerted families are 3.6 times more likely to be healthy compared to children in the loose families. Including child gender and willingness to participate in model 2 does not change the precedent coefficients greatly. A female child, however, is more likely to be healthy (OR = 1.67, $p < 0.05$). Finally, several variables measuring family characteristics were introduced to model 3. Among them, the relational conflict among parents is negatively associated with health (OR = 0.62, $p < 0.001$). A one-unit increase in parental conflict is associated with a 38% lower chance of reporting a healthy child. Family characteristics accounted for the association between family type and child health, as its coefficients turned non-significant at an alpha level of 5%. The association between child health and social participation remains significant (OR = 1.84, $p < 0.05$).

Table 5. Logistic regression results in odds ratios with standard errors and 95% confidence intervals.

| Criterion Variable = Healthy | Model 1 (n = 891) | | Model 2 (n = 891) | | Model 3 (n = 891) | |
|---|---|---|---|---|---|---|
| Family type (ref = loose) | | | | | | |
| -free | 0.96 (0.40) | 0.43–2.16 | 0.97 (0.41) | 0.43–2.20 | 0.82 (0.35) | 0.36–1.88 |
| -pressed | 1.27 (0.33) | 0.76–2.13 | 1.28 (0.34) | 0.76–2.14 | 1.16 (0.31) | 0.69–1.96 |
| -concerted | 3.60 (2.23) * | 1.07–12.2 | 3.60 (2.24) * | 1.06–12.18 | 2.97 (1.86) | 0.87–10.2 |
| Social participation | 1.94 (.49) ** | 1.18–3.20 | 1.93 (0.50) * | 1.16–2.30 | 1.84 (0.50) * | 1.08–3.12 |
| Participation willing | | | 0.93 (0.21) | 0.60–1.44 | 0.97 (0.22) | 0.62–1.51 |
| Child sex (ref = male) | | | 1.67 (0.41) * | 1.03–2.69 | 1.69 (0.41) * | 1.04–2.73 |
| Parent subjective class | | | | | 1.21 (0.24) | 0.82–1.79 |
| Parent education | | | | | 0.92 (0.08) | 0.77–1.10 |
| Household size | | | | | 0.97 (0.13) | 0.74–1.27 |
| Parent relation | | | | | 0.62 (0.09) *** | 0.46–0.83 |
| Pseudo R2 | 0.03 | | 0.04 | | 0.07 | |
| Correctly classified † | 90.8% | | 90.8% | | 90.6% | |

† Pr(D | +) + Pr(~D | −), Pr > 50%. * $p < 0.05$, ** $p < 0.01$, *** $p < 0.001$.

## 4. Discussion

The current study employed a structural functionalist theoretical framework to understand the intricate role of children's health in the functioning and integration of the family, as well as in children's participation in social activities outside the family domain. This model builds upon a tradition in medical sociology that contrasts against the prevailing biomedical model of health as an independent agent in the causal chain from social determinants to individual health outcomes. Instead, medical sociology views health not only as a product of social determinants in the multilevel ecological layers full of risk factors but also emphasizes health as a function and organic part that enables the integration and solidarity of a societal unit, such as a family or a corporate [21]. People with a satisfactory level of health perform daily tasks defined by their social role; thus, their health is an essential component of a functional social role.

The literature on family and child development has touched base on how the style and intensity of integration and regulation within a family are associated with behavioral and social outcomes among children. Studies have elaborated the typology of parenting; for example, into authoritative, authoritarian, permissive, and uninvolved [11]. Authoritative parenting that combines child agency and certain levels of regulation may benefit the child in terms of deviant behaviors and academic outcomes. Recent studies on concerted parenting point to a similar finding that underlies our argument: the functional operation of a family organization in a competitive environment requires the active participation of multiple actors, including parents and children [18,35,36]. Therefore, in line with the Durkheimian tradition, we argue that both integrations of children in the family and regulation by parents towards children are necessary components in understanding the family as a functional unit.

Based on the functionalist perspective of family, this study argued that family could be conceptually classified into four types based on the levels of integration and regulation: the loose, the free, the pressed, and the concerted type. These conceptional ideal types are validated with empirical data from 891 parental reports of family relations in a 2018 Chinese sample. In the subsequent regression analyses, we found that reported health is positively associated with the concerted type of family compared to the loose type, with a very large odds ratio of 3.6. Only the coefficient was reduced to being non-significant after controlling for family characteristics. Social participation is significantly associated with the reported health of children throughout all models. These findings indicate that children's health is an integral component for the functional operation of the family in both domestic and extra-family activities. A child with above average health lives in a concerted family where the child's agency is encouraged and actively incorporated into family decisions; meanwhile, parents' regulation on the child is also maintained at a considerable level. The same child with good health also participates in more social activities, and more intensively so.

The overall level of child health tends to be stable in a society, but children with a bad health condition make their families sacrifice more resources and energy in maintaining their wellbeing. Furthermore, the family will suffer more than physical and material loss as it reorients its organizational structure and change the types of regulation and integration among family members. In the Chinese context, predominant single-child households with a sick child face serious challenges regarding their own integration into the broader society. In short, families with a sick child may not perform their full function and risk the cohesion between different social components.

One must bear in mind that this study employs a functional theory in regard to the relationship between children's health and their social integration, instead of a causal mechanism. The functional analysis is concerned with the constitution of a family organization by certain integral components each contributing a function to the operation of the family; thus, it is not preoccupied with the direction of an effect. Each functional component of the family, including the children's health, family finance, and spousal relation, is topologically connected to other components so that they synergistically form the functions of a family. Children's health may lead to a more concerted family type and more active social participation, but it may well be the reverse causality that a concerted family improves its children's health outcome. However, this study has no intention to engage in the mechanism discussion on what causes or is caused by children's health. Overall, this study adds to the child development literature by revealing that children's health is functionally necessary for a family with higher levels of integration and regulation and for closer social engagement through social participation.

## 5. Limitations

The current study was subjected to several limits that restrained the generalizability of the results to all contexts. First, this study employed the functionalist perspective that regards health wellbeing as a functional element for the maintenance and performance of the family unit. Scholars from a different theoretical tradition may see health only as an outcome caused by the structure and wellbeing of the family institution. Second, this study was based on a cross-sectional survey, and does not intend to inform readers of the causality between children's health and family structure. Third, the sample came from a specific cultural region of China and cannot extrapolate the results to the heterogenous country.

## 6. Conclusions

Adopting a functionalist analytic framework, the current study investigates children's health as a necessary component for the functioning of the family institution and argues that children's health is closely integrated in how parents interact with the children. Using a 2018 sample from the southern Jiangsu province of China, we employed a latent class analysis to categorize four types of a parent–child relationship: the loose, free, pressed, and concerted types. Multivariate logistic regressions showed that the concerted type, in which parents moderately regulate the behavior of the children, is associated with a better level of children's health. The results suggest that children with good health render it possible for a family to develop a concerted parent–child relationship and function as an integrated unit. Such a finding calls for policymakers to consider that children's health has consequences beyond medical and healthcare relevancy. Children's health may further matter for a functioning family institution and, ultimately, a well-balanced and integrated society in which individuals find solidarity and cohesion among themselves.

**Author Contributions:** Conceptualization, X.Y. and C.Z.; methodology: X.Y.; Validation, C.Z.; data curation: C.Z.; writing: X.Y.; visualization: X.Y.; funding acquisition: C.Z. All authors have read and agreed to the published version of the manuscript.

**Funding:** This study was funded by the MOE (Ministry of Education in China) Project of Humanities and Social Sciences (Grant No. 18YJC840053) and the National Natural Science Foundation of China (Grant No. 71804120).

**Institutional Review Board Statement:** The study was approved by Soochow University Ethics Committee (2018033), the date for the approval #2018033 is 3 March 2018.

**Informed Consent Statement:** Informed consent was obtained from all subjects involved in the study. No individual participants can be identified and tracked by the collected data.

**Data Availability Statement:** Data sharing not applicable.

**Conflicts of Interest:** The authors declare no conflict of interest.

## References

1. Song, C.; Zhang, C. The Public's Supportive Attitude towards the Social Inclusion of Children with Special Needs: Theory and Experience. *China Nonprofit Rev.* **2021**, *12*, 213–232. [CrossRef]
2. Durkheim, E. *De la Division du Travail Social: Étude sur L'organisation des Sociétés Supérieures*; Félix Alcan: Paris, French, 1893.
3. Cherlin, A.J. *Labor's Love Lost: The Rise and Fall of the Working-Class Family in America*; Russell Sage Foundation: New York, NY, USA, 2014.
4. Maccoby, E.E. *The Role of Parents in the Socialization of Children: An Historical Overview*; American Psychological Association: Washington, DC, USA, 1994; pp. 589–615.
5. Grusec, J.E.; Lytton, H. Socialization and the family. In *Social Development*; Springer: Berlin, Germany, 1988; pp. 161–212.
6. Hay, C.; Forrest, W. The Development Of Self-Control: Examining Self-Control Theory's Stability Thesis*. *Criminology* **2006**, *44*, 739–774. [CrossRef]
7. Kalmijn, M.; De Graaf, P.M. Life Course Changes of Children and Well-being of Parents. *J. Marriage Fam.* **2012**, *74*, 269–280. [CrossRef]
8. Zhang, C. 'Nothing about us without us': The emerging disability movement and advocacy in China. *Disabil. Soc.* **2017**, *32*, 1096–1101. [CrossRef]
9. Silverstein, M.; Gans, D.; Lowenstein, A.; Giarrusso, R.; Bengtson, V.L. Older parent–child relationships in six developed nations: Comparisons at the intersection of affection and conflict. *J. Marriage Fam.* **2010**, *72*, 1006–1021. [CrossRef]
10. Sawyer, S.M.; Azzopardi, P.S.; Wickremarathne, D.; Patton, G.C. The age of adolescence. *Lancet Child Adolesc. Health* **2018**, *2*, 223–228. [CrossRef]
11. Dhingra, P. *Hyper Education: Why Good Schools, Good Grades, and Good Behavior Are Not Enough*; NYU Press: New York, NY, USA, 2020.
12. Bengtson, V.; Giarrusso, R.; Mabry, J.B.; Silverstein, M. Solidarity, Conflict, and Ambivalence: Complementary or Competing Perspectives on Intergenerational Relationships? *J. Marriage Fam.* **2002**, *64*, 568–576. [CrossRef]
13. Silverstein, M.; Bengtson, V.L.; Lawton, L. Intergenerational solidarity and the structure of adult child-parent relationships in American families. *Am. J. Sociol.* **1997**, *103*, 429–460. [CrossRef]
14. Kirkpatrick, L.A.; Davis, K.E. Attachment style, gender, and relationship stability: A longitudinal analysis. *J. Pers. Soc. Psychol.* **1994**, *66*, 502. [CrossRef]
15. Shaver, P.R.; Brennan, K.A. Attachment Styles and the "Big Five" Personality Traits: Their Connections with Each Other and with Romantic Relationship Outcomes. *Personal. Soc. Psychol. Bull.* **1992**, *18*, 536–545. [CrossRef]
16. Hirschi, T. Causes and Prevention of Juvenile Delinquency. *Sociol. Inq.* **1977**, *47*, 322–341. [CrossRef]
17. Morton, P.M.; Ferraro, K.F. Early Social Origins of Biological Risks for Men and Women in Later Life. *J. Health Soc. Behav.* **2020**, *61*, 503–522. [CrossRef]
18. Schroeder, R.D.; Higgins, G.E.; Mowen, T.J. Maternal Attachment Trajectories and Criminal Offending By Race. *Am. J. Crim. Justice* **2014**, *39*, 155–171. [CrossRef]
19. Yu, T.; Pettit, G.S.; Lansford, J.E.; Dodge, K.A.; Bates, J.E. The interactive effects of marital conflict and divorce on parent–adult children's relationships. *J. Marriage Fam.* **2010**, *72*, 282–292. [CrossRef]
20. Yang, X.Y.; Anderson, J.G.; Yang, T. Impact of Role Models and Policy Exposure on Support for Tobacco Control Policies in Hangzhou, China. *Am. J. Health Behav.* **2014**, *38*, 275–283. [CrossRef] [PubMed]
21. Parsons, T. *Action Theory and the Human Condition*; Free Press: New York, NY, USA, 1978.
22. Shilling, C. Culture, the 'sick role' and the consumption of health. *Br. J. Sociol.* **2002**, *53*, 621–638. [CrossRef]
23. Williams, K.D. Ostracism. *Annu. Rev. Psychol.* **2007**, *58*, 425–452. [CrossRef] [PubMed]
24. Parsons, T. The Sick Role and the Role of the Physician Reconsidered. In *Action Theory and the Human Condition*; Free Press: New York, NY, USA, 1975; pp. 17–33.

25. Kawachi, I.; Berkman, L.F. Social ties and mental health. *J. Urban Health* **2001**, *78*, 458–467. [CrossRef] [PubMed]
26. Yang, X.Y.; Hendley, A. The gendered effects of substance use on employment stability in transitional China. *Health Sociol. Rev.* **2018**, *27*, 312–329. [CrossRef]
27. Yang, X.Y.; Kelly, B.; Yang, T. Peer Association and Routine Activities in Sex Worker Patronage among Male Migrant Workers. *Deviant Behav.* **2020**, *43*, 322–339. [CrossRef]
28. Yang, X.Y.; Yang, T. Nonmedical Prescription Drug Use Among Adults in Their Late Twenties: The Importance of Social Bonding Trajectories. *J. Drug Issues* **2017**, *47*, 665–678. [CrossRef]
29. Crowley, A.A. Sick child care: A developmental perspective. *J. Pediatr. Health Care* **1994**, *8*, 261–267. [CrossRef] [PubMed]
30. Yang, X.Y. Marijuana Use at Early Midlife and the Trajectories of Social Bonds. *J. Dev. Life-Course Criminol.* **2017**, *3*, 284–303. [CrossRef]
31. De Silva, M.J.; McKenzie, K.; Harpham, T.; Huttly, S.R.A. Social capital and mental illness: A systematic review. *J. Epidemiol. Community Health* **2005**, *59*, 619–627. [CrossRef]
32. Kawachi, I.; Berkman, L. Social cohesion, social capital, and health. In *Social Epidemiology*; Kawachi, I., Berkman, L., Eds.; Oxford University Press: Oxford, UK, 2000; pp. 174–190.
33. Zhao, X.; Zhang, C. From isolated fence to inclusive society: The transformational disability policy in China. *Disabil. Soc.* **2018**, *33*, 132–137. [CrossRef]
34. Nylund-Gibson, K.; Choi, A.Y. Ten frequently asked questions about latent class analysis. *Transl. Issues Psychol. Sci.* **2018**, *4*, 440. [CrossRef]
35. Matthews, S.H. A window on the 'new' sociology of childhood. *Sociol. Compass* **2007**, *1*, 322–334. [CrossRef]
36. Moran-Ellis, J. Reflections on the sociology of childhood in the UK. *Curr. Sociol.* **2010**, *58*, 186–205. [CrossRef]

**Disclaimer/Publisher's Note:** The statements, opinions and data contained in all publications are solely those of the individual author(s) and contributor(s) and not of MDPI and/or the editor(s). MDPI and/or the editor(s) disclaim responsibility for any injury to people or property resulting from any ideas, methods, instructions or products referred to in the content.

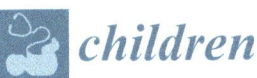 

*Article*

# The Mealtime Behavior Problems of Children with Developmental Disabilities and the Teacher's Stress in Inclusive Preschools

Chen-Ya Juan

Center of Teacher Education, Minghsin University of Science and Technology, Hsinchu 30401, Taiwan; chenyajuan@must.edu.tw

**Abstract:** With an increasing number of children with developmental disabilities entering inclusive preschools, preschool teachers face more behavioral problems in class. Preschool teachers typically attempt to address mealtime behavior problems of children with and without developmental disabilities simultaneously in class. This study used qualitative research to identify the stress triggers of preschool teachers addressing the mealtime behavior problems of children with developmental disabilities. Five preschool teachers attended semi-structured interviews. The results indicated that most children with developmental disabilities had problems with eating only preferred foods, using eating utensils appropriately during mealtime, becoming distracted from eating, and becoming frustrated with the classroom routine. Although solving these problems triggered stress in the preschool teachers, their stress was mainly in response to the children's parents, other children's imitation of inappropriate mealtime behaviors, and classroom schedule time management. Most of the preschool teachers stated that they had insufficient support. Preschool teachers require specialized information and strategies for improving the mealtime behaviors of children with developmental disabilities.

**Keywords:** mealtime behavior problems; children with developmental disabilities; inclusive preschool; preschool teacher's stress

**Citation:** Juan, C.-Y. The Mealtime Behavior Problems of Children with Developmental Disabilities and the Teacher's Stress in Inclusive Preschools. *Children* **2023**, *10*, 441. https://doi.org/10.3390/children10030441

Academic Editor: Tingzhong Yang

Received: 30 November 2022
Revised: 8 February 2023
Accepted: 20 February 2023
Published: 24 February 2023

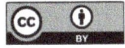

**Copyright:** © 2023 by the author. Licensee MDPI, Basel, Switzerland. This article is an open access article distributed under the terms and conditions of the Creative Commons Attribution (CC BY) license (https://creativecommons.org/licenses/by/4.0/).

## 1. Introduction

Many children with special needs have behavior-related eating problems, including having particular food preferences, exhibiting aggression during mealtime, and becoming distracted from eating [1,2]. Many exhibit behavior problems during mealtime, including eating only small quantities of food, spitting out food, eating too quickly without chewing, eating too slowly without swallowing; chewing insufficiently, exhibiting rumination syndrome, pushing away food, and demanding specific feeders, specific food settings, or food with particular textures [3]. These inappropriate mealtime behaviors (IMBs) impede children from receiving the necessary nourishment from food, which may cause serious health problems or developmental obstacles [4].

Mealtime behavior problems are one of preschool teachers' most common daily challenges. According to my on-site observations, the stress that preschools teacher experience in relation to children's mealtime behavior problems typically results from the children's parents, time pressure, other children's imitation of misbehaviors, and the preschool administrator's concern. Some parents in Asia have a tendency to be overinvolved in their children's eating in preschool out of concern that their children are receiving insufficient food and nutrition to support them developmentally. Parents might review the school menu monthly and request that the teacher feed their children during mealtime. Instead of teaching their children appropriate mealtime behaviors at home, parents believe that teachers must become more efficient and trained in improving their children's mealtime behaviors. Laws and regulations in Taiwan also address the importance of nutrition for children with disabilities [5,6]. Many children with developmental disabilities demonstrate

IMBs in preschools, which may result in insufficient nutritional intake. Some children wanted to watch cartoons or play with mobile devices while eating, to wait for teachers to feed them, or to run around and eat in the classroom, and others were unable to spoon-feed themselves. These problem behaviors increase teachers' stress levels and directly impede the children's food intake.

With 1 to 15 children per class, managing all children's mealtime behaviors is challenging for teachers. Before mealtime, the teachers would remind the children to tidy up their toys and clean their table, take their lunch bowls and spoons from their bags, wash their hands, line up to receive food, and return to their seats carefully. Sometimes, children fail to tidy up their toys and clean their tables, are unable to find their lunch bags, push others when lining up, and make noise in class. During mealtime, the preschool teachers must monitor the children's eating to ensure they have eaten all the food, not only eating their preferred food, holding their lunch bowls and spoons correctly, and remain in their seats. When children are finished eating, the teachers would remind them to clean their lunch bowls, spoons, teeth, hands, and table. Children who demonstrate inappropriate behaviors delay the class routine, increasing the teachers' stress. During mealtime, the teachers are concerned that the IMBs of children with disabilities may prevent them from obtaining proper nutrition but are also concerned that the children cannot participate in all scheduled class activities if they have spent too much time eating. Therefore, time management is critical for preschool teachers during mealtime.

The imitation of misbehaviors is a major challenge for preschool teachers. Children aged 3 to 6 years often imitate each other's behaviors at this developmental stage. Therefore, when one child demonstrates inappropriate behaviors in class, other children may attempt to imitate those misbehaviors to obtain attention. If preschool teachers are unable to address these problem behaviors, such behaviors can quickly spread among children in the class, further disrupting class management. Therefore, when teachers observe inappropriate behaviors, they must immediately correct the misbehavior by introducing an alternative behavior.

The preschool administrator's concern is another source of stress for preschool teachers. When children repeatedly exhibit problem behaviors in class, such as crying loudly, screaming, and attacking others, administrators may be concerned about the teacher's ability to manage their class. The more behavioral problems that occur, the more concerns the administrator has about the teacher. The teacher may lose the support of the administrator, leaving the teacher in an isolated position. Because preschool administrators often monitor classes during lunchtime, the children's mealtime behaviors are part of the administrator's assessment of the teacher's class management and problem-solving ability.

Although researchers have formulated strategies to improve IMBs, few were concerned about preschool teachers' stress when dealing with these problem behaviors [7–9]. I speculated that the more stress preschool teachers experience, the less self-efficacy they have in teaching children with developmental disabilities. To understand how preschool teachers feel about children mealtime behavior problems, this study applied qualitative research to analyze the stress triggers of five preschool teachers who had intervened to address IMBs of children with developmental disabilities. The interview questions included the following:

1. What mealtime problem behavior of children with disabilities in the class have you observed in class, and how did you deal with these problem behaviors?
2. How did you felt when you were dealing with the children's IMBs?
3. What are the factors you think might influence children's mealtime behaviors?

## 2. Literature Review

Children require sufficient nutrition to grow and remain healthy. For children with developmental disabilities, nutrition can somewhat compensate for their developmental disabilities and provide them with the energy required to participate in all preschool activities [10]. Sufficient and balanced nutrition assists children with developmental disabilities in participating in the same activities as children without disabilities in an inclusive learning environment [5,6,11]. However, mealtime behavior problems seriously impede the nutrition intake of children with developmental disabilities. Therefore, assisting these children in eating correctly enables them to obtain sufficient and balanced nutrition from food. Furthermore, sufficient energy and health can benefit the cognition of children with developmental disabilities, because playing and learning with children without disabilities increases the self-esteem, self-confidence, and personal value of children with developmental disabilities [12].

Emphasizing the critical nature of the nutrition of children with disabilities, the Individuals with Disabilities Education Act, Part H (1990) [5], regulates that schools or parents must provide nutrition that meets the children's needs. Parents should be committed to supporting their children's development and learning, respecting individual differences, and promoting their children's self-awareness, competence, self-worth, resiliency, and physical well-being [11]. Article 1 of Taiwan's Protection of Children and Youths Welfare and Rights Act (2021) [6] also regulates that schools and parents must promote the healthy development of children's bodies and minds, protect their interests, and increase their welfare. Although the development and health of children in schools have been emphasized in different countries, the nutrition of children with developmental disabilities in preschools in Taiwan has not been explored. Research examining how schools can be supported to ensure children with and without disabilities have their nutritional needs met in preschools is lacking.

Children with, and without, disabilities often do not obtain sufficient nutrients [13]; many experience eating problems during mealtime at home or in school. Researchers have conducted studies and large-scale surveys and have reported parental concerns about their children's problem behaviors at different ages. For example, parents of children aged between 6 weeks and 4.5 years primarily worried about their children's sleeping, eating, and crying behaviors [13]. For children aged 1 and 2 years, parents were mostly concerned about their eating and sleeping difficulties. The number and intensity of parental concerns peaked when their children were aged 3 years and were related to difficulties with management and discipline. Other researchers reported that toileting, eating habits, and sleeping problems are common concerns for parents of 3-year-old children [14,15]. Because the development of children with developmental disabilities lags considerably relative to children without disabilities, the frequency, forms, and severity of their feeding problem behaviors are more apparent and more difficult to solve.

Secrist-Mertz et al. [16] argued that feeding problems for children with disabilities are complex and depend on the physical characteristics and nutritional needs of the child, the interactions between the child and feeders, and the child's eating behaviors. The child's physical condition may influence whether the child can successfully eat food. Children who have difficulty chewing and swallowing food, have particular feeding approaches, require dietary modifications, have low activity levels, or are treated using medications, may not have adequate nutrient intake. Parent-child interactions also influence children's eating behaviors and may be affected by unique caregiving demands, particular feeding preferences, and pressure to eat [17]. Additionally, when the child demonstrates problem behaviors such as refusing to eat and having inflexible food preferences, ensuring the child receives adequate nutrition is difficult.

Common mealtime behavior problems of children with developmental disabilities include a low level of independent eating, food refusal, inflexible food preferences, and distraction from eating. Some children exhibit aggressive problem behaviors when they refuse to eat, including spitting food, pushing the table, breaking the chair, and other destructive behaviors. When children with developmental disabilities exhibit challenging behaviors, these problem behaviors become a source of stress for preschool teachers.

Alvarez [18] and Stormont [19] have observed that stressed teachers spend more than 20% of their class time engaged in negative interactions with children who exhibit problem behaviors, and only 5% of their class time in positive interactions with children. The USA

National Prekindergarten study of 2003–2004 also indicated that 10.4% of state-funded prekindergarten teachers expelled at least one preschool child from their program, which was 3.2 times higher than that of children of other school grades. Amstad and Müller [20] noted that problem behaviors of children with disabilities are a source of stress for teachers, with kicking, hitting, and biting behaviors rated as the most stressful for teachers. Disruptive and antisocial behaviors were also reported as the most stressful behaviors in class [21]. Gebbie et al. [22] investigated the needs of preschool teachers in a North Carolina county in the United States. They noted that most teachers requested training on managing children's challenging behaviors; those teachers who received training and mentoring in classroom behavior management strategies felt competent in managing challenging behaviors and increased their self-efficacy. When teachers can successfully solve problem behaviors, their stress is reduced.

Researchers have argued that Applied Behavioral Analysis strategies and techniques could successfully alleviate problem behaviors of children with disabilities, especially IMBs. ABA strategies include negative reinforcement, positive reinforcement, and escape extinction, which can assist teachers in modifying children's mealtime behaviors [7–9]. Ahearn et al. [7] used negative reinforcement contingencies to physically guide children to accept food, whereby the feeder did not remove the spoon until the child accepted the presented food. Through this method, the children's food acceptance increased. Hoch et al. [9] used positive reinforcement procedures and contingency contracting strategies and successfully increased children's food acceptance. However, the children's negative vocalization and class disruption behaviors did not change. Cooper et al. [8] also reported that using positive reinforcers increased the number of bites of food children took. Researchers revealed that reinforcement and escape extinction methods improved mealtime behavior problems in children with disabilities. The feeder used reinforcers to increase children's appropriate eating behaviors and escape extinction to avoid children distancing themselves from the food they did not want to eat during mealtime [23–25].

Other educators claimed that the mealtime period presents an excellent opportunity to train children in positive social skills by teaching new techniques or replacement behaviors. Lalli et al. [26] used a behavioral consultation approach to reduce children's problem behaviors and to increase their appropriate verbal behaviors during mealtime. Gaverea and Schwartz [27] used "snack talk" cards to increase appropriate social interaction among children with and without disabilities during mealtime. Therefore, I proposed that teaching appropriate techniques or behaviors successfully reduces children's problem behaviors and increased proper behaviors during mealtime. As described in related research, children's challenging behaviors are a source of teachers' stress. The present study was conducted to determine how teachers feel when they are faced with children's IMBs, the support they require, and the factors they believe are related to children's mealtime behavior problems.

## 3. Research Method

### 3.1. Research Method

Semi-structured interviews were conducted with five preschool teachers who had experience with managing the IMBs of children with developmental disabilities in separate classes. Semi-structured interviews can provide rich and detailed perspectives on such children's problem behaviors and how the teacher feels when dealing with those problems. Semi-structured interviews involve open-ended questions that allow teachers to provide in-depth and spontaneous responses [28]. This research approach was appropriate for collecting in-depth information to examine preschool teachers' stress, problem-solving skills, and desired support.

### 3.2. Subjects

The sample consisted of five preschool teachers who had experience with managing IMBs of children with developmental disabilities in a classroom setting. The participating teachers were recruited through snowball sampling and were referred by collaborative preschool principles. Each teacher attended one-on-one interviews that each lasted at least 2 h. The interviews were held in a private room in the interviewer's preschool. If required, the teachers attended multiple interviews. A total of 15 h of interviews were recorded. The interviewees were sent the questions before the interviews and the transcripts after the interviews. The background information of the five teachers is presented in Table 1.

Table 1. The Background Information of the Interviewees.

| Teacher | Age | Major | Seniority | Children's Name | Children's Age | Children's Mealtime Problem |
|---------|-----|-------|-----------|-----------------|----------------|------------------------------|
| A | 35 | Bachler's in Education | 9 years | Andy | 5 | Selecting food. |
| B | 28 | Master in dept. of social and local development | 6 years | Bill | 2 | Eat rice only, eating distractions. |
| C | 28 | Master's in special education | 4 years | Cody | 4.5 | Eating without using spoons properly, eating distractions. |
| D | 40 | Bachelor's in early childhood care and education | 8 years | David | 8 | Eat white toast only. |
| E | 22 | Bachelor's in Early childhood care and education | 4 years | Emily | 4 | Selecting food. |

As reported in Table 1, all interviewees were currently working as preschool teachers. All interviewees graduated with a bachelor's degree in education, early childhood care, or special education. The average age of the children who exhibited mealtime problems was 3.7 (range: 2–5) years. The mealtime behavior problems included eating only preferred foods, eating only rice, eating only white toast, becoming distracted from eating, and not using eating utensils properly. All children had been identified as having developmental disabilities.

*3.3. Interview Procedure*

During a 2-h session, I trained a bachelor-level clinician in interview techniques to enable them to conduct the teacher interviews. I developed the interview questions, and the interviewer was informed of the study purpose and research design before the interviews.

The interviewer applied a semi-structured interview protocol, which outlined essential topics to generate rapport, gather information, and close the interview [29,30]. In addition, this study investigated the teachers' problem-solving skills, stress triggers, effects, and factors influencing the effects. I used open-ended questions to facilitate in-depth discussion; if the discussion on a subject was incomplete, follow-up questions were used to collect additional information. I received all interviewees' consent before audio-recording the interviews.

*3.4. Interview Credibility*

Epoché is crucial in qualitative research to prevent researchers' preconceived ideas and beliefs about the phenomenon under investigation from biasing the results. To avoid personal beliefs influencing the outcomes, I trained the interviewer to conduct the interviews and developed the credibility process for this study.

Three primary methods were used to establish the credibility of the interviews. First, I examined the transcripts to ensure the interview content was relevant to the purpose of this study. Second, I conducted a triangulation process with two independent experts to reach a consensus on the themes extracted from the interviews that could be further analyzed. Third, I provided the interviewees with the interview transcripts to confirm their content.

*3.5. Data Analysis*

The data analysis process involved coding and breaking the data into segments. First, I used inductive coding to transcribe the recordings into numbered statements. I then clustered and identified themes that reflected each interviewee's experiences and feelings. I employed the horizontalization process to identify relevant horizons [31], removing repetitive and irrelevant statements. The initial list of horizons was verified by comparing the interviews in sequence. I used the strategy of bracketing the data when reviewing the interview transcripts, in which the interviewees' experiences were "bracketed" by adopting an "outsider" perspective and focusing on data that could be examples of the research topic. Finally, I compared the textural descriptions to develop a group composite textural descriptions to examine the phenomenon of teacher stress in the context of addressing children's mealtime behavior problems in class.

**4. Findings**

The analysis of the semi-structured interviews revealed the following four major themes related to the interviewees' experiences and feelings about addressing IMBs of children with developmental disabilities: (a) the identification of children's mealtime behavior problems, (b) the application of problem-solving skills to address such problems, (c) the stress of solving such problems, and (d) the factors influencing children's IMBs. In addition to sharing their experiences, reactions, strategies, and feelings when managing children's mealtime behavior problems, the teachers also provided suggestions for improving the IMBs of children with developmental disabilities.

*4.1. Theme 1: Identification of Children's Mealtime Problems: "Different from and More Complicated Than How I Imagined."*

The preschool teachers had not expected that addressing the IMBs of children with developmental disabilities would be much different from, and more complicated than, addressing those of children without disabilities. Some teachers indicated that each child with a developmental disability had distinct eating problems during mealtime.

*"Andy has a problem with picking out his preferred food. If he sees something he does not like in the lunch bowl, he gets angry, cries, and screams in class. He even became so mad that he pushed the table away so the bowl and spoon fell to the floor."* (Teacher A: 50–52)

*"Bill only eats white rice. Although he does not eat much, he picks out the white rice to eat. After eating, he plays with his toy without noticing what's happening in the classroom, including cleaning up. He does not eat breakfast if there is no white rice. He refuses to eat everything else, including dessert, if there is no white rice."* (Teacher B: 43–49)

*"Cody enjoys eating lunch and dessert in preschool but does not like vegetables. His major mealtime problem is that he uses his hands to grab food instead of using a spoon, and sometimes he eats while putting one foot on the chair, leaves his seat without permission, or drops rice on the table. He would also use his dirty hand to touch everything near him, and he would get distracted from eating. He throws the food he does not like on the table or leaves it in the bowl."* (Teacher C: 29–41)

*"David has a severe problem with picking out his preferred food. He only likes toast with strawberry jam and white rice with meat floss topping. When he comes across food he does not like, he will stop eating, leave the lunch on the table, or spit out the food. He also has a distraction problem; he becomes distracted from eating when other children are chatting or doing other things after they have completed the clean-up routine during mealtime. He also does not like chewing food when he is eating."* (Teacher D: 28–47)

*"Emily likes to eat meat or fried meat. She eats fast when she finds food she likes, but she picks food out if she does not like it. Moreover, she uses her bare hands to grab things she wants to eat and throws food away or on the floor if she does not like it. Sometimes, she just sits still refusing to eat, or spits out the food she does not like. She also gets distracted*

*from eating during mealtime. Another problem is using a spoon. She cannot hold a spoon correctly, so she sometimes drops rice on the table or floor."* (Teacher E: 38–69)

According to the interviews, children's IMBs include picking out preferred foods, refusing to eat, using hands instead of a spoon to grab food from the lunch bowl, putting one foot on the chair when eating, dropping rice on the table or floor, becoming distracted from eating, and purposefully spitting out food. Picking out preferred food is the most common problem with mealtime behavior of children with developmental disabilities. Children may demonstrate various misbehaviors when they encounter food they do not enjoy, such as screaming, crying, pushing the food away, picking out food, refusing to move, vomiting, and leaving the table. The teachers observed that IMBs are more severe and complex in children with developmental disabilities than in children without disabilities.

*4.2. Theme 2: Problem-Solving Skills: Persuading or Direct Teaching?*

When faced with children's IMBs, most preschool teachers preferred not to deal with the problem behaviors immediately when the child demonstrating such behaviors is in a non-compliant mood. If the child was not angry or violent, some of the teachers would intervene directly and teach the child the appropriate behaviors. Some attempted to communicate with the child first before applying any strategy.

*"When Andy sees food he does not like in his bowl, he gets angry. First, I help him pick out the food he does not like and put it on the bowl cover. Then, I try to talk to him to slowly persuade him to accept the food. It takes a long time, but I will not force him to eat everything."* (Teacher A: 50–64)

*"Bill eats only white rice, and when he is finished eating, he plays with his toys without following the class routine. I tell other children in the class that he can play with his toy because he has finished eating. Because this situation has been ongoing for a while, I know he likes a particular car. So, I put the car he likes in front of his lunch and tell him, 'If you can try a little bit of food other than the white rice, I will let you play with the car.'"* (Teacher B: 102–107)

*"Cody has a variety of behavioral problems. I applied for a special education teaching assistant. This teaching assistant and I are jointly responsible during mealtime. For example, I help prepare the children's meals, and the assistant helps the children to get ready to line up for lunch. The teaching assistant sets the IEP objectives to help the child learn to have lunch while seated, use a spoon correctly, and clean up after mealtime. When he is finished, he is allowed to play with the children. I also use related picture books to teach the children which utensils we use to eat, and we all discuss them in class. Then, I use the pictures to remind the children to eat with proper manners."* (Teacher C:237–272)

*"David has a problem with picking out his preferred foods, but I insist he finishes the food in the bowl without running away. I encourage him to go to the corner of the room he likes if he finishes the meal. If he does not finish the meal, he is not allowed to play in his favorite corner. I continually remind him to eat without picking out his preferred food and to improve his communication skills. I believe that each child has individual differences. If we give children more time, they can do well."* (Teacher D: 58–75)

*"Because Emily has a problem with becoming distracted from eating, she needs to learn and practice concentration. I have to watch her eating all the time during mealtime. When she tries to use her hand to grab food, I tell her to use a spoon to eat. There are two teachers trying to fix her mealtime problems. One teacher asks her to finish the food in the bowl, even if it is only one bite of food left. The other teacher does not have time to watch Emily constantly during mealtime, so if Emily does not finish the meal, the teacher feeds her. When Emily spits out the food, the teacher simply gives her another spoonful so she understands that spitting out the food is no use. We also ask her to finish all her food*

*before brushing her teeth, because some children keep the food in their mouths without swallowing it."* (Teacher E: 82–94)

The preschool teachers applied different techniques to persuade or teach the children to eat appropriately, such as discussion, feeding, and the use of reinforcement procedures. Teacher B used Bill's favorite car toy as a reinforcer to encourage him to eat, and Teacher D used David's favorite playing corner to encourage him to improve his mealtime behavior problems. Some of the teachers applied the extinction strategy to prevent children from escaping from their meals, such as Teacher D and Teacher E. Teacher C used a more systematic procedure to teach Cody correct mealtime behaviors. For example, the special education teacher developed IEP goals, and Teacher C and the assistant collaboratively assisted Cody in achieving these goals.

*4.3. Theme 3: The Stress of Solving Problems: Powerless and Self-Doubt*

When dealing with the children's IMBs, the preschool teachers tended to feel powerless and self-doubting, because they may not see the positive and successful outcome of the intervention. Furthermore, they must also deal with the children's other problem behaviors during class time. The preschool teachers described the characteristics of each child with special needs, revealing their stress and concerns from managing these children's problem behaviors.

*"Andy cannot express his emotions. Therefore, when he is doing an activity and is interrupted, he becomes angry. He only does activities he likes, and I feel very stressed when changing activities. There are six children with special needs in the school, and we have three children with special needs in my class but only two teachers. I teach Andy when he listens to me, but I cannot do anything if Andy is so angry that he refuses to listen."* (Teacher A: 23–48)

*"Most private preschools do not accept children with disabilities. Two young children in my class were diagnosed after they enrolled. I feel a little stressed because, at school, I was training Bill to feed himself without picking out food, but his grandmother usually feeds him at home and tells me nothing about his food or eating behaviors. Therefore, he does whatever he wants in class, and it is difficult for me to teach him proper mealtime behaviors."* (Teacher B: 77–96)

*"So, the assistant and I help Cody with many tasks that he should complete during mealtime. Because if we do not help him, he will disrupt the whole class schedule. Besides, I also worry that his bad eating behaviors might make him sick during mealtime. Cody does not live with his parents; he is an aboriginal resident of a rural area and lives with his aunt, and his parents work in another city. Therefore, it is challenging to meet and communicate with his parents. I have to teach Cody all behaviors in school."* (Teacher C: 48–58)

*"Emily has a developmental disability that affects her speech and communication, and she has a problem with self-care and emotional stability. She has undergone speech therapy. Because she spits out the food on the floor when the other children are eating, I ask the other children to leave and clean it up. She also has a problem with concentrating on tasks. When we ask her to do something, she looks at what the other children are doing and forgets to do what she was told. Therefore, I feel stressed when I must constantly watch and remind her what she should be doing. I also feel stressed when parents do not cooperate with the teacher. Although I teach Emily to eat everything in her bowl without picking out food, her parents allow her to pick out the food she does not like. Inevitably, she becomes angry and demonstrates inappropriate mealtime behaviors when she cannot do whatever she wants in school."* (Teacher E: 82–101)

The preschool teachers' stress resulted primarily from the children's problem behaviors and a lack of support for the teachers from the children's families. The problem behaviors of the children have exceeded the scope of the preschool teachers' understanding, and parents' inconsistent discipline and laissez-faire attitude further negatively affect the results of the teachers' interventions in school.

*4.4. Theme 4: Factors Influencing Children's Mealtime Behaviors: Family Support Is the Key*

The preschool teachers believed that several factors affect the children's IMBs, including health problems, emotional status, motor development, disabilities, parental socioeconomic status, and inconsistent discipline. However, some of the preschool teachers indicated that family support is critical in addressing and educating children on mealtime behaviors.

> "When Andy was sick, he ate less. He takes longer than the other children to eat during mealtime, and I have to try different methods to improve his mealtime behaviors. When he can express his emotion, his is less aggressive." (Teacher A: 55–73)

> "His problem with picking out food was so serious when I first met him, and he was still sucking on the pacifier at 2 years old. His grandparents let him do whatever he wants, and I believe that his mealtime behavior problems are related to his eating habits at home." (Teacher B: 109–144)

> "Cody was diagnosed with a developmental disability and was not the only one with a disability in the class. Therefore, I feel powerless when I have to deal with many similar situations at the same time. If other children have ADHD problems, managing the class is more challenging. Cody's parents are of a low socioeconomic status and have to work outside the village to earn a living to support their family. I believe the characteristics of Cody's disability and his family support are primary factors influencing his mealtime behaviors." (Teacher C: 154–169)

> "David has a developmental disability affecting his cognitive and language abilities, but he can understand simple commands. He does not like to chew and does not like to eat when he feels sick." (Teacher D: 15–38)

> "I think different disciplinary methods influence each child's mealtime behaviors. I ask Emily to finish what she has in her lunch bowl, but Emily can decide the amount she wants to eat. However, when another teacher uses different disciplinary methods to address Emily's inappropriate mealtime behaviors, such as feeding her, I found Emily's problem behavior is worse than before." (Teacher E: 72–79)

Some of the preschool teachers believed that IMBs of children with developmental disabilities are attributable to their developmental limitations, and others maintained that such behaviors are influenced by the children's family support.

## 5. Discussion

The purpose of the interviews was to explore the experience of five preschool teachers with experience in addressing IMBs of children with developmental disabilities in class. The research focused on identifying the main IMBs of children with developmental disabilities, teachers' strategies or levels of support for managing such behaviors, teachers' stress, and factors contributing to children's IMBs. Four major themes emerged during the study: (a) the identification of children's mealtime behavior problems, (b) the application of problem-solving skills to address such problems, (c) the stress of solving such problems, and (d) the factors influencing children's IMBs. As the number of children with developmental disabilities enrolling in inclusive preschool classrooms increases, the need for preschool teachers to understand the children's individual needs and characteristics also grows. When addressing IMBs, teachers experienced stress through feelings of uncertainty, isolation, and powerlessness. Because the problem behaviors of children with developmental disabilities are different from those without disabilities, identifying an effective intervention strategy to improve children's behaviors is difficult for teachers. Even with the extra support provided in Teacher C's case, where a teaching assistant assisted in improving children's IMBs, the outcome was still limited. Therefore, what form of support can be helpful and practical for solving IMBs of children with developmental disabilities in preschools must be determined.

Because children with developmental disabilities demonstrate mealtime behavior problems that are more difficult and complex than children without disabilities, addressing these behavioral problems through discussions or commands only may be ineffective. The form, intensity, and frequency of IMBs of children with developmental disabilities differ from those of children without disabilities and can generate more stress for teachers

This study has several limitations, which must be considered before generalizing the findings to other preschool teachers. First, the sample was small, representing the views of only five preschool teachers; they thus may not reflect most preschool teachers' experiences in inclusive classrooms. Therefore, more preschool teachers must be recruited in further studies to investigate the IMBs of children with developmental disabilities by using a quantitative research method or mixed-method approach to establish reliable information. Second, the findings of this study were obtained primarily from preschool teacher interviews; thus, this study lacked additional data resources, such as observation records of children's behaviors, IEPs, and classroom management notes. Future research is required to further examine the effectiveness of the support and strategies provided by preschools. Such research could assist preschools in developing well-designed and practical supportive models to reduce preschool teachers' stress. Furthermore, future studies could focus on successful interventions for addressing IMBs of children with developmental disabilities to increase preschool teachers' self-advocacy and advocacy of inclusive classes.

## 6. Recommendations for Future Preschools

Preschools should implement measures to reduce the stress of teachers managing IMBs of children with disabilities. First, preschools can assign a mobile support teacher to classrooms in which support is required immediately. Second, preschools must hire experienced professionals to effectively address children's problem behaviors in class. Third, to increase intervention success, preschools can develop a support system to assist teachers in determining when and for whom interventions or strategies are implemented, what the intervention or strategy is, and how the intervention or strategy can be continually evaluated and modified as necessary. Fourth, communication with children's families is critical for influencing children's eating behaviors. Therefore, preschool teachers must learn to effectively communicate with the children's families to gain the families' support. Finally, preschool teachers must regularly communicate with preschool principals or directors to ensure that the principals or directors understand the preschool teachers' stress and the difficulties of managing children's behavior problems.

The findings of this study indicate that many preschool teachers do not know how to quickly and effectively solve the mealtime behavior problems of children with developmental disabilities, which increases teachers' stress. Therefore, the practical approaches taught in higher education must focus on teaching teachers how to identify, manage, and change children's problematic behaviors to ensure that the teachers are well-prepared for classroom settings.

The IMBs of children with developmental disabilities cannot be ignored because they directly relate to the children's health, development, and educational activities in preschool. Developing an effective support system for preschool teachers to improve their skills in solving children's mealtime behavior problems is imperative. This research provided valuable insight into preschool teachers' experiences when encountering mealtime behavior problems of children with developmental disabilities, and the results provide a starting point for examining the curriculum of higher education teacher training and the need to provide preschool teachers with adequate class management skills.

**Funding:** This research received no external funding.

**Institutional Review Board Statement:** This study was approved by the Research Ethics Review Committee National Tsing Hua University (ethic code: 11106ET072; date: 15 September 2021).

**Informed Consent Statement:** Informed consent was obtained from all subjects involved in the study.

**Data Availability Statement:** I confirmed that the data supporting the findings of this study are available within the article. The descriptive data will be available upon reasonable request.

**Conflicts of Interest:** The author declares no conflict of interest.

## References

1. Kerwin, M.E.; Eicher, P.; Gelsinger, J. Parental report of eating problems and gastrointestinal symptoms in children with pervasive developmental disorders. *Child. Health Care* **2005**, *34*, 217–234. [CrossRef]
2. Palmer, S.; Thompson, R.J.; Linscheid, T.R. Applied behavior analysis in the treatment of childhood feeding problems. *Dev. Med. Child Neurol.* **1975**, *17*, 333–339. [CrossRef] [PubMed]
3. Matson, J.L.; Kuhn, D.E. Identifying feeding problems in mentally retarded persons: Development and reliability of the screening tool of feeding problems (STEP). *Res. Dev. Disabil.* **2001**, *22*, 165–172. [CrossRef] [PubMed]
4. Rogers, L.G.; Magill-Evans, J.; Rempel, G.R. Mothers' challenges in feeding their children with autism spectrum disorder—Managing more than just picky eating. *J. Dev. Phys. Disabil.* **2012**, *24*, 19–33. [CrossRef]
5. Disabilities Education Act, Part H. 1990. Available online: https://www.eeoc.gov/americans-disabilities-act-1990-original-text (accessed on 10 May 2022).
6. The Protection of Children and Youths Welfare and Rights Act of Taiwan, Article 1. 2021. Available online: https://law.moj.gov.tw/ENG/LawClass/LawParaDeatil.aspx?pcode=D0050001&bp=5 (accessed on 10 May 2022).
7. Ahearn, W.H.; Kerwin, M.E.; Eicher, P.S.; Shantz, J.; Swearingin, W. An alternating treatment comparison of two intensive interventions for food refusal. *J. Appl. Behav. Anal.* **1996**, *29*, 321–332. [CrossRef]
8. Cooper, L.J.; Wacker, D.P.; Brown, K.; McComas, J.J.; Peck, S.M.; Drew, J.; Asmus, J.; Kayser, K. Use of a concurrent operants paradigm to evaluate positive reinforcers during treatment of food refusal. *Behav. Modif.* **1999**, *23*, 3–40. [CrossRef]
9. Hoch, T.A.; Babbitt, R.L.; Coe, D.A.; Krell, D.M.; Hackbert, L. Contingency contacting: Combining positive reinforcement and escape extinction procedures to treat persistent food refusal. *Behav. Modif.* **1994**, *18*, 106–128. [CrossRef]
10. Harris, J.R. *The Nurture Assumption: Why Children Turn out the Way They Do*; Free Press: New York, NY, USA, 1998.
11. Parent Manual, Rev.03. 2013. Available online: http://kidscoopnurseryschool.com/KIDS%20Parent%20Orien%20Manual,%20rev%20MARCH%202015.pdf (accessed on 10 May 2022).
12. Kumari, S. Nurturing values in disabled children: Role of psychology. *Indian J. Health Wellbeing* **2017**, *8*, 361–364.
13. Jenkins, S.; Bax, M.; Hart, H. Behaviour problems in preschool children. *J. Child Psychol. Psychiatry* **1980**, *21*, 5–18. [CrossRef]
14. Earls, F. The prevalence of behavior problems in 3-year-old children. *Arch. Gen. Psychiatry* **1980**, *37*, 1153–1159. [CrossRef]
15. Richman, N.; Stevenson, J.; Graham, P.J. *Preschool to School: A Behavioural Study*; Academic Press: London, UK, 1982.
16. Secrist-Mertz, C.; Brotherson, M.J.; Oakland, M.J.; Litchfield, R. Helping families meet the nutritional needs of children with disabilities: An integrated model. *Child. Health Care* **1997**, *26*, 151–168. [CrossRef]
17. De-Souzae, F.J.; Paul, P. Perceived parental parenting style and social competence. *J. Indian Acad. Appl. Psychol.* **2013**, *39*, 103–109.
18. Alvarez, H.K. The impact of teacher preparation on responses to child aggression in the classroom. *Teach. Teach. Educ.* **2007**, *23*, 1113–1126. [CrossRef]
19. Stormont, M. Externalizing behavior problems in young children: Contributing factors and early intervention. *Psychol. Sch.* **2002**, *39*, 127–138. [CrossRef]
20. Amstad, M.; Müller, C.M. Students' problem behaviors as sources of teacher stress in special needs schools for individuals with intellectual disabilities. *Front. Educ.* **2020**, *4*, 159. [CrossRef]
21. Koot, H.M. *Problem Behavior in Dutch Preschoolers*; Erasmus University: Rotterdam, The Netherlands, 1993.
22. Gebbie, D.H.; Ceglowski, D.; Taylor, L.K.; Miels, J. The role of teacher efficacy in strengthening classroom support for preschool children with disabilities who exhibit challenging behaviors. *Early Child. Educ. J.* **2012**, *40*, 35–46. [CrossRef]
23. Hanley, G.P.; Iwata, B.A.; McCord, B.E. Functional analysis of problem behavior: A review. *J. Appl. Behav. Anal.* **2003**, *36*, 147–185. [CrossRef]
24. Hodges, A.; Gerow, S.; Davis, T.N.; Radhakrishnan, S.; Feind, A.; OGuinn, N.; Prawira, C. An Initial Evaluation of Trial-Based Functional Analyses of Inappropriate Mealtime Behavior. *J. Dev. Phys. Disabil.* **2018**, *30*, 391–408. [CrossRef]
25. LeGray, M.W.; Dufrene, B.A.; Mercer, S.; Olmi, D.J.; Sterling, H. Differential reinforcement of alternative behavior in center-based classrooms: Evaluation of pre-teaching the alternative behavior. *J. Behav. Educ.* **2013**, *22*, 85–102. [CrossRef]
26. Lalli, J.S.; Browder, D.M.; Mace, F.C.; Brown, D.K. Teachers use descriptive analysis data to implement interventions to decrease students' problem behavior. *J. Appl. Behav. Anal.* **1993**, *26*, 227–238. [CrossRef]
27. Gaverea, A.N. Using "Snack Talk" to support social communication in the inclusive preschool classroom. *Young Except. Child.* **2017**, *22*, 187–197. [CrossRef]

28. Ryan, F.; Michael, C.; Cronin, P. Interviewing in qualitative research: The one-to-one interview. *Int. J. Ther. Rehabil.* **2009**, *16*, 309–314. [CrossRef]
29. McFarlance, K.; Krebs, S. Techniques for interviewing and evidence gathering. In *Sexual Abuse of Young Children*; Guilford Publication: New York, NY, USA, 1986; pp. 62–100.
30. Wood, S.; Orsak, C.; Murphy, M.; Cross, H.J. Semistructured child sexual abuse interviews: Interview and child characteristics related to credibility of disclosure. *Child Abuse Negl.* **1992**, *20*, 81–92. [CrossRef] [PubMed]
31. Moustakas, C. *Phenomenological Research Methods*; Sage Publications: Newbury Park, CA, USA, 1994.

**Disclaimer/Publisher's Note:** The statements, opinions and data contained in all publications are solely those of the individual author(s) and contributor(s) and not of MDPI and/or the editor(s). MDPI and/or the editor(s) disclaim responsibility for any injury to people or property resulting from any ideas, methods, instructions or products referred to in the content.

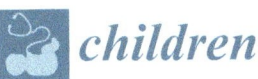 

Article

# Examining the Contributions of Parents' Daily Hassles and Parenting Approaches to Children's Behavior Problems during the COVID-19 Pandemic

Ibrahim H. Acar [1,*], Sevval Nur Sezer [1], İlayda Uculas [1] and Fatma Ozge Unsal [2]

1 Department of Psychology, Faculty of Social Sciences, Çekmeköy Campus, Ozyeğin University, 34794 Istanbul, Turkey
2 Department of Early Childhood Education, Faculty of Education, Göztepe Campus, Marmara University, 34722 Istanbul, Turkey
* Correspondence: ibrahim.acar@ozyegin.edu.tr

**Abstract:** The present study was designed to examine the direct and indirect contributions of parenting daily hassles and approaches to children's externalizing and internalizing behavior problems during the COVID-19 pandemic. The sample for this study was 338 preschool children (53.6% girls, $M_{age}$ = 56.33 months, $SD$ = 15.14) and their parents in Turkey. Parents reported their daily hassles, parenting approaches, and children's behavior problems. Findings from the structural equation model showed that higher levels of parenting daily hassles predicted higher levels of externalizing and internalizing behavior problems. In addition, we found an indirect effect of daily hassles on children's internalizing behaviors via positive parenting. Further, there was an indirect path from parenting daily hassles to children's externalizing behaviors through the negative parenting approach. Results are discussed in the context of the COVID-19 pandemic.

**Keywords:** parenting daily hassles; the COVID-19 pandemic; parenting approaches; behavior problems

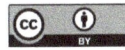

## 1. Introduction

Unprecedented times and contexts, such as the COVID-19 pandemic, procreate adverse effects for specific groups, such as parents with young children because of their fragility, exacerbated burden in childcaring and sustaining within-family functioning [1,2]. Further, more than 1.6 billion children were out of school because of lockdown policies [3], which placed an additional burden on parents with young children. As a natural consequence of home confinement and within-family dysfunctions (e.g., juggling between childcare and work, dealing with children's needs) due to the COVID-19 pandemic, children's behavior problems have increased [4,5]. From this perspective, we aimed to investigate the daily hassles of parents related to parenting practices within the family and how this within-family functioning undermined children's behavior problems.

Behavior problems in children can be grouped into internalizing (e.g., anxiety and depression) and externalizing behaviors (e.g., aggression and hyperactivity) [6]. As a consequence of the COVID-19 pandemic, children have experienced a lack of social interactions and movement restrictions, which have adversely affected their development [3]. For example, Jiao et al. [7] found that children felt insecure, frightened, and lonely during the pandemic, and also experienced sleep disturbances, nightmares, eating problems, agitation, inattention, and separation anxiety. Overall, young children have mainly been affected by the COVID-19 pandemic, as developmentally making sense of the situation could be more challenging for them [8–10].

As children experience the pandemic in a family context, within-family functioning reflecting parenting approaches and daily routines naturally affect children's behavioral outcomes [2]. The change, stress, restrictions, and financial problems that came with the pandemic have increased the burden on parents and overall within-family interactions [1,11]. Because children require support from their parents in daily functioning to a large extent in the preschool period, parents with the burdens of the pandemic may lack support for their children, which could lead children to display behavior problems [1,2]. Considering the importance of parenting approaches and parenting stress within the family context on the development of children's behavior problems, it is essential to examine the impacts of parents' daily hassles and parenting approaches on children's behavior problems during the COVID-19 pandemic.

## 1.1. Parents' Socialization and Children's Behavior Problems

The family context is the first social environment for children where they begin socializing [12]. Child-rearing approaches as part of the family social context play a critical role in the socialization of children, leading them to display culturally accepted behaviors. While positive child-rearing practices may contribute positively to the socialization of children, negative child-rearing approaches may prevent children's socialization and pave the way for behavioral problems for children [13]. Parents utilize positive child-rearing practices such as inductive reasoning and warmth and negative practices such as punishment and obedience-demanding [14]. Practicing negative child-rearing approaches (i.e., punishment and obedience-demanding) may increase children's risk of developing behavioral problems. For example, using physical punishment as a discipline and demanding obedience (e.g., expecting compliance without explanation) by parents has been positively linked to child behavior problems such as aggression [15]. On the other hand, using inductive reasoning (e.g., providing explanations to children) and warmth (e.g., showing acceptance and sensitivity to a child's needs) has been linked to a decrease in children's behavior problems [15]. Further, children whose interests and needs were not considered expressed anger by crying, stomping, and holding their breath to get what they wanted, reflecting behavior problems [15,16]. Overall, using overprotection and strict discipline as child-rearing approaches is associated with having children with internalizing and externalizing behavioral problems such as introversion, withdrawal, anxiety, and self-harm; on the other hand, adopting warmth and a positive parent–child relationship as child-rearing approaches was associated positively with the social development of children [16].

Grounded on the findings of previous studies, we can speculate that the child-rearing approaches adopted by the parents are effective in the development of behavioral problems of the children. However, the nature of the child-rearing approaches may have changed due to the adverse effects of the COVID-19 pandemic [17,18]. Confinement of parents may have placed an additional burden on parents with young children, leading them to display negative parenting practices [1].

## 1.2. Roles of Parenting Daily Hassles on Children's Behavior Problems

Parents with young children have juggled multiple tasks during the pandemic, mainly dealing with daily routines. Hassles in daily functioning may have undermined parental well-being and the quality of parent–child interactions [19]. Daily parenting hassles refer to experiences of common day-to-day burdens that emerge from caring for children [20]. In detail, daily parenting hassles could be both the burdens that parents experience in parenting-related chores (e.g., running errands) and their children's behaviors (e.g., picky eater) [19,21]. For example, the major daily hassles could be arranging bedtime routines, meal-time difficulties, cleaning toys, or sibling arguments, as well as other minor stressors in day-to-day living. Daily parenting hassles could undermine children's internalizing and externalizing behavior problems. Results from previous studies showed that daily parenting hassles contributed to children's behavior problems concurrently and longitudinally [22–24].

The COVID-19 pandemic may have increased daily hassles for parents, particularly parents with young children [25]. Knowing that daily hassles are critical underlying predictors of child-rearing practices and children's well-being, it is important to examine their role in child behavior problems during the COVID-19 pandemic.

*1.3. Link from Daily Hassles to Children's Behavior Problems through Parenting Approaches*

Understanding the needs of the children and responding to them appropriately is very important in terms of the psychological well-being of children and the quality of the bond they establish with their parents. The nature of parenting approaches could provide a socialization context for children to develop both positive and negative social outcomes [26,27]. Evidence is clear that positive parenting approaches, such as parental warmth, can make children feel secure and help children to display fewer behavior problems [28,29]. On the other hand, negative parenting approaches are often accompanied by punishment and obedience-demanding, which can increase children's behavior problems [15,23].

Daily hassles in parenting may deplete the resources of parents and undermine their regulatory capacity, which may lead them to display negative parenting approaches [20,30]. In detail, daily hassles emerging from parenting roles and demands, affecting the psychological well-being of parents, may be associated with disruptive and less optimal parenting approaches, which in turn lead their children to display behavior problems [23]. For example, parents with high levels of hassles showed negative parenting approaches (e.g., less tolerance towards their children, over-controlling), which were naturally found to be associated with internalizing and externalizing behavior problems in children (e.g., anxiety, depression, withdrawal, hyperactivity, and aggression [24,31]. Furthermore, a study with Turkish families showed an indirect effect of daily parenting hassles on children's social and aggressive behaviors through parenting approaches [23]. More specifically, parents with higher levels of daily hassles tended to display more physical punishment towards their children, which in turn predicted greater aggressive behavior in children. Everything considered, these findings highlight the social-contextual notion that children's behavior problems can be influenced by parenting context [32].

Study Purpose and Hypotheses

The pandemic may have brought additional hassles in parents' daily functioning, which may have undermined their capability to attune children's needs, which could lead their children to display more behavioral problems. To our knowledge, there has been no research examining the roles of daily hassles and parenting approaches on children's behavior problems during the COVID-19. Therefore, the purpose of the current study was to investigate the contributions of association parenting daily hassles parenting approaches to child behavior problems during the COVID-19 pandemic. We first hypothesized that daily hassles would be positively associated with children's behavior problems. Second, we hypothesized that daily hassles would be positively associated with negative parenting approaches and inversely associated with positive parenting approaches. Third, we hypothesized that positive parenting approaches would be negatively and that negative parenting approaches would be positively associated with children's behavior problems. Fourth, we hypothesized that daily hassles would undermine positive parenting and exacerbate negative parenting, leading children to display higher levels of behavior problems.

## 2. Materials and Methods

*2.1. Participants*

The sample for the current study was 338 Turkish preschool children (53.6% girls, $M_{age}$ = 56.33 months, $SD$ = 15.14). Only 11 of the participants were fathers; the remaining were mothers. Mothers' age ranged from 24 to 47 years ($M$ = 35.01, $SD$ = 4.14) and fathers' age ranged from 28 to 50 ($M$ = 37.64, $SD$ = 4.46). A total of 43.5% of mothers were employed, while 98.8% of fathers were employed during the pandemic. Family income was reported in blocks of TRY 1000 (Turkish liras) (~USD 117) and ranged from TRY 1000–2000 to more than TRY 7000/month, with a mode of TRY 7000 and higher. Employed mothers reported higher levels of parenting daily chores ($M = 2.04$, $SD = 0.44$; $M = 1.91$, $SD = 0.45$), $t(336) = 2.67$, $p < 0.01$) and behaviors ($M = 2.13$, $SD = 0.56$; $M = 1.99$, $SD = 0.54$, respectively, $t(336) = 2.34$, $p < 0.01$) compared to unemployed parents. The socioeconomic (SES) variable was created by averaging standardized (z-transformations) family income and education levels.

*2.2. Materials*

2.2.1. Behavior Problems

Parents reported on the Child Behavior Checklist (CBCL) [6]. The CBCL has 100 items and is rated on a 3-point Likert-like scale (0 = Not True, 1 = Somewhat or Sometimes True, 2 = Very True or Often True). The CBCL has been validated and used with Turkish children [33,34]. The CBCL consists of internalizing behaviors (e.g., "unhappy, sad, or depressed") and externalizing behaviors (e.g., "destroys things belonging to his/her family or other children") subscales. Cronbach's alpha was $\alpha = 0.87$ for externalizing behaviors and $\alpha = 0.91$ for internalizing behaviors. We summed items to create subscales where higher scores indicated higher levels of the construct.

2.2.2. Parenting Approaches

Parents reported on the Child-Rearing Questionnaire (CRQ) [14]. The CRQ is a 30-item scale rated on a 5-point Likert-type scale (1 = Never and 5 = Always). The CRQ has been validated and used with Turkish parents [23,26,35]. The CRQ has four subscales measuring warmth (e.g., "*My child and I have warm, intimate times together*"), inductive reasoning (e.g., "*I try to explain to my child why certain things are necessary*"), punishment (e.g., "*I use physical punishment, e.g., smacking, for very bad behavior*"), and obedience-demanding (e.g., "*I expect my child to do what he/she is told to do, without stopping to argue about it*"). Internal consistency scores (Cronbach's alpha) for inductive reasoning, punishment, obedience-demanding, and warmth were 0.80, 0.68, 0.79, and 0.87, respectively. We created positive (inductive reasoning and warmth) and negative (punishment and obedience-demanding) parenting latent constructs. See the Section 3 for the measurement model and factor loading values.

2.2.3. Parenting Daily Hassles

Parents reported on the Parenting Daily Hassles Scale (PDHS) [19]. The PDHS is a 20-item scale rated on a 4-point Likert-type scale (1 = Rarely and 4 = Constantly). The PDHS has been validated and used with Turkish parents [23,36]. Taylor [21] reexamined the structure of the 20-item PDHS and recommended using two subscales: behaviors (e.g., "*Need to keep a constant eye on what kids are doing*") and parenting chores (e.g., "*Kids get dirty and need to have clothes changed*"). Correspondingly, we used these two subscales in the current study to assess parents' daily hassles. Internal consistency scores (Cronbach's alpha) for behaviors and parenting chores were 0.82 and 0.80, respectively. We averaged items to create subscales where higher scores indicated higher levels of the construct.

2.2.4. Fear of COVID-19

We used the Fear of COVID-19 Scale (FCV-19S). [36]. The FCV-19S is a 7-item scale rated on a 5-point Likert-type scale (1 = Strongly disagree and 5 = Strongly agree) (e.g., "*It makes me uncomfortable to think about coronavirus-19*"). The FCV-19S has been validated and used with Turkish participants [37,38]. The internal consistency score (Cronbach's alpha) for the scale was 0.85. We averaged items to create a composite score where higher scores indicated higher levels of the construct. We used this construct as a covariate in our analyses.

*2.3. Procedure*

Following the University Human Subjects Ethics Committee's approval on 22 March 2021(code: 2021/06/03), we created two data collection methods. First, we distributed consent forms and questionnaires to parents through child-care centers and parenting groups. Parents who voluntarily wanted to participate in this study returned their consent forms and completed questionnaires. Second, we created an online survey through Qualtrics. This step helped us reach out to more parents during the COVID-19 pandemic. In online data collection, aligned with paper-pencil data collection procedures, participants signed their consent before completing the questionnaires. We utilized the chain-referral sampling technique in both methods, where primarily contacted participants enabled us to find additional participants.

### 2.4. Data Analysis

We tested normality assumptions by using the criteria of +3 and −3 for skewness and +10 and −10 for kurtosis [39]. Our variables were within the acceptable range; therefore, no transformation was employed. See Table 1. Multivariate analyses were conducted in *Mplus 8.4* [40], using structural equation modeling (SEM) with maximum likelihood estimation. We followed the two-step model-building approach [40]. First, we tested the measurement model where we created latent factors of parenting daily hassles and parenting approaches (positive and negative). Once the measurement model fit the data, we tested the hypothesized structural model to examine whether there is an indirect effect of parenting daily hassles on children's internalizing and externalizing behaviors through parenting approaches. We utilized top-down model building, where we included all possible covariates, including age, child sex, SES, and fear of COVID-19 in the model. We then removed the nonsignificant ones by considering the model fit improvement. We tested the significance of the indirect effects by using the bootstrapping technique (2000 resampling) with 95% confidence intervals [41]. We utilized a 95% bias-corrected bootstrap method, providing parsimonious results [40,41]. In line with Kline's [40] recommendations, comparative fit index (CFI) and Tucker–Lewis index (TLI) values greater than 0.90, root mean square error of approximation (RMSEA) values of 0.08 or below, and standardized root means square residual (SRMR) values of 0.08 or below were employed to indicate a good fit [41,42]. Finally, we collected the data from the same respondents by using self-reported surveys at one point in time, and some measures could involve similar notional items, which may have created a common method bias [43] We used Harman's single-factor test to see whether common method variance was present or not. The post hoc Harman's single-factor test was used to check if a single factor is accountable for variance in the data [44]. The results from Harman's single-factor test showed that only 18.23% of the variance was captured with the first unrotated factor (<50%), indicating that common method variance was not an issue in this study [44].

**Table 1.** Bivariate correlations and descriptive statistics for the study variables.

| | Variables. | 1 | 2 | 3 | 4 | 5 | 6 | 7 | 8 | 9 | 10 | 11 | 12 | 13 |
|---|---|---|---|---|---|---|---|---|---|---|---|---|---|---|
| 1. | Externalizing Beh | - | | | | | | | | | | | | |
| 2. | Internalizing Beh | 0.64 ** | - | | | | | | | | | | | |
| 3. | Warmth | −0.36 ** | −0.39 ** | - | | | | | | | | | | |
| 4. | Inductive Reasoning | −0.38 ** | −0.35 ** | 0.75 ** | - | | | | | | | | | |
| 5. | Obedience | 0.11 * | 0.24 ** | −0.12 * | −0.10 | - | | | | | | | | |
| 6. | Punishment | 0.51 ** | 0.45 ** | −0.49 ** | −0.43 ** | 0.34 ** | - | | | | | | | |
| 7. | DH_Behaviors | 0.63 ** | 0.51 ** | −0.32 ** | −0.27 ** | 0.15 ** | 0.48 ** | - | | | | | | |
| 8. | DH_Chores | 0.54 ** | 0.47 ** | −0.24 ** | −0.21 ** | 0.04 | 0.34 ** | 0.68 ** | - | | | | | |
| 9. | COVID Fear | −0.03 | 0.09 | 0.18 ** | 0.14 ** | 0.31 ** | 0.01 | −0.02 | 0.02 | - | | | | |
| 10. | Child Age | 0.21 ** | −0.04 | 0.02 | 0.14 ** | 0.03 | −0.01 | −0.15 ** | −0.23 ** | 0.03 | - | | | |

Table 1. Cont.

| | Variables. | 1 | 2 | 3 | 4 | 5 | 6 | 7 | 8 | 9 | 10 | 11 | 12 | 13 |
|---|---|---|---|---|---|---|---|---|---|---|---|---|---|---|
| 11. | Mother Age | −0.21 ** | −0.10 | 0.07 | 0.17 ** | 0.02 | −0.07 | −0.18 ** | −0.15 ** | 0.09 | 0.54 ** | - | | |
| 12. | Father Age | −0.19 ** | −0.09 | 0.06 | 0.15 ** | 0.01 | −0.09 | −0.16 ** | −0.13 * | 0.09 | 0.45 ** | 0.81 ** | - | |
| 13. | Family SES | −0.19 ** | −0.18 * | 0.01 | 0.15 ** | −0.01 | −0.01 | −0.08 | −0.15 ** | −0.04 | 0.06 | 0.26 ** | 0.11 * | - |
| 14. | Child Sex | −0.12 * | −0.04 | 0.01 | −0.01 | 0.03 | 0.04 | −0.08 | −0.18 ** | 0.01 | 0.02 | 0.01 | −0.02 | 0.04 |
| | n | 338 | 338 | 338 | 338 | 338 | 338 | 338 | 338 | 338 | 338 | 338 | 338 | 338 |
| | Mean | 9.59 | 11.13 | 4.76 | 4.64 | 2.54 | 1.43 | 2.05 | 1.97 | 2.59 | 56.33 | 35.01 | 37.64 | 0.00 |
| | SD | 6.07 | 7.09 | 0.32 | 0.42 | 0.73 | 0.32 | 0.55 | 0.45 | 0.78 | 15.14 | 4.14 | 4.46 | 0.82 |
| | Range | 0–31 | 0–39 | 3.67–5 | 3.14–5 | 1–4.83 | 1–2.75 | 1–3.86 | 1–3.33 | 1–4.71 | 21–89 | 24–47 | 28–50 | −3.20–2.23 |
| | Skewness | 0.882 | 0.795 | −1.428 | −1.123 | 0.200 | 1.218 | 0.392 | 0.018 | 0.068 | −0.106 | −0.038 | 0.159 | −1.252 |
| | Kurtosis | 0.659 | 0.304 | 1.333 | 0.405 | −0.180 | 2.057 | 0.018 | 0.018 | −0.323 | −0.327 | −0.979 | −0.345 | −0.402 | 2.792 |

Note. * $p < 0.05$, two-tailed. ** $p < 0.01$, two tailed. Sex: 1 = Girl, 0 = Boy. Beh: Behaviors. DH = Daily Hassles.

## 3. Results

Initially, we analyzed the bivariate correlations (Pearson) among study variables. Results showed that externalizing and internalizing behaviors were correlated with inductive reasoning, warmth, obedience, and punishment as part of the parenting approaches as well as parenting daily hassles. See Table 1 for complete correlation results.

### 3.1. Measurement Model

We tested the measurement model in *Mplus 8.4* [40] by creating latent variables of positive parenting, which consisted of warmth and inductive reasoning subscales; negative parenting, which consisted of obedience and punishment subscales; and parenting daily hassles, which consisted of behaviors and chores subscales. The results from the CFA showed that the measurement model fit the data very well, $\chi^2(9) = 37.71$, $p < 0.01$, CFI = 0.96, TLI = 0.93, RMSEA = 0.09, 90% CI [0.06–0.13], SRMR = 0.08. The standardized item loadings ranged from 0.41 to 0.97 across latent variables, meaning that all loadings were acceptable. Once the measurement model fit the data well, we moved forward with the structural model [40].

### 3.2. Structural Model

As we followed a top-down model-building approach, in the first model we included all possible covariates, including child age, child sex, family SES, mother employment status during the pandemic, and fear of COVID-19 in the model. The results of SEM were as follows: $\chi^2(30) = 139.294$, $p < 0.001$, CFI = 0.91, RMSEA = 0.10, 90% CI [0.08, 0.12], SRMR = 0.07. As seen from the model fit indices, there was room for model improvement. In the competing nested model, we removed the nonsignificant paths from the covariates in the model. Results from the final structural model showed a better fit to the data: $\chi^2(44) = 152.448$, $p < 0.001$, CFI = 0.92, RMSEA = 0.08, 90% CI [0.71, 0.10], SRMR = 0.07. In the second model, the RMSEA value was better, indicating the model was improved [42]. In the parsimonious model, parenting daily hassle was positively related to children's internalizing behaviors ($B = 7.06$ ($SE = 1.15$), $\beta = 0.41$, $p < 0.001$) and externalizing behaviors ($B = 7.60$ ($SE = 1.08$), $\beta = 0.51$, $p < 0.001$). Furthermore, the positive parenting approach was negatively related to children's internalizing behaviors ($B = -4.53$ ($SE = 1.78$), $\beta = -0.20$, $p < 0.01$), and the negative parenting approach was positively related to children's externalizing behaviors ($B = 4.85$ ($SE = 2.05$), $\beta = 0.24$, $p < 0.05$). The final model is depicted in Figure 1.

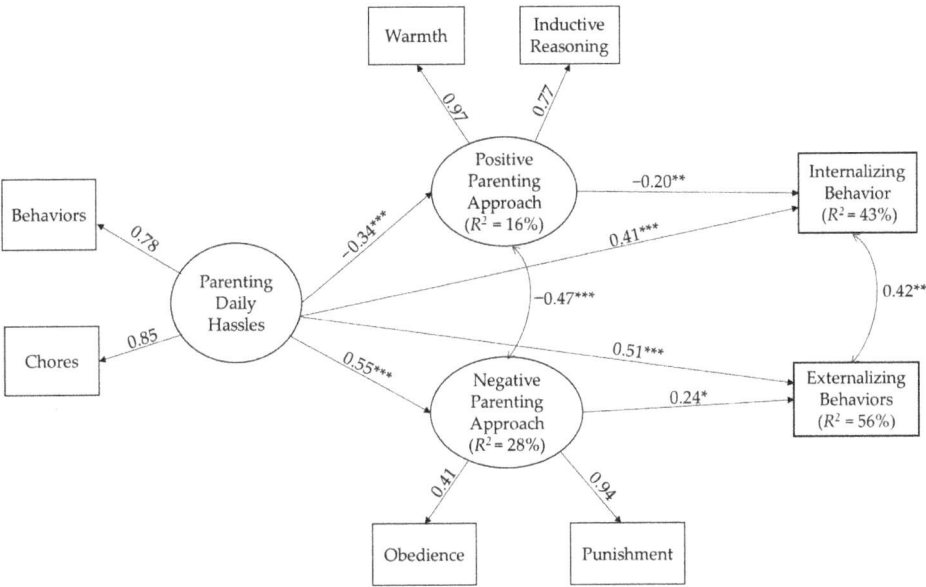

**Figure 1.** Parenting daily hassles predicting children's internalizing and externalizing behaviors through positive and negative parenting approaches. *** $p < 0.001$, ** $p < 0.01$, * $p < 0.05$. Note. Only significant paths are depicted for brevity. Child sex (B = −0.13, $\beta$ = −0.16, $p < 0.01$, favoring boys), child age (B = −0.006, $\beta$ = −0.21, $p < 0.001$), family SES (B = −0.07, $\beta$ = −0.15, $p = 0.01$), mother employment status (B = 0.15, $\beta$ = 0.19, $p < 0.01$, favoring employed mothers) as a covariate was controlled for daily hassles. Child sex (B = 0.06, $\beta$ = 0.11, $p < 0.05$, favoring girls) and child age (B = 0.002, $\beta$ = 0.10, $p < 0.05$) as a covariate was controlled for the negative parenting approach. Fear of COVID-19 (B = 0.08, $\beta$ = 0.19, $p < 0.001$) as a covariate was controlled for the negative parenting approach. Family SES (B = −0.82, $\beta$ = −0.11, $p < 0.05$) and child age (B = −0.04, $\beta$ = −0.10, $p < 0.01$) as a covariate was controlled for externalizing behaviors. Family SES (B = −0.97, $\beta$ = −0.11, $p < 0.05$) and fear of COVID-19 (B = 1.27, $\beta$ = 0.14, $p < 0.01$) as a covariate was controlled for internalizing behaviors.

There was a significant indirect path from parenting daily hassles to children's internalizing behaviors through the positive parenting approach ($\beta$ = 0.07 (SE = 0.02), [95% CI: 0.01, 0.13]). In addition, there was an indirect path from parenting daily hassles to children's externalizing behaviors through a negative parenting approach ($\beta$ = 0.13 (SE = 0.05), [95% CI: 0.03, 0.25]). Nevertheless, testing mediating effect in the absence of longitudinal data would be problematic [45]; therefore, our significant result from this model could be interpreted as an indirect effect rather than a pure mediation. Overall, parents with higher levels of daily hassles showed lower positive parenting; in turn, their children showed higher levels of internalizing behaviors. In addition, parents with higher levels of daily hassles showed higher negative parenting; in turn, their children showed higher externalizing behaviors. See Supplementary Material (Figures S1 and S2) for graphical depictions of bootstrap distributions with bias-corrected 95% credible confidence intervals.

## 4. Discussion

We aimed to examine the contributions of parenting daily hassles and parenting approaches to child behavior problems during the COVID-19 pandemic with a particular interest in testing the indirect effect of daily hassles on children's behavior problems via parenting approaches. We found a significant indirect effect of daily hassles on children's internalizing behaviors via positive parenting. In addition, there was an indirect path from parenting daily hassles to children's externalizing behaviors through the negative parenting approach. In the following sections, we discussed each result in turn.

### 4.1. Parenting Daily Hassles and Children's Behavior Problems

Our first research question was to discover associations between parenting daily hassles and children's behavior problems. In light of this question, we hypothesized that daily hassles would be positively associated with children's behavior problems. The findings from the current study confirmed our expectations by showing that daily parenting hassles were positively related to children's internalizing and externalizing behavior problems. In other words, parents' experiences of day-to-day burdens stemming from caring for children contributed to children's behavior problems. Consistent with our findings, previous studies also indicated that the daily hassles that emerge through parenting tasks undermine children's behavior problems [22–24]. For instance, in a longitudinal study, Stone and her colleagues [46] found that parenting daily hassles when children were four years old were predictors of children's internalizing and externalizing behavior problems for the next two subsequent years. Based on the previous studies and the current results, it may be suggested that parents with high levels of daily hassles could unintentionally or intentionally lead children to display higher levels of behavior problems.

### 4.2. Parenting Approaches and Children's Behavior Problems

In another research question, we aimed to examine the association between parenting approaches and children's behavior problems. We hypothesized that positive parenting approaches would lead children to display fewer behavior problems, and negative parenting approaches would lead them to exhibit higher levels of behavior problems. Results from the current study confirmed our hypothesis by revealing a statistically significant direct effect of parenting approaches on children's behavior problems. Aligned with the present findings, previous studies also found that negative parenting approaches, such as punishment, were related to the frequency of children's externalizing and internalizing behavior problems [23,45,47]. One possible explanation for why positive parenting practices (e.g., inductive reasoning and warmth) inhibit children from showing behavior problems, while negative parenting practices (e.g., punishment and obedience-demanding) could trigger children to display more frequent behavior problems may be that children model their parents in their behavior patterns [48]. Children exposed to negative parenting approaches may model their parents' behavior and show it in different contexts, which may be the signs of externalizing behavior problems. Another possible explanation may be that using negative parenting approaches, such as demanding obedience and punishment, may hinder children from internalizing the parents' messages, resulting in violation of rules and expressing externalizing behavior problems [49,50]. On the other hand, practicing positive parenting approaches has been consistently related to positive child outcomes [47]. Compared to negative parenting approaches, positive parenting practices, such as showing warmth and inductive reasoning, may help children understand the parents' social messages and internalize their values, supporting children to practice positive behaviors and reducing their behavior problems.

Considering the cross-sectional nature of the current study, correlational results could be interpreted the other way around too, which is that children's behavior problems may induce harsh parenting styles. Consistent with previous work [26,33], children who are temperamentally difficult (e.g., lack of self-regulation and higher reactivity) could lead parents to use negative parenting practices.

### 4.3. Indirect Effect of Parenting Daily Hassles on Children's Behavior Problems through Parenting Approaches

Consistent with prior research, parents with high levels of daily hassles were likely to report higher levels of behavior problems in their children [22,24]. High parenting daily hassles may be seen as an environmental risk factor for children's behavioral outcomes [23].

Although the evidence is clear that children of parents with high parenting daily hassles are likely to report frequent behavior problems in their children [22], the mechanism behind why daily hassles undermine children's behavior problems can be explained more precisely by considering the parenting approach in the association between daily parenting hassles and children's behavior problems.

In the current research, we examined the relationship between parenting daily hassles and children's behavior problems through parenting approaches. Firstly, our findings showed the indirect effect of parenting daily hassles on children's externalizing behaviors through negative parenting approaches. In detail, parents with more parenting daily hassles exhibited more negative parenting behaviors, which in turn tended to predict more externalizing behaviors in children. Thus, the association between parenting daily hassles and children's externalizing behaviors grew to be accounted for by negative parenting approaches. This suggests that daily parenting hassles may have a worsening effect on externalizing behaviors through an association with negative parenting approaches [23].

Secondly, our findings showed the indirect effect of parenting daily hassles on children's internalizing behaviors through positive parenting approaches. Parents with higher parenting daily hassles showed less positive parenting approaches, and in turn, their children showed higher levels of internalizing behaviors. This finding is congruent with previous studies, showing parenting daily hassles reflect stress and burden that could undermine positive parenting approaches [51,52]. In the current study, we found that when parents reported higher parenting daily hassles, they were more likely to report less positive parenting approaches, such as providing fewer explanations (inductive reasoning) and showing less warmth to their children, which naturally resulted in children displaying internalizing behavior problems. We should consider the fact that negative and positive parenting approaches in the same research model showed differential outcomes on children's behavior problems. Based on the current study's findings, we can suggest that positive and negative parenting approaches have differential roles in children's behavior problems. These differential paths from parenting daily hassles to children's behavioral problems are consistent with previous work with Turkish parents and children [23].

*4.4. Practical Implications*

Even though there are studies examining the relationship between parenting stress and child adjustment through an indirect path via parenting, the current study is unique to our knowledge in examining the pattern by focusing on parenting daily hassles, which include the daily parenting stress of parents as well as other minor stressors in day-to-day living. Our findings suggest that interventions focusing on stress management may be effective in reducing daily parenting hassles, which may lead to a decrease in practicing negative parenting strategies and, in turn, lead to a reduction in children's behavior problems.

Given the indirect relationship between parenting daily hassles and children's externalizing behavior problems, we can propose that in intervention programs aiming to reduce children's externalizing behavior problems, it may be more effective to study parenting daily hassles and parents' negative parenting approaches, such as punishment and obedience-demanding practices. On the other hand, in interventions aiming to reduce children's internalizing behavior problems focusing on parenting daily hassles and positive parenting approaches may be more effective.

Furthermore, the current study provided evidence addressing the indirect effect of parenting daily hassles on children's behavior problems through parenting approaches during the COVID-19 outbreak. During the COVID-19 lockdown, some parents may have faced an increased amount of parenting daily hassles compared to before the pandemic [53]. In order to overcome the adverse effects of the COVID-19 pandemic on parents, intervention studies may focus on reducing the parenting daily hassles in their day-to-day interactions with children. In addition, studying the family interactions and both parents' support for each other in their role as parents might be explored in this model as it can reduce the perception of parenting daily hassles. Recent studies have shown that a spouse's support in child-rearing issues during the COVID-19 was related to adaptive parenting behaviors [53]. Therefore, parents' interaction during the COVID-19 might be crucial as it may be related to parenting daily hassles and, in turn to parents' parenting approaches.

## 5. Study Limitations

There were some limitations to the present study. First, the nature of this study was cross-sectional, which limits making causal inferences from the results. Second, we solely relied on one mother's reports for children's behavior problems. In addition to maternal reports, direct observations and taking multi-informant reports may be more reliable in measuring children's behavior problems [53]. Third, the present research only considered the maternal parenting approaches and parenting daily hassles in studying children's behavior problems. There are studies showing the relationship between paternal parenting styles and children's behavior problems [54]. Studying paternal parenting daily hassles in this model might be a unique contribution to the literature. Comparing the fathers' perception of parenting daily hassles to that of the mothers and examining how it may affect their parenting behavior and, in turn, the children's behavior problems, might be more explanatory in understanding the mediation mechanism. Fourth, including parents' mental health in the study could provide a comprehensive picture of the baseline of parents' and children's behavioral outcomes.

## 6. Conclusions

In the current study, we examined the contributions of parenting daily hassles and parenting approaches to child behavior problems during the COVID-19 pandemic with a particular interest in testing the indirect effect of daily hassles on children's behavior problems via parenting approaches. Daily hassles of the parents contributed to both their parenting and children's behavior problems. Positive parenting practices negatively predicted internalizing behaviors, and negative parenting practices positively predicted externalizing behaviors. Finally, the daily hassles of parents undermined their positive parenting practices, which in turn negatively predicted children's internalizing behaviors. In addition, the daily hassles of parents exacerbated negative parenting practices, which in turn increased children's externalizing behaviors.

**Supplementary Materials:** The following supporting information can be downloaded at: https://www.mdpi.com/article/10.3390/children10020312/s1, Bootstrap distributions of indirect effects; Figure S1: Parenting daily hassles to internalizing behaviors via positive parenting approach; Figure S2: Parenting daily hassles to eternizing behaviors via negative parenting approach.

**Author Contributions:** Conceptualization, I.H.A. and İ.U.; methodology, I.H.A.; software, I.H.A.; validation, I.H.A. and S.N.S.; formal analysis, I.H.A.; investigation, İ.U. and F.O.U.; resources, I.H.A., S.N.S., İ. U. and F.O.U.; data curation, İ.U., I.H.A. and F.O.U.; writing—original draft preparation, İ.U. and S.N.S.; writing—review and editing, I.H.A. and S.N.S.; visualization, I.H.A.; supervision, I.H.A.; project administration, I.H.A., İ.U. and F.O.U. All authors have read and agreed to the published version of the manuscript.

**Funding:** This research received no external funding.

**Institutional Review Board Statement:** This study was approved by the Institutional Review Board at Özyeğin University with the code number 2021/06/03 on 22 March 2021.

**Informed Consent Statement:** Informed consent was obtained from all subjects involved in this study.

**Data Availability Statement:** The datasets generated during and/or analyzed during the current study are available from the corresponding author upon reasonable request.

**Conflicts of Interest:** The authors declare no conflict of interest.

## References

1. Spinelli, M.; Lionetti, F.; Pastore, M.; Fasolo, M. Parents' Stress and Children's Psychological Problems in Families Facing the COVID-19 Outbreak in Italy. *Front. Psychol.* **2020**, *11*, 1713. [CrossRef]
2. Whittle, S.; Bray, K.O.; Lin, S.; Schwartz, O. Parenting, child and adolescent mental health during the COVID-19 pandemic. *PsyArXiv* **2020**. [CrossRef]
3. UNICEF. The State of the World's Children 2021. UNICEF. Available online: https://www.unicef.org/reports/state-worlds-children-2021 (accessed on 22 October 2021).
4. Brown, S.M.; Doom, J.; Lechuga-Peña, S.; Watamura, S.E.; Koppels, T. Stress and parenting during the global COVID-19 pandemic. *Child Abus. Negl.* **2020**, *110*, 104699. [CrossRef]
5. Sun, J.; Singletary, B.; Jiang, H.; Justice, L.M.; Lin, T.-J.; Purtell, K.M. Child behavior problems during COVID-19: Associations with parent distress and child social-emotional skills. *J. Appl. Dev. Psychol.* **2021**, *78*, 101375. [CrossRef] [PubMed]
6. Achenbach, T.M.; Rescorla, L.A. *Manual for the ASEBA Preschool Forms & Profiles: An Integrated System of Multi-İnformant Assessment*; Child behavior checklist for ages 1 1/2-5; Language development survey; Caregiver-teacher report form; The University of Vermont: Burlington, VT, USA, 2000.
7. Jiao, W.Y.; Wang, L.N.; Liu, J.; Fang, S.F.; Jiao, F.Y.; Pettoello-Mantovani, M.; Somekh, E. Behavioral and Emotional Disorders in Children during the COVID-19 Epidemic. *J. Pediatr.* **2020**, *221*, 264–266.e1. [CrossRef]
8. Barata, Ö.; Acar, I.H. Turkish children's bedtime routines during the COVID-19 pandemic: Preliminary evaluation of the bedtime routines questionnaire. *Child. Health Care* **2022**, 1–20. [CrossRef]
9. Ghosh, R.; Dubey, M.J.; Chatterjee, S.; Dubey, S. Impact of COVID -19 on children: Special focus on the psychosocial aspect. *Minerva Pediatr.* **2020**, *72*, 226–235. [CrossRef] [PubMed]
10. Liu, W.; Zhang, Q.; Chen, J.; Xiang, R.; Song, H.; Shu, S.; Chen, L.; Liang, L.; Zhou, J.; You, L.; et al. Detection of Covid-19 in Children in Early January 2020 in Wuhan, China. *N. Engl. J. Med.* **2020**, *382*, 1370–1371. [CrossRef]
11. Gadermann, A.C.; Thomson, K.C.; Richardson, C.G.; Gagné, M.; McAuliffe, C.; Hirani, S.; Jenkins, E. Examining the impacts of the COVID-19 pandemic on family mental health in Canada: Findings from a national cross-sectional study. *BMJ Open* **2021**, *11*, e042871. [CrossRef]
12. Axpe, I.; Rodríguez-Fernández, A.; Goñi, E.; Antonio-Agirre, I. Parental Socialization Styles: The Contribution of Paternal and Maternal Affect/Communication and Strictness to Family Socialization Style. *Int. J. Environ. Res. Public Health* **2019**, *16*, 2204. [CrossRef]
13. Maccoby, E.E. The role of parents in the socialization of children: An historical overview. *Dev. Psychol.* **1992**, *28*, 1006–1017. [CrossRef]
14. Paterson, G.; Sanson, A. The Association of Behavioural Adjustment to Temperament, Parenting and Family Characteristics among 5-Year-Old Children. *Soc. Dev.* **2001**, *8*, 293–309. [CrossRef]
15. Chen, X.; Chen, H.; Wang, L.; Liu, M. Noncompliance and child-rearing attitudes as predictors of aggressive behaviour: A longitudinal study in Chinese children. *Int. J. Behav. Dev.* **2002**, *26*, 225–233. [CrossRef]
16. Rubin, K.H.; Burgess, K.B. Parents of aggressive and withdrawn children. In *Handbook of Parenting: Children and Parenting*; Bornstein, M.H., Ed.; Lawrence Erlbaum Associates Publishers: Hillsdale, NJ, USA, 2002; pp. 383–418.
17. Loth, K.; Ji, Z.; Wolfson, J.; Berge, J.; Neumark-Sztainer, D.; Fisher, J. COVID-19 pandemic shifts in food-related parenting practices within an ethnically/racially and socioeconomically diverse sample of families of preschool-aged children. *Appetite* **2021**, *168*, 105714. [CrossRef]
18. Prime, H.; Wade, M.; Browne, D.T. Risk and resilience in family well-being during the COVID-19 pandemic. *Am. Psychol.* **2020**, *75*, 631–643. [CrossRef] [PubMed]
19. Crnic, K.A.; Greenberg, M.T. Minor Parenting Stresses with Young Children. *Child Dev.* **1990**, *61*, 1628. [CrossRef]
20. Crnic, K.A.; Low, C. *Everyday stresses and parenting.*, In *Handbook of Parenting: Vol. 5. Practical İssues in Parenting*, 2nd ed.; Bornstein, M.H., Ed.; Lawrence Erlbaum Associates: Hillsdale, NJ, USA, 2002; pp. 243–267.
21. Taylor, J. Structural validity of theParenting Daily Hassles Intensity Scale. *Stress Health J. Int. Soc. Investig. Stress* **2019**, *35*, 176–186. [CrossRef]
22. Coplan, R.J.; Bowker, A.; Cooper, S.M. Parenting daily hassles, child temperament, and social adjustment in preschool. *Early Child. Res. Q.* **2003**, *18*, 376–395. [CrossRef]
23. Gülseven, Z.; Carlo, G.; Streit, C.; Kumru, A.; Selçuk, B.; Sayıl, M. Longitudinal relations among parenting daily hassles, child rearing, and prosocial and aggressive behaviors in Turkish children. *Soc. Dev.* **2017**, *27*, 45–57. [CrossRef]
24. Tanner, S.M. The Relation Between Parenting Daily Hassles And Child Behavior Problems Among Low-Income Families: Examining The Role Of Caregiver Positive Expressiveness. Master's Thesis, Wayne State University, Detroit, MI, USA, 2017.
25. Alonzi, S.; Park, J.; Pagán, A.; Saulsman, C.; Silverstein, M. An Examination of COVID-19-Related Stressors among Parents. *Eur. J. Investig. Health Psychol. Educ.* **2021**, *11*, 838–848. [CrossRef]
26. Acar, I.H.; Veziroğlu-Çelik, M.; Çelebi, Ş.; Ingeç, D.; Kuzgun, S. Parenting styles and Turkish children's emotion regulation: The mediating role of parent-teacher relationships. *Curr. Psychol.* **2019**, *40*, 4427–4437. [CrossRef]
27. Bakermans-Kranenburg, M.J.; van Ijzendoorn, M.H.; Juffer, F. Less is more: Meta-analyses of sensitivity and attachment interventions in early childhood. *Psychol. Bull.* **2003**, *129*, 195–215. [CrossRef] [PubMed]

28. Hastings, P.; McShane, K.; Parker, R.; Ladha, F. Ready to Make Nice: Parental Socialization of Young Sons' and Daughters' Prosocial Behaviors With Peers. *J. Genet. Psychol.* **2007**, *168*, 177–200. [CrossRef]
29. Laible, D.; Carlo, G.; Torquati, J.; Ontai, L. Children's Perceptions of Family Relationships as Assessed in a Doll Story Completion Task: Links to Parenting, Social Competence, and Externalizing Behavior. *Soc. Dev.* **2004**, *13*, 551–569. [CrossRef]
30. Muraven, M.; Baumeister, R.F. Self-regulation and depletion of limited resources: Does self-control resemble a muscle? *Psychol. Bull.* **2000**, *126*, 247–259. [CrossRef] [PubMed]
31. Platt, R.; Williams, S.R.; Ginsburg, G.S. Stressful Life Events and Child Anxiety: Examining Parent and Child Mediators. *Child Psychiatry Hum. Dev.* **2015**, *47*, 23–34. [CrossRef]
32. Crnic, K.A.; Gaze, C.; Hoffman, C. Cumulative parenting stress across the preschool period: Relations to maternal parenting and child behaviour at age 5. *Infant Child Dev.* **2005**, *14*, 117–132. [CrossRef]
33. Acar, I.H.; Ahmetoğlu, E.; Özer, I.B.; Yağlı, Ş.N. Direct and indirect contributions of child difficult temperament and power assertive parental discipline to Turkish children's behaviour problems. *Early Child Dev. Care* **2019**, *191*, 2232–2245. [CrossRef]
34. Erol, N.; Simsek, Z.; Oner, O.; Munir, K. Behavioral and Emotional Problems Among Turkish Children at Ages 2 to 3 Years. *J. Am. Acad. Child Adolesc. Psychiatry* **2005**, *44*, 80–87. [CrossRef]
35. Yagmurlu, B.; Sanson, A. Parenting and temperament as predictors of prosocial behaviour in Australian and Turkish Australian children. *Aust. J. Psychol.* **2009**, *61*, 77–88. [CrossRef]
36. Ahorsu, D.K.; Lin, C.-Y.; Imani, V.; Saffari, M.; Griffiths, M.D.; Pakpour, A.H. The Fear of COVID-19 Scale: Development and Initial Validation. *Int. J. Ment. Health Addict.* **2020**, *20*, 1537–1545. [CrossRef]
37. Bakioğlu, F.; Korkmaz, O.; Ercan, H. Fear of COVID-19 and Positivity: Mediating Role of Intolerance of Uncertainty, Depression, Anxiety, and Stress. *Int. J. Ment. Health Addict.* **2020**, *19*, 2369–2382. [CrossRef] [PubMed]
38. Satici, B.; Gocet-Tekin, E.; Deniz, M.E.; Satici, S.A. Adaptation of the Fear of COVID-19 Scale: Its Association with Psychological Distress and Life Satisfaction in Turkey. *Int. J. Ment. Health Addict.* **2020**, *19*, 1980–1988. [CrossRef] [PubMed]
39. Kline, R.B. *Principles and Practice of Structural Equation Modeling*, 3rd ed.; Guilford Publications: New York, NY, USA, 2010.
40. Muthén, L.K.; Muthén, B. *Mplus User's Guide*; Muthén & Muthén: Los Angeles, CA, USA, 2017.
41. Mackinnon, D.; Fairchild, A.; Fritz, M. Mediation Analysis. *Annu. Rev. Psychol.* **2007**, *58*, 593–614. [CrossRef] [PubMed]
42. Jin, Y. A note on the cutoff values of alternative fit indices to evaluate measurement invariance for ESEM models. *Int. J. Behav. Dev.* **2019**, *44*, 166–174. [CrossRef]
43. Podsakoff, P.M.; MacKenzie, S.B.; Lee, J.-Y.; Podsakoff, N.P. Common method biases in behavioral research: A critical review of the literature and recommended remedies. *J. Appl. Psychol.* **2003**, *88*, 879–903. [CrossRef]
44. Chang, S.-J.; Van Witteloostuijn, A.; Eden, L. From the Editors: Common method variance in international business research. *J. Int. Bus. Stud.* **2010**, *41*, 178–184. [CrossRef]
45. Agler, R.; De Boeck, P. On the Interpretation and Use of Mediation: Multiple Perspectives on Mediation Analysis. *Front. Psychol.* **2017**, *8*, 1984. [CrossRef]
46. Stone, L.L.; Mares, S.H.W.; Otten, R.; Engels, R.C.M.E.; Janssens, J.M.A.M. The Co-Development of Parenting Stress and Childhood Internalizing and Externalizing Problems. *J. Psychopathol. Behav. Assess.* **2015**, *38*, 76–86. [CrossRef]
47. Braza, P.; Carreras, R.; Muñoz, J.M.; Braza, F.; Azurmendi, A.; Pascual-Sagastizábal, E.; Cardas, J.; Sánchez-Martín, J.R. Negative Maternal and Paternal Parenting Styles as Predictors of Children's Behavioral Problems: Moderating Effects of the Child's Sex. *J. Child Fam. Stud.* **2013**, *24*, 847–856. [CrossRef]
48. Serbin, L.A.; Kingdon, D.; Ruttle, P.L.; Stack, D.M. The impact of children's internalizing and externalizing problems on parenting: Transactional processes and reciprocal change over time. *Dev. Psychopathol.* **2015**, *27*, 969–986. [CrossRef] [PubMed]
49. Davies, P.T.; Woitach, M.J. Children's Emotional Security in the Interparental Relationship. *Curr. Dir. Psychol. Sci.* **2008**, *17*, 269–274. [CrossRef]
50. Gershoff, E.T. Spanking and Child Development: We Know Enough Now to Stop Hitting Our Children. *Child Dev. Perspect.* **2013**, *7*, 133–137. [CrossRef] [PubMed]
51. Chen, X.; Liu, M.; Li, D. Parental warmth, control, and indulgence and their relations to adjustment in Chinese children: A longitudinal study. *J. Fam. Psychol.* **2000**, *14*, 401–419. [CrossRef]
52. Flannery, A.J.; Awada, S.R.; Shelleby, E.C. Influences of Maternal Parenting Stress on Child Behavior Problems: Examining Harsh and Positive Parenting as Mediators. *J. Fam. Issues* **2021**. advance online publication. [CrossRef]
53. Fontanesi, L.; Marchetti, D.; Mazza, C.; Di Giandomenico, S.; Roma, P.; Verrocchio, M.C. The effect of the COVID-19 lockdown on parents: A call to adopt urgent measures. *Psychol. Trauma Theory, Res. Pract. Policy* **2020**, *12*, S79–S81. [CrossRef]
54. Uzun, H.; Karaca, N.H.; Metin, Ş. Assesment of parent-child relationship in Covid-19 pandemic. *Child. Youth Serv. Rev.* **2020**, *120*, 105748. [CrossRef]

**Disclaimer/Publisher's Note:** The statements, opinions and data contained in all publications are solely those of the individual author(s) and contributor(s) and not of MDPI and/or the editor(s). MDPI and/or the editor(s) disclaim responsibility for any injury to people or property resulting from any ideas, methods, instructions or products referred to in the content.

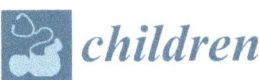 

Article

# Maternal and Paternal Authoritarian Parenting and Adolescents' Impostor Feelings: The Mediating Role of Parental Psychological Control and the Moderating Role of Child's Gender

Yosi Yaffe

Tel-Hai Academic College, Department of Education, Upper Galilee, Qiryat Shemona 12208, Israel; yaffeyos@telhai.ac.il

**Abstract:** Introduction: Recent systematic reviews about the impostor phenomenon unveil a severe shortage of research data on adolescents. The present study aimed at reducing this gap in the literature by investigating the association between maternal and paternal authoritarian parenting and impostor feelings among adolescents, while testing the mediating role played by parental psychological control and the moderating role of the child's gender in this context. Methods: Three hundred and eight adolescents took part in an online survey, in which they reported anonymously on their impostor feelings and their parents' parenting styles via several valid psychological questionnaires. The sample consisted of 143 boys and 165 girls, whose age ranged from 12 to 17 ($M = 14.67$, $SD = 1.64$). Results: Of the sample's participants, over 35% reported frequent to intense impostor feelings, with girls scoring significantly higher than boys on this scale. In general, the maternal and paternal parenting variables explained 15.2% and 13.3% (respectively) of the variance in the adolescents' impostor scores. Parental psychological control fully mediated (for fathers) and partially mediated (for mothers) the association between parental authoritarian parenting and the adolescents' impostor feelings. The child's gender moderated solely the maternal direct effect of authoritarian parenting on impostor feelings (this association was significant for boys alone), but not the mediating effect via psychological control. Conclusions: The current study introduces a specific explanation for the possible mechanism describing the early emergence of impostor feelings in adolescents based on parenting styles and behaviors.

**Keywords:** impostor phenomenon; parenting styles; psychological control; adolescent

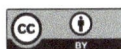

## 1. Introduction

### 1.1. Impostor Phenomenon

The concept of impostor phenomenon refers to talented and successful individuals according to external and objective standards, who are prone to doubt their own competence as if they were a fraud who has fooled everybody else's impression about them [1]. Rather than their personal qualities (such as intelligent and skills), people who experience impostor feelings attribute their accomplishments to external factors, such as luck, and to other factors unrelated to actual talent and ability, such as manipulation and charm [2]. The most common impostor symptoms include reluctance to accept credit for accomplishments and to internalize the sense of being talented and competent, feelings of self-doubt, a propensity to attribute success to external causes, and a chronic fear that success will not be possible to maintain [2,3]. Indeed, the impostor phenomenon construct was originally divided into three theoretical dimensions, including self-doubts about one's own intelligence and abilities (fake), the tendency to attribute success to chance/luck (luck), and the inability to admit a good performance (discount) [4,5]. When first clinically identified and conceptualized [1], the impostor phenomenon was thought to be a gender-specific disturbance, whose origins are rooted in feminine social role stereotypes and early experiences of gender-based family dynamics. Later data, however, failed to support the phenomenon's gender-specific premise, indicating that the impostor phenomenon is a more general problem that may similarly occur in men [2]. Indeed, the impostor phenomenon is no longer considered a gender-typical psychological issue [6]. A recent systematic review on the prevalence and predictors of the impostor phenomenon [7,8], counted 16 articles (a little less than 50% out of 33 articles that considered gender differences) that found greater symptoms of imposter feelings among women, while the majority of works (17 articles) found no gender differences. Whilst these meta-analytic data clearly indicate that the phenomenon affects both genders [7], it may imply that, subject to certain conditions, women could be somewhat more predisposed to experience impostor feelings than men. This information mostly relies on research data about adult participants, while there is a serious shortage in research studies with adolescents [9,10]. This is despite the fact that the "Impostor phenomenon feelings are already well established by adolescence and that there may be earlier ethology of impostor phenomenon" [11] (p. 402).

To date, there is growing evidence suggesting that moderate to intense impostor feelings are very prevalent phenomena in individuals of both genders [8,12–16], with their ratio among personnel and students varying from 9% to 82%, and on average exceeding 40%. According to Bravata and colleagues [8], the prevalence of the impostor phenomenon varies widely depending on several factors, especially the study participants (or population-based evaluation), the screening tool employed, and cut-off points used to assess symptoms. At any rate, in a view of the growing empirical information about the impostor phenomenon in recent years, it is clear now that we are facing a concerning phenomenon with potentially detrimental psychological consequences to various populations. In this regard, more and more concerned scholars are calling for the inclusion of impostor syndrome as a specific diagnostic category in the next edition of the Diagnostic and Statistical Manual (DSM) of the American Psychiatric Association [7,8].

According to the research literature, the prominent personality correlations and psychological conditions with which the impostor phenomenon often occurs as comorbid are low self-esteem, anxiety, and depression [7]. Langford and Clance (1993) [2] explained that "impostor feelings are frequently accompanied by worry, depression, and anxiety resulting from pressure to live up to one's successful image and the fear that one will be exposed as unworthy and incompetent" (p. 495). In terms of the big five personality traits, the impostor phenomenon was found to be associated with high neuroticism and low conscientiousness, as well as with high introversion [2,5,17]. Indeed, these psychological conditions and other emotional distresses later described in the literature (such as somatic problems, emotional exhaustion, burnout, and more) may be the toll that a heightened fear over performance and intense effort spent at masking inadequacy take from those who cope with impostor feelings [18,19]. Yet, it is unclear whether the impostor phenomenon is caused by these factors, affects them, or whether they are simply co-occurring [16].

*1.2. Parenting Styles*

Parenting style is a broad construct describing stable attitudes and behaviors regarding child-rearing [20]. In her early work, Baumrind [21,22] proposed three types of parental control in child-rearing (i.e., authoritative, permissive, and authoritarian), which later became known as patterns or styles of parental authority [23]. These types of parental control generally vary by the way the parents set and enforce rules, exert power, grant autonomy, encourage verbal negotiation over decisions, use reasoning, and regulate the child's behavior. Baumrind's typology [23,24] also distinguishes between the three patterns or styles of parenting according to the degree and quality to which they project emotional warmth and acceptance toward the child. Later salient conceptualization of parenting styles introduced two orthogonal, independent, parental dimensions known as responsiveness and demandingness [25], from which four parenting styles were composed. These dimensions generally depict parental aspects such as warmth, affection, sensitivity, autonomy granting, reasoned communication, behavior regulation, control, confrontation, protection, and monitoring [26,27]. Responsiveness refers to the extent to which the parent shows the child love, acceptance, and affection, and giving his/her support when dealing with the child's good and bad behaviors [26,28]. Demandingness, however, is aimed at socializing the child as part of imparting behavioral norms and maintaining the parent's authority, which is reflected in the parent's usage of discipline, control, and regulation of the child's behavior [28,29]. The compositions of the responsiveness (also known as warmth) and demandingness (also known as strictness) dimensions yields four distinctive types of parenting attitudes and behaviors in child rearing (partially corresponding with Baumrind's typology), which can reflect the family climate and the quality of parent–child relations [25,29,30]. Authoritative (i.e., warm and strict) and authoritarian (i.e., strict but not warm) parents vary on responsiveness variables such as warmth and support, whereas authoritative and indulgent (i.e., warm but not strict, similar to the labeled permissive style in the present study) parents vary on demandingness variables such as control and monitoring [24,25]. Neglectful parents are neither warm nor strict.

Research on parental socialization indicates that authoritative parenting constitutes the optimal style in affinity to psychological well-being and educational functioning of children and adolescents [27,31], especially in middleclass families from Anglo-Saxon European and north American countries. Recent research evidence from other nationalities and ethnic samples suggests, however, that the parental effect on the child's well-being may vary by cultural contexts [30]. Indeed, the most recent evidence conducted in European and Latin American countries support the idea that the indulgent style is associated with the best child psychosocial adjustment [32,33]. Contrary to authoritative parenting, authoritarian parenting is consistently associated in the research literature with adverse psychological outcomes in children and adolescents, including externalizing and internalizing problems, and academic and psychoeducational impairments in students [31,34–36]. Unlike the authoritative parent, the authoritarian parent uses coercive power and assertive disciplinary practices, which include verbal hostility, arbitrary discipline, and psychological control [37]. The latter pattern was explicitly mentioned by Baumrind as parental behaviors of coercive practices, whose consequences on the child were found to be uniquely detrimental and especially predictive of internalizing problems and poor self-efficacy [38]. Parental psychological control is a form of parental control typically manifested by excessive practices of manipulation, coercion, and disrespect that intrude on the child's psychological development [38,39]. This maladaptive pattern has been specifically associated in past research with various detrimental emotional outcomes of child development, especially anxiety and depression [40,41], and may be the concrete mechanism explaining the aversive effects of authoritarian parenting on the child's psychological well-being reported in the literature. Indeed, some researchers have proposed that parental psychological control mediates the relationship between over-controlling parenting (such as the authoritarian style) and emotional functioning in children and adolescents [42]. Finally, a considerable body of research suggests that mothers and fathers may differ in their dominant parenting styles and practices, with the former being more supportive, responsive, and behaviorally controlling in their child-rearing orientation (i.e., authoritative parenting) and the latter being more coercive, punitive, and psychologically controlling in their child-rearing orientation (i.e., authoritarian parenting) [43]. Gender differences in parenting were also accounted for in relation to children's and adolescents' psychological outcomes, with somewhat more evidence suggesting possible precedence for maternal parenting over paternal parenting in both predicting externalizing and internalizing problems [44–49]. While this trend was not sufficiently consistent across studies to establish a definitive conclusion regarding the differential parental-gender effect on the child's outcomes [35,36,50], it does warrant discrete measurements for mothers and fathers. Particularly in the context of the gender-dyadic in parent–child relations (i.e., in consideration of both parent's and child's gender), the findings in regard to children's and adolescents' psychological outcomes are considerably inconsistent across studies and require further examination in various respects [44].

### 1.3. Parenting and the Impostor Phenomenon

One of the phenomenon's most studied etiology factors is early family relations and dynamics. The family background of people with impostor feelings has been described as unsupportive, non-expressive, conflictual, and overcontrolling [2,51]. In a recent systematic review work focusing on this very topic [10], four forms of familial and parental factors were identified as associated with the impostor phenomenon. This included parental rearing styles and behaviors, attachment styles, maladaptive parenting and parent–child relations, and familial achievement orientation. The noticeable and more promising group of studies, however, dealt with the role of parental rearing styles and behaviors in the context of the impostor phenomenon, especially parental (low) care and over-protectiveness [14,19,52]. The effects observed for these parental variables on the offspring's impostor feelings in these studies were of relatively small to moderate size (especially when simultaneously accounting for other socio-emotional variables) and the extent of research evidence was limited. Therefore, while this review work concluded that parent–child relations and parental child-rearing behaviors could play a substantial role in the emergence of the impostor feelings in the offspring, its conclusion was subject to a few considerable limitations and to the acute need for more research evidence. First, it is essential to broaden the limited framework of the familial and parental variables used in previous research to predict impostor feelings, in an attempt to identify patterns that may be more specific to the phenomenon's context. Based on previous research, it can be assumed that authoritarian parenting could be generally predictive of the child's impostor feelings, due to its configuration of low care/acceptance and high control. As a specific authoritarian pattern, however, parental psychological control may serve as the mechanism specifically explaining the emergence of impostor feelings (i.e., as a mediator), because of its notorious detrimental nature in affinity to the child's emotional well-being (as discussed earlier). Indeed, a recent study was the first to demonstrate specifically the unique association between maternal psychological control and students' impostor feelings [53], both directly and indirectly through low-self-efficacy. Surprisingly, this compelling prediction hypothesis of the impostor phenomenon based on the constellations of these particular parental constructs (i.e., authoritarian parenting and psychological control as mediators) has not yet been tested empirically. Moreover, in light of the acute shortage in studies conducted with adolescents (as the vast majority of studies in this body of research employed adults' retrospective reports on their family and parents' patterns), it is also necessary to examine some of the research questions regarding the relationship between parenting factors and the impostor phenomenon with young populations in the present time. Indeed, some highly cited research works have been interested in the long-term effects of past family and parental patterns on the impostor feelings at the present time of adult students or professional workers. In this regard, Sonnak and Towell (2001) [14] demonstrated that perceived past parental over-protectiveness and low care during childhood and adolescence in their original families, along with some aspects of mental health, significantly explained undergraduate adult students' present impostor feelings. Subject to excluding the participants' self-esteem as a co-predictor, the findings suggested that parental rearing styles, especially parental (low) care, may play an essential role in the emergence of offspring's impostor feelings, which persists into adulthood. This implies the existence of long-term consequences of parenting on offspring's impostor feelings. However, recollections of such patterns are at great risk of inaccuracy and must not be interpreted in longitudinal terms but rather in contemporaneous terms (that is, to treat these retrospective reports as current perceived parenting) [19,54]. Using adolescent participants to test some relative empirical issues could partially overcome this methodological obstacle. Not only could testing etiological-based questions regarding the impostor phenomenon with young populations help illuminate the possible effects of some familial and psycho-social factors during adolescence [11,55], but it could also lay the foundation for testing the longitudinal long-term effects. To date, there have been very few studies in this body of research addressing these crucial needs.

*1.4. The Current Study*

In light of the shortcomings in the etiological research literature about the impostor phenomenon, the current study aimed to test the association between overall maternal and paternal parenting styles (i.e., authoritative, authoritarian, and permissive) and psychological control and impostor feelings among adolescent boys and girls. Surprisingly, these specific parental constructs have not been used in previous research in the empirical context of the impostor phenomenon, despite their terminological centrality and great importance in the body of knowledge of child socialization and parent–child relations in the family. Specifically, the study sought to examine the unique role played by the authoritarian parenting style and psychological control (i.e., when permissive and authoritative parenting are taken into account) in predicting impostor feelings among adolescents. (1) We hypothesized that authoritarian parenting would significantly predict impostor feelings among adolescents, in a form of positive associations between these variables. (2) In addition, since psychological control constitutes a distinct authoritarian parenting pattern that may by particularly detrimental to the child's emotional well-being, we hypothesized that it would partially mediate the positive association between authoritarian parenting and impostor feelings. Moreover, given the possible differentiation in maternal and paternal parenting styles and practices, as well as in their unique effects on the child's well-being, the study's hypotheses were tested separately for fathers and mothers while accounting for the child's gender. Specifically, the direct and indirect associations (as mediated by parental psychological control) between maternal and paternal authoritarian parenting and adolescents' impostor feelings were tested for moderation of the child's gender (in accordance with the model described in Figure 1). The gender of adolescents may have an impact on how they perceive parental authoritarian parenting and psychological control specifically [56]. (3) Therefore, it was expected that the direct and indirect (via parental psychological control) associations between authoritarian parenting and impostor feelings would at least partially vary across adolescent boys and girls (i.e., a moderation and moderated mediation effects by the child's gender). Yet, the literature on parenting styles provides inconsistent and inconclusive evidence regarding the impact of parenting in parent–adolescent gender dyads [44]. Hence, gender-specific hypotheses (i.e., specifying parent–child gender dyads) on the associations between parenting and impostor feelings cannot be established.

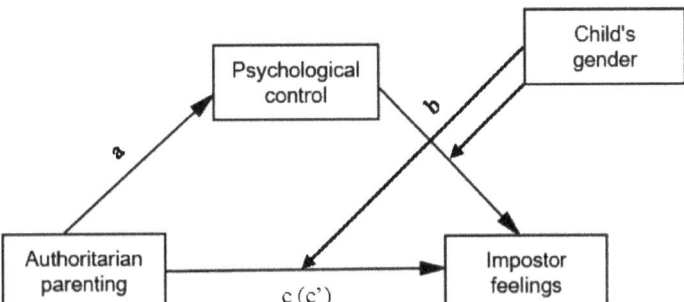

**Figure 1.** Hypothesized moderation and moderated mediation model for adolescents' impostor feelings. Direct effect of authoritarian parenting on psychological control (a); direct effect of parental psychological control on adolescents' impostor feelings (b); total effect of authoritarian parenting on adolescents' impostor feelings (c); direct effect of authoritarian parenting on adolescents' impostor feelings, controlling for parental psychological control (c′).

## 2. Methods

*2.1. Participants and Procedure*

Three hundred and eight adolescents took part in an online survey where they reported anonymously on themselves and their parents via several valid psychological questionnaires. The sample consisted of 143 boys and 165 girls whose age ranged from 12 to 17 ($M = 14.67$, $SD = 1.64$). Age was distributed equally across the gender groups ($F = 0.12$, $p = 1.64$), while boys and girls did not differ by age (Mean differences = 0.31; $t(306) = 1.642$, $p = 0.10$). Based on a convenience sampling method, the participants (minor adolescents) were recruited by a professional Israeli survey provider through their parents, who read the research information, perused the questionnaires, and gave their signed consent for their children to take part in an online survey. The participants who received the online link to the survey, subject to their parents' permission, were introduced to the research details and were presented with an informed consent form, which they were asked to sign prior to filling out the questionnaires. The research procedure and data collection according to this framework were approved beforehand by the author's institutional review board (IRB) of Tel-Hai academic college (ref. 10-10/2022).

## 2.2. Instruments

Parental Authority Questionnaire (PAQ). The PAQ [57] contains 30 items and is used to classify parents into one of Baumrind's three parenting styles (Baumrind, 1971), based on the child's report on a 5-point Likert scale (ranging from 1—strongly disagree to 5—strongly agree): Authoritative (10 items, e.g., "As I was growing up, once family policy had been established, my parents discussed the reasoning behind the policy with the children in the family"), Authoritarian (10 items, e.g., "As I was growing up my parents did not allow me to question any decision they had made"), and Permissive (10 items, e.g., "As I was growing up my parents seldom gave me expectations and guidelines for my behavior"). The index for each of the three parenting styles is the sum of the items of each scale. Thus, the total score for each scale ranges from 10 to 50, with a higher score indicating a higher specification of the parenting style. The questionnaire is widely used internationally for various research purposes. It is a valid questionnaire to assess Baumrind's (1971) [23] three styles of parenting using adolescents' reports, with adequate evidence of internal consistency and test–retest reliabilities (0.74 to 0.78) [57,58]. In the current study, we recorded Cronbach's Alpha coefficients for the permissive, authoritarian, and authoritative scales of 0.77, 0.83, and 0.80 (respectively for father), and 0.77, 0.84, and 0.75 (respectively for mother), consistent with the reliability data reported for the instrument in past research. The scales' scores appear in Table 1, separately for mothers and fathers.

**Table 1.** Descriptive statistics and zero-order correlations between the study variables ($N = 308$).

|  | 1 | 2 | 3 | 4 | 5 | Mean (Mother) | SD (Mother) |
|---|---|---|---|---|---|---|---|
| 1. Impostor feelings | - | 0.28 *** | 0.03 | 0.21 *** | 0.24 *** | 54.47 | 15.97 |
| 2. Permissive parenting | 0.29 *** | - | 0.15 ** | 0.02 | 0.07 | 25.76 | 5.96 |
| 3. Authoritative parenting | 0.01 | 0.20 *** | - | −0.18 *** | −0.31 *** | 38.18 | 4.18 |
| 4. Authoritarian parenting | 0.16 ** | 0.10 | −0.07 | - | 0.36 *** | 29.30 | 7.05 |
| 5. Psychological control | 0.26 *** | 0.19 *** | −0.32 *** | 0.38 *** | - | 1.80 | 0.67 |
| Mean (father) | 54.47 | 25.84 | 36.98 | 29.98 | 1.88 | - | - |
| SD (father) | 15.97 | 6.23 | 5.80 | 7.24 | 0.70 | - | - |

Note: Figures above diagonal represent mothers' data and figures below diagonal represent fathers' data. ** $p \leq 0.005$, *** $p \leq 0.001$.

Impostor Phenomenon Scale (CIPS; Clance, 1985) [5]. The scale contains 20 items designed for self-report, in which the response for an item is given on a 5-point Likert scale. The scale gauges impostor feelings and cognitions, such as fear of evaluation (e.g., "I avoid evaluations if possible and have a dread of others evaluating me"), self-doubt regarding one's abilities (e.g., "I rarely do a project or task as well as I'd like to do it"), and expressions of phoniness with fears of being exposed by others as a fraudster (e.g., "I'm afraid people important to me may find out that I'm not as capable as they think I am"). The impostor phenomenon construct was originally divided into three theoretical dimensions [5], including self-doubts about one's own intelligence and abilities (Fake), a tendency to attribute success to chance/luck (Luck), and the inability to admit a good performance (Discount). However, due to the limited support for the three-factor model and the lack of a clearly identifiable factorial structure [59], currently the scoring methodology is commonly used as a unidimensional construct. The Hebrew version of the CIPS (HCIPS) has been validated against external variables, while demonstrating its psychometric properties [60]. Consistent with this evidence, the Cronbach's Alpha recorded in the current study for the overall scale was 0.92. The scale's scores appear in Table 1.

Psychological Control Scale–Disrespect (PCDS; Barber et al., 2012) [38]. The parental psychological control of the participants' mothers and fathers was measured using Barber's new Psychological Control Scale–Disrespect. Participants were instructed to think about the relationship with their parents during their childhood and adolescence in the family and to determine the extent to which each of the scale's eight statements (e.g., "my parents try to make me feel guilty for something I've done or something they thought I should do") describe them well (separately for mother and father). The scale was validated against several measures of parenting and child's outcome, including the child's antisocial behavior and depression [38]. In the current study, the response for an item was given on a 5-point Likert-type scale ranging from 1—Not like her/him at all to 5—Very much like her/him, with a higher response representing a higher expression of maternal/paternal psychological control. Considering the scale's relatively small items number, in the current study we obtained good indexes of internal consistency reliability both for the mother ($\alpha = 0.82$) and father ($\alpha = 0.81$). The scale's scores appear in Table 1. The translation and adaptation process of the English PCDS into Hebrew was carried out by the author and a professional bi-lingual English translator, using the three steps back–forward translation procedure.

## 3. Data Analysis

Missing data were handled by employing the listwise deletion method. IBM SPSS statistical package version 28 was used to perform the descriptive and correlational statistics for the sample's data. For the mediation, moderation, and moderated mediation regression analyses, SPSS macro PROCESS [61] was utilized while applying the bootstrapping method based on the recommendations provided by Preacher and Hayes (2008) [62].

## 4. Results

### 4.1. Preliminary Correlational Analysis and Descriptive Statistics

Table 1 displays the means, standard deviations, and the correlations between the study's main variables. As expected, adolescents' impostor feelings were significantly and positively correlated with maternal and paternal authoritarian parenting and with the pattern of psychological control. Impostor feelings were also positively associated with maternal and paternal permissive parenting, but not with authoritative parenting. Parenting styles were intercorrelated significantly, with the authoritative and authoritarian styles inversely associated for mothers and the authoritative and permissive styles positively associated for both parents. Finally, the maternal and paternal parenting styles were correspondingly associated with psychological control, with the latter pattern inversely related to the authoritative style and positively related to the authoritarian style.

### 4.2. Impostor Feelings: Sample Scores and Gender Differences

The sample's mean score of impostor feelings was below 60, which represents a moderate impostor feelings level [5,63]. Girls reported significantly higher impostor feelings than boys did ($t(306) = 2.76$, $p < 0.001$), with the former scoring on average $56.79 \pm 14.83$ and the latter scoring on average $51.80 \pm 16.85$. Further, about 18.8% of the sample's adolescents scored below 40 (few impostor characteristics), 45.6% scored between 40 and 60 (moderate impostor characteristics), 29.6% scored between 61 and 80 (frequent impostor characteristics), and the rest (about 6%) scored higher than 80 (intense impostor characteristics).

### 4.3. Predicting Impostor Feelings from Parenting Styles and Psychological Control (H1,2)

First, we tested the predictability of the maternal and paternal variables of the impostor feelings in adolescents using a hierarchical multiple regression analysis. At first, the three parenting styles were entered into the regression model as one block, and then the psychological control variable was entered in a subsequent step. This allowed us to weigh the unique contribution added by the latter variable in predicting the adolescents' impostor feelings from the parental styles and to establish and test its mediating effect in this context. Table 2 presents the results of the regression analysis predicting impostor feelings from the parenting styles (Equation (1)) and psychological control (Equation (2)) for mothers and fathers separately. Consistent with hypothesis 1, the maternal and paternal parenting styles explained a significant proportion of the impostor feelings variance (12.1% and 10.4% respectively), with the authoritarian and permissive parenting styles uniquely and positively correlated with the latter variable. Maternal psychological control predicted an extra significant proportion of 3% of the variance in the child's impostor feelings ($F(1, 303) = 11.06$, $p < 0.001$), above and beyond the variance explained by the maternal parenting styles. Paternal psychological control predicted an extra significant proportion of 2.9% of the variance in the child's impostor feelings ($F(1, 303) = 10.04$, $p = 0.002$), above and beyond the variance explained by the paternal parenting styles. Taken together, the maternal and paternal parenting variables explained 15.2% and 13.3% (respectively) of the variance in the adolescents' impostor scores.

**Table 2.** Regression analysis predicting the child's impostor feelings from the parental variables.

|  | Maternal | | | | Paternal | | | |
|---|---|---|---|---|---|---|---|---|
|  | B | SE | t | p | B | SE | t | p |
| *Direct effect—Equation (1)* | | | | | | | | |
| Permissive style | 0.73 | 0.15 | 5.01 | <0.001 | 0.73 | 0.14 | 5.12 | <0.001 |
| Authoritative style | 0.09 | 0.18 | 0.48 | 0.63 | −0.11 | 0.15 | −0.73 | 0.47 |
| Authoritarian style | 0.48 | 0.12 | 3.84 | <0.001 | 0.30 | 0.12 | 2.45 | 0.015 |
| $R^2$ | 0.121 | | | | 0.104 | | | |
| F | $F(3, 304) = 13.97$ | | | $p < 0.001$ | $F(3, 304) = 11.81$ | | | $p < 0.001$ |
| *Direct effect—Equation (2)* | | | | | | | | |
| Permissive style | 0.68 | 0.15 | 4.67 | <0.001 | 0.62 | 0.15 | 4.28 | <0.001 |
| Authoritative style | −0.25 | 0.18 | −1.39 | 0.16 | 0.08 | 0.16 | 0.48 | 0.63 |
| Authoritarian style | 0.34 | 0.13 | 2.62 | 0.009 | 0.150 | 0.14 | 1.18 | 0.24 |
| Psychological control | 4.69 | 1.41 | 3.33 | <0.001 | 4.56 | 1.44 | 3.17 | 0.002 |
| $R^2$ | 0.152 | | | | 0.133 | | | |
| F | $F(4, 303) = 13.59$ | | | $p < 0.001$ | $F(4, 303) = 11.63$ | | | $p < 0.001$ |

Following the regression analysis, we tested the indirect effect of authoritarian parenting on the impostor feelings via psychological control as a mediator, using a bootstrapping method of a 95% confidence interval. Accordingly, maternal psychological control partially mediated the positive association between maternal authoritarian parenting and adolescents' impostor feelings, as, after controlling for psychological control, the regression coefficient of authoritarian parenting decreased but was still significant (Equations (1) and (2), Table 2). The positive CI estimate values confirmed the significance of the indirect effect via psychological control as a mediator ($b = 0.14$; CI = 0.04, 0.27). The positive association between paternal authoritarian parenting and adolescents' impostor feelings was fully mediated by paternal psychological control, as, after controlling for the latter variable, the regression coefficient of the authoritarian parenting decreased and became insignificant (Equations (1) and (2), Table 2). The positive CI estimate values confirmed that the indirect effect via psychological control as a mediator was significant ($b = 0.15$; CI = 0.05, 0.25). Partially consistent with hypothesis 2, the findings indicated that adolescents whose parents are more authoritarian experience greater impostor feelings partially (regarding mothers) and fully (regarding fathers) due to their parents being more psychologically controlling.

*The relationship between authoritarian parenting and adolescent's impostor feelings: Testing the moderating role of the child's gender and the moderated mediating role of parental psychological control (H3)*

In this section, we examined whether the main effect of authoritarian parenting and the mediating effect of parental psychological control on the adolescents' impostor feelings were moderated by the child's gender (see Figure 1). According to the procedure suggested by Hayes (2013) [61], we used the SPSS macro-PROCESS to test the moderation and moderated mediation for authoritarian parenting on the child's impostor feelings. The results (Table 3) revealed that the direct positive association between maternal authoritarian parenting and adolescents' impostor feelings was moderated by the child's gender ($b = -0.62$, $p = 0.012$), indicating that maternal authoritarian parenting was significantly associated with adolescents' impostor feelings only among boys ($b = 0.64$, $p \leq 0.001$) but not among girls ($b = 0.02$, $p = 0.91$). The direct association between paternal authoritarian parenting and adolescents' impostor feelings was not moderated by the child's gender ($b = -0.31$, $p = 0.20$), as this association was insignificant among both boys ($b = 0.36$, $p = 0.06$) and girls ($b = 0.04$, $p = 0.80$).

**Table 3.** Moderation and moderated mediation analysis for impostor feelings: Regression model predicting impostor feelings from authoritarian parenting and psychological control as a mediator with child's gender as a moderator.

|  | Maternal | | | | Paternal | | | |
| --- | --- | --- | --- | --- | --- | --- | --- | --- |
|  | B | SE | t | p | B | SE | t | p |
| Authoritarian style | 1.26 | 0.40 | 3.17 | 0.002 | 0.67 | 0.40 | 1.68 | 0.09 |
| Parental-psychological control | 4.66 | 1.28 | 3.38 | <0.001 | 0.53 | 1.35 | 3.90 | <0.001 |
| Child's gender | 23.25 | 7.36 | 3.16 | 0.002 | 14.76 | 7.45 | 1.98 | 0.049 |
| Authoritarian style X Child's gender | −0.62 | 0.24 | −2.53 | 0.012 | −0.31 | 0.24 | −1.29 | 0.20 |
| Psychological control X Child's gender | −0.56 | 2.76 | −0.20 | 0.84 | −0.92 | 2.72 | −0.34 | 0.74 |

However, the indirect association between maternal authoritarian parenting and impostor feelings was not significantly moderated by the child's gender ($b = -0.56$, $p = 0.84$), which means that maternal psychological control played a similar mediating role in this association for boys and girls. This was also the case for father–child relations (i.e., the absence of a significant moderated mediation effect for psychological control by the child's gender; $b = -0.92$, $p = 0.74$), where the association between paternal authoritarian parenting and adolescents' impostor feelings was fully mediated by psychological control (namely, the paternal effect of authoritarian parenting on impostor feelings, which was only significant through psychological control as mediator, applied equally to boys and girls). Hence, the findings partially support hypothesis 3 embodied in the model (Figure 1) solely for mothers, with the direct effect, but not the indirect effect (as mediated by psychological control), of authoritarian parenting on adolescents' impostor feelings being moderated by the child's gender.

## 5. Discussion

Despite the massive growing interest in the impostor phenomenon during the last decade [7], surprisingly little research work has investigated the phenomenon with adolescents [9], and most of it not recently. This is especially peculiar given the knowledge about the phenomenon's familial roots [1,2] and prior evidence suggesting that impostor feelings in adolescence may be as prevalent and intense as in adulthood [11,64]. Indeed, the current data about adolescent boys and girls recorded similar rates of impostor feelings in comparison with data reported in previous research with adult students [60], with about 36% of the participants reporting experiencing frequent to intense impostor feelings. The present study aimed at reducing this gap in the body of research by testing the association between maternal and paternal authoritarian parenting and impostor feelings among adolescents, while accounting for the mediation effect of parental psychological control and the moderation effect of the child's gender in this context.

In general, the findings demonstrated the importance of parenting styles and behaviors in concurrently explaining impostor feelings in adolescents, with the permissive and the authoritarian parenting styles uniquely predicting a significant proportion of variance of the adolescents' impostor scores. Our findings generally accord with previous research data linking between non-authoritative parenting styles (i.e., permissive and authoritarian) and emotional difficulties in adolescents [35]. In the specific emotional context of impostor feelings, these findings could be attributed to the parental properties of care and control [19]. This evidence, however, is the first and the only evidence in the research literature linking between overall parenting styles, according to Baumrind's typology [23,24] and the impostor phenomenon. The study's main finding demonstrated the mediating role played by parental psychological control in the association between authoritarian parenting and the impostor phenomenon. While previous research addressed the role played by overcontrolling parenting, including lack of parental care, in the context of the impostor phenomenon [14,19,52], the current findings suggest a more specific explanation regarding the possible mechanism describing the early emergence of impostor feelings in adolescents. In this regard, our data suggest that adolescents whose parents are more authoritarian experience greater impostor feelings due to their parents being more psychologically controlling. Indeed, parental psychological control is described in the parenting literature as a uniquely hazardous pattern to the child's emotional well-being, normally asserted by the authoritarian parent, whose presence in child-rearing is shown to be associated with several internalized and externalized behavior problems [37,38,40,65] mostly anxiety, depression, and a poor sense of the self. Perhaps the exposure to the prolonged disrespectful, rejecting, conditional, and criticizing nature of psychological control treatment from the parent undermines the child's self-confidence and self-worth, which, in turn, evokes the dependency on external approval for maintaining a good self-worth. The continuous necessity to conform with the psychologically controlling parent's expectation to gain approval for the self as worthy in early relations within the family [39,66] could be projected and generalized later in life onto various social and relationship contexts, as the impostor relies on others' approval and admiration to validate their self-esteem and feelings of self-worth [2].

Interestingly, psychological control as an explaining mechanism of the relationship between authoritarian parenting and the child's impostor feelings was telling the whole story for fathers but only part of the story for mothers, whose authoritarian parenting effects on impostor feelings was merely partially mediated by psychological control. In other words, relative to mothers, other aspects of authoritarian parenting beyond psychological control per se were relevant to explaining adolescents' impostor feelings. Along with our finding of a greater proportion of variance of the participants' impostor feelings explained by the maternal variables compared with the paternal variables (15.2% and 13.3%, respectively), this evidence reinforces the assumption of the gender differential parental effect on the child's outcome. Specifically, it somewhat reflects a priority of the maternal effects over the paternal effects in predicting impostor feelings (especially concerning authoritarian parenting), as found in some previous research in several contexts of internalizing and externalizing outcomes in adolescents [44–47,49], but not yet specifically in the context of impostor feelings [10]. Perhaps the fact that mothers are primary caregivers who still play more central and involved roles in child-rearing within the family [10,67] makes the negative influence of maladaptive maternal parenting (especially over psychological control and lack of care) on the child more significant. In the absence of a conclusive picture regarding the impact of parenting in a parent–adolescent dyad by gender in the research literature [44], this generic explanation and more specific ones will need to be further empirically inspected. Based on a hypothesized moderated and moderated mediation model (Figure 1), we also tested the direct and indirect (via psychological control) associations between parental styles and adolescents' impostor feelings for moderation of the child's gender. In this regard, a child's gender moderation was found solely for the maternal direct effect of authoritarian parenting on impostor feelings (i.e., the association between the variables was significant only for boys), but not for the indirect effect through psychological control. Boys may be at greater risk of being more exposed to parental maladaptive behaviors such as severe punishment [68], which can partially explain why only boys' impostor feelings were affected by mothers' authoritarian parenting in the current sample. Another explanation could be that boys perceive a higher level of parental psychological control than girls [65]. Importantly, psychological control seemed to have a similar effect across both genders and gender dyads, suggesting that this parental behavior plays a unique, distinct role in the context of adolescents' impostor feelings, regardless of the child's gender. Indeed, many researchers have maintained that psychologically controlling parenting has a negative effect on the child's internal powers such as their sense of self [40,66].

Finally, inconsistent with the data reported in two previous studies with adolescents [11,69], we found gender differences in impostor feelings rates among the sample's participants, in which girls scored significantly higher than boys. This inconsistency in gender differences across studies could be explained, however, by the lack of uniformity in the research tools used for screening the impostor phenomenon [7]. However, our data are in line with at least 16 previous studies that recorded a gender difference in impostor feelings (mostly with emerging adults) [8], suggesting that, in certain conditions, women rather than men may be more vulnerable to impostor feelings during their lifetime. The question of whether gender differences in impostor feelings are stronger at a younger developmental period (i.e., in adolescence) should be further examined in more studies with young populations, most importantly based on longitudinal data.

The findings of this cross-sectional design study are limited in several respects. First and foremost, these findings and suggested conclusions are not to be interpreted in causal terms, as if parenting styles and behaviors necessarily influence the child's impostor feelings. Indeed, perhaps the best theoretical way of understanding the current findings regarding the associations between the parenting variables and adolescents' impostor feelings is in terms of the parental effect on the child. Yet, the study's data can also suggest the reverse explanation, according to which impostor feelings affect adolescents' perceptions of their parents' authoritarian parenting and psychological control. To resolve this possible confounding situation, more longitudinal data must be obtained as part of future research. In that case, it would also be useful to examine the influence of other parenting styles on adolescents' impostor feelings, which were not measured or considered in the current study. Moreover, the parenting indexes in the current study rely solely on the child's reports, which reflect their subjective perception and may not match the parent's self-perceived parenting style nor reflect their actual parenting style [70]. In addition, with the adolescents filling out all the measures, a correlational inflation may potentially be caused by the shared methods measurement [71]. While this could confine the validity of the study findings, there is great merit in the child's point of view on parental characteristics, due to its importance and close relevance to their behavior and emotion [39,70]. Finally, the study was conducted with Israeli adolescents, hence the generalizability of its findings is limited to the culture and ethnical characteristics in which the current study took place.

**Funding:** This research received no external funding.

**Institutional Review Board Statement:** The study was conducted in accordance with the Declaration of Helsinki, and approved by the Institutional Review Board of Tel-Hai College (ref. 10-10/2022, in October 2022).

**Informed Consent Statement:** Informed consent was obtained from all subjects involved in the study.

**Data Availability Statement:** Data is available from the author upon reasonable request.

**Conflicts of Interest:** The authors declare no conflict of interest.

## References

1. Clance, P.R.; Imes, S.A. The imposter phenomenon in high achieving women: Dynamics and therapeutic intervention. *Psychother. Theory Res. Pract.* **1978**, *15*, 241–247. [CrossRef]
2. Langford, J.; Clance, P.R. The imposter phenomenon: Recent research findings regarding dynamics, personality and family patterns and their implications for treatment. *Psychother. Theory Res. Pract. Train.* **1993**, *30*, 495. [CrossRef]
3. Robinson, S.L.; Goodpaster, S.K. The effects of parental alcoholism on perceptions of control and impostor phenomenon. *Curr. Psychol.* **1991**, *10*, 113–119. [CrossRef]
4. Chrisman, S.M.; Pieper, W.A.; Clance, P.R.; Holland, C.L.; Glickauf-Hughes, C. Validation of the Clance Imposter Phenomenon Scale. *J. Personal. Assess.* **1995**, *65*, 456–467. [CrossRef]
5. Clance, P.R. *The Impostor Phenomenon: Overcoming the Fear That Haunts Your Success*; Peachtree Publishers: Atlanta, GA, USA, 1985; Volume 209.
6. Leonhardt, M.; Bechtoldt, M.N.; Rohrmann, S. All impostors aren't alike—Differentiating the impostor phenomenon. *Front. Psychol.* **2017**, *8*, 1505. [CrossRef]
7. Bravata, D.M.; Watts, S.A.; Keefer, A.L.; Madhusudhan, D.K.; Taylor, K.T.; Clark, D.M.; Nelson, R.S.; Cokley, K.O.; Hagg, H.K. Prevalence, predictors, and treatment of impostor syndrome: A systematic review. *J. Gen. Intern. Med.* **2020**, *35*, 1252–1275. [CrossRef] [PubMed]
8. Bravata, D.M.; Madhusudhan, D.K.; Boroff, M.; Cokley, K.O. Commentary: Prevalence, predictors, and treatment of impostor syndrome: A systematic review. *J. Ment. Health Clin. Psychol.* **2020**, *4*, 12–16. [CrossRef]
9. Bernard, D.; Neblett, E. A culturally informed model of the development of the impostor phenomenon among African American youth. *Adolesc. Res. Rev.* **2017**, *3*, 279–300. [CrossRef]
10. Yaffe, Y. The Association between Familial and Parental Factors and the Impostor Phenomenon—A Systematic Review. *Am. J. Fam. Ther.* **2022**, 1–19. [CrossRef]
11. Caselman, T.D.; Self, P.A.; Self, A.L. Adolescent attributes contributing to the imposter phenomenon. *J. Adolesc.* **2006**, *29*, 395–405. [CrossRef]
12. Clark, M.; Vardeman, K.K.; Barba, S.E. Perceived inadequacy: A study of the imposter phenomenon among college and research librarians. *Coll. Res. Libr.* **2014**, *75*, 255–271. [CrossRef]
13. Hutchins, H.M. Outing the imposter: A study exploring imposter phenomenon among higher education faculty. *New Horiz. Adult Educ. Hum. Resour. Dev.* **2015**, *27*, 3–12. [CrossRef]
14. Sonnak, C.; Towell, T. The impostor phenomenon in British university students: Relationships between self-esteem, mental health, parental rearing style and socioeconomic status. *Personal. Individ. Differ.* **2001**, *31*, 863–874. [CrossRef]
15. Tigranyan, S.; Byington, D.R.; Liupakorn, D.; Hicks, A.; Lombardi, S.; Mathis, M.; Rodolfa, E. Factors related to the impostor phenomenon in psychology doctoral students. *Train. Educ. Prof. Psychol.* **2021**, *15*, 298. [CrossRef]
16. Urwin, J. Imposter phenomena and experience levels in social work: An initial investigation. *Br. J. Soc. Work.* **2018**, *48*, 1432–1446. [CrossRef]
17. Bernard, N.S.; Dollinger, S.J.; Ramaniah, N.V. Applying the big five personality factors to the impostor phenomenon. *J. Personal. Assess.* **2002**, *78*, 321–333. [CrossRef]
18. Hutchins, H.M.; Penney, L.M.; Sublett, L.W. What imposters risk at work: Exploring imposter phenomenon, stress coping, and job outcomes. *Hum. Resour. Dev. Q.* **2018**, *29*, 31–48. [CrossRef]
19. Yaffe, Y. Students' recollections of parenting styles and impostor phenomenon: The mediating role of social anxiety. *Personal. Individ. Differ.* **2021**, *172*, 110598. [CrossRef]
20. Smetana, J.G. Current research on parenting styles, dimensions, and beliefs. *Curr. Opin. Psychol.* **2017**, *15*, 19–25. [CrossRef]
21. Baumrind, D. Effects of authoritative parental control on child behavior. *Child Dev.* **1966**, *37*, 887–907. [CrossRef]
22. Baumrind, D. Authoritarian vs. authoritative parental control. *Adolescence* **1968**, *3*, 255–272.
23. Baumrind, D. Current patterns of parental authority. *Dev. Psychol. Monogr.* **1971**, *4*, 1–103. [CrossRef]
24. Baumrind, D. Patterns of Parental Authority and Adolescent Autonomy. *New Dir. Child Adolesc. Dev.* **2005**, *108*, 61–69. [CrossRef]
25. Maccoby, E.E.; Martin, J.A. Socialization in the context of the family: Parent–child interaction. In *Handbook of Child Psychology*; Mussen, P.H., Ed.; Wiley: New York, NY, USA, 1983; Volume 4, pp. 1–101.
26. Climent-Galarza, S.; Alcaide, M.; Garcia, O.F.; Chen, F.; Garcia, F. Parental socialization, delinquency during adolescence and adjustment in adolescents and adult children. *Behav. Sci.* **2022**, *12*, 448. [CrossRef]
27. Steinberg, L. We know something: Parent-adolescent relationships in retrospect and prospect. *J. Res. Adolesc.* **2001**, *11*, 1–19. [CrossRef]
28. Gimenez-Serrano, S.; Garcia, F.; Garcia, O.F. Parenting styles and its relations with personal and social adjustment beyond adolescence: Is the current evidence enough? *Eur. J. Dev. Psychol.* **2022**, *19*, 749–769. [CrossRef]
29. Darling, N.; Steinberg, L. Parenting Style as Context: An Integrative Model. *Psychol. Bull.* **1993**, *113*, 487–496. [CrossRef]
30. Garcia, O.F.; Fuentes, M.C.; Gracia, E.; Serra, E.; Garcia, F. Parenting warmth and strictness across three generations: Parenting styles and psychosocial adjustment. *Int. J. Environ. Res. Public Health* **2020**, *17*, 7487. [CrossRef]
31. Pinquart, M.; Kauser, R. Do the associations of parenting styles with behavior problems and academic achievement vary by culture? Results from a meta-analysis. *Cult. Divers. Ethn. Minor. Psychol.* **2018**, *24*, 75. [CrossRef] [PubMed]

32. Fuentes, M.C.; Garcia, O.F.; Alcaide, M.; Garcia-Ros, R.; Garcia, F. Analyzing when parental warmth but without parental strictness leads to more adolescent empathy and self-concept: Evidence from Spanish homes. *Front. Psychol.* **2022**, *13*, 7612. [CrossRef] [PubMed]
33. Palacios, I.; Garcia, O.F.; Alcaide, M.; Garcia, F. Positive parenting style and positive health beyond the authoritative: Self, universalism values, and protection against emotional vulnerability from Spanish adolescents and adult children. *Front. Psychol.* **2022**, *13*, 1066282. [CrossRef] [PubMed]
34. Chen, W.W.; Yang, X.; Jiao, Z. Authoritarian parenting, perfectionism, and academic procrastination. *Educ. Psychol.* **2022**, *42*, 1145–1159. [CrossRef]
35. Pinquart, M. Associations of parenting dimensions and styles with externalizing problems of children and adolescents: An updated meta-analysis. *Dev. Psychol.* **2017**, *53*, 873. [CrossRef]
36. Pinquart, M. Associations of parenting dimensions and styles with internalizing symptoms in children and adolescents: A meta-analysis. *Marriage Fam. Rev.* **2017**, *53*, 613–640. [CrossRef]
37. Baumrind, D. Differentiating between confrontive and coercive kinds of parental power-assertive disciplinary practices. *Hum. Dev.* **2012**, *55*, 35–51. [CrossRef]
38. Barber, B.K.; Xia, M.; Olsen, J.A.; McNeely, C.A.; Bose, K. Feeling disrespected by parents: Refining the measurement and understanding of psychological control. *J. Adolesc.* **2012**, *35*, 273–287. [CrossRef]
39. Barber, B.K. Parental psychological control: Revisiting a neglected construct. *Child Dev.* **1996**, *67*, 3296–3319. [CrossRef]
40. Chyung, Y.J.; Lee, Y.A.; Ahn, S.J.; Bang, H.S. Associations of perceived parental psychological control with depression, anxiety in children and adolescents: A meta-analysis. *Marriage Fam. Rev.* **2022**, *58*, 158–197. [CrossRef]
41. Gorostiaga, A.; Aliri, J.; Balluerka, N.; Lameirinhas, J. Parenting styles and internalizing symptoms in adolescence: A systematic literature review. *Int. J. Environ. Res. Public Health* **2019**, *16*, 3192. [CrossRef]
42. Winner, N.A.; Nicholson, B.C. Overparenting and narcissism in young adults: The mediating role of psychological control. *J. Child Fam. Stud.* **2018**, *27*, 3650–3657. [CrossRef]
43. Yaffe, Y. Systematic review of the differences between mothers and fathers in parenting styles and practices. *Curr. Psychol.* **2020**. [CrossRef]
44. Bolkan, C.; Sano, Y.; De Costa, J.; Acock, A.C.; Day, R.D. Early adolescents' perceptions of mothers' and fathers' parenting styles and problem behavior. *Marriage Fam. Rev.* **2011**, *46*, 563–579. [CrossRef]
45. Gryczkowski, M.R.; Jordan, S.S.; Mercer, S.H. Differential relations between mothers' and fathers' parenting practices and child externalizing behavior. *J. Child Fam. Stud.* **2010**, *19*, 539–546. [CrossRef]
46. Niditch, L.A.; Varela, R.E. Perceptions of Parenting, Emotional Self-Efficacy, and Anxiety in Youth: Test of a Mediational Model. *Child Youth Care Forum* **2012**, *41*, 21–35. [CrossRef]
47. Tur Porcar, A.; Mestre Escrivá, M.V.; Samper García, P.; Malonda Vidal, E. Upbringing and aggressiveness of minors: Is the influence of the father and mother different? *Psicothema* **2012**, *24*, 284–288.
48. Szkody, E.; Steele, E.H.; McKinney, C. Effects of parenting styles on sychological problems by self esteem and gender differences. *J. Fam. Issues* **2021**, *42*, 1931–1954. [CrossRef]
49. Verhoeven, M.; Bögels, S.M.; van der Bruggen, C.C. Unique roles of mothering and fathering in child anxiety: Moderation by child's age and gender. *J. Child Fam. Stud.* **2012**, *21*, 331–343. [CrossRef]
50. Waite, P.; Whittington, L.; Creswell, C. Parent-child interactions and adolescent anxiety: A systematic review. *Psychopathol. Rev.* **2014**, *1*, 51–76. [CrossRef]
51. Bussotti, C. *The Impostor Phenomenon: Family Roles and Environment*; Georgia State University-College of Arts and Sciences: Atlanta, GA, USA, 1990.
52. Want, J.; Kleitman, S. Imposter phenomenon and self-handicapping: Links with parenting styles and self-confidence. *Personal. Individ. Differ.* **2006**, *40*, 961–971. [CrossRef]
53. Yaffe, Y. How do impostor feelings and general self-efficacy co-explain students' test-anxiety and academic achievements: The preceding role of maternal psychological control. *Soc. Psychol. Educ.* **2023**, 1–19. [CrossRef]
54. Haverson, C.E. Remembering your parents: Reflections on the retrospective method. *J. Personal.* **1988**, *56*, 435–443. [CrossRef] [PubMed]
55. Grenon, E.; Bouffard, T.; Vezeau, C. Familial and personal characteristics profiles predict bias in academic competence and impostorism self-evaluations. *Self Identity* **2020**, *19*, 784–803. [CrossRef]
56. Lu, M.; Walsh, K.; White, S.; Shield, P. Influence of perceived maternal psychological control on academic performance in Chinese adolescents: Moderating roles of adolescents' age, gender, and filial piety. *Marriage Fam. Rev.* **2018**, *54*, 50–63. [CrossRef]
57. Buri, J.R. Parental authority questionnaire. *J. Personal. Assess.* **1991**, *57*, 110–119. [CrossRef] [PubMed]
58. Smetana, J.G. Parenting styles and conceptions of parental authority during adolescence. *Child Dev.* **1995**, *66*, 299–316. [CrossRef] [PubMed]
59. French, B.F.; Ullrich-French, S.C.; Follman, D. The psychometric properties of the Clance Impostor Scale. *Personal. Individ. Differ.* **2008**, *44*, 1270–1278. [CrossRef]
60. Yaffe, Y. Validation of the Clance Impostor Phenomenon Scale with female Hebrew-speaking students. *J. Exp. Psychopathol.* **2020**, *11*, 2043808720971341. [CrossRef]

61. Hayes, A.F. *Introduction to Mediation, Moderation, and Conditional Process Analysis: A Regression-Based Approach*; Guilford Press: New York, NY, USA, 2013. [CrossRef]
62. Preacher, K.J.; Hayes, A.F. Asymptotic and resampling strategies for assessing and comparing indirect effects in multiple mediator models. *Behav. Res. Methods* **2008**, *40*, 879–891. [CrossRef]
63. Vaughn, A.R.; Taasoobshirazi, G.; Johnson, M.L. Impostor phenomenon and motivation: Women in higher education. *Stud. High. Educ.* **2020**, *45*, 780–795. [CrossRef]
64. Cromwell, B.; Brown, N.; Adair, F.L. The impostor phenomenon and personality characteristics of high school honor students. *J. Soc. Behav. Personal.* **1990**, *5*, 563.
65. Cascio, V.L.; Guzzo, G.; Pace, F.; Pace, U.; Madonia, C. The relationship among paternal and maternal psychological control, self-esteem, and indecisiveness across adolescent genders. *Curr. Psychol.* **2016**, *35*, 467–477. [CrossRef]
66. Barber, B.K.; Harmon, E.L. Violating the self: Parental psychological control of children and adolescents. In *Intrusive Parenting: How Psychological Control Affects Children and Adolescents*; Barber, B.K., Ed.; American Psychological Association Press: Washington, DC, USA, 2002; pp. 15–52.
67. Pleck, J.H.; Mascaidrelli, B.P. Parental involvement: Levels, sources and consequences. In *The Role of the Father in Child Development*; Lamb, M.E., Ed.; John Wiley and Sons: Hoboken, NJ, USA, 2004; pp. 66–103.
68. Gershoff, E.T. Corporal punishment by parents and associated child behaviors and experiences: A meta-analytic and theoretical review. *Psychol. Bull.* **2002**, *128*, 539–579. [CrossRef] [PubMed]
69. Lester, D.; Moderski, T. The impostor phenomenon in adolescents. *Psychol. Rep.* **1995**, *76*, 466. [CrossRef] [PubMed]
70. Varvil-Weld, L.; Turrisi, R.; Scaglione, N.; Mallett, K.A.; Ray, A.E. Parents' and students' reports of parenting: Which are more reliably associated with college student drinking? *Addict. Behav.* **2013**, *38*, 1699–1703. [CrossRef]
71. Campbell, D.T.; Fiske, D.W. Convergent and discriminant validation by the multitrait-multimethod matrix. *Psychol. Bull.* **1959**, *56*, 81–105. [CrossRef] [PubMed]

**Disclaimer/Publisher's Note:** The statements, opinions and data contained in all publications are solely those of the individual author(s) and contributor(s) and not of MDPI and/or the editor(s). MDPI and/or the editor(s) disclaim responsibility for any injury to people or property resulting from any ideas, methods, instructions or products referred to in the content.

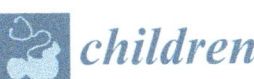 

Article

# Association between Family Environment and Adolescents' Sexual Adaptability: Based on the Latent Profile Analysis of Personality Traits

Rui Zhao [1,2], Jun Lv [3], Yan Gao [4], Yuyan Li [2], Huijing Shi [1], Junguo Zhang [5], Junqing Wu [2,*] and Ling Wang [1,*]

[1] Key Laboratory of Public Health Safety, Ministry of Education, Department of Maternal, Child and Adolescent Health, School of Public Health, Fudan University, Shanghai 200032, China
[2] NHC Key Laboratory of Reproduction Regulation, Shanghai Institute for Biomedical and Pharmaceutical Technologies, Fudan University, Shanghai 200237, China
[3] Key Laboratory of Health Technology Assessment, National Health Commission, China Research Center on Disability Issues, School of Public Health, Fudan University, Shanghai 200032, China
[4] Division of Biostatistics, Medical College of Wisconsin, Milwaukee, WI 53226, USA
[5] Department of Epidemiology, School of Public Health, Sun Yat-sen University, Guangzhou 510080, China
* Correspondence: wujunqing@sibpt.com (J.W.); lingwang@fudan.edu.cn (L.W.); Tel.: +86-21-6477-1237 (J.W.); +86-21-5423-7982 (L.W.)

**Abstract:** Sexual adaptation plays an important role in psychosexual health. Our study aimed to investigate the relationship between the family environment and sexual adaptability among adolescents with different personality traits. A cross-sectional study was conducted in Shanghai and Shanxi province. A total of 1106 participants aged 14–19 was surveyed in 2019, including 519 boys and 587 girls. Univariate analyses and mixed regression models were performed to assess the association. Girls had a significantly lower average score of sexual self-adaptation compared to boys (4.01 ± 0.77 vs. 4.32 ± 0.64, $p < 0.001$). We found that the family environment did not impact boys' sexual adaptation in different personality groups. For girls in a balanced group, expressiveness factors improved their sexual adaptability ($p < 0.05$), intellectual–cultural orientation and organization promoted social adaptability ($p < 0.05$) and active–recreational orientation and control decreased their social adaptability ($p < 0.05$). In the high-neuroticism group, cohesion facilitated sexual control ($p < 0.05$), while conflict and organization reduced sexual control ability, and active–recreational orientation decreased sexual adaptation ($p < 0.05$). No factors associated with the family environment were found to influence sexual adaptability in groups with low neuroticism and high ratings in other personality factors. Compared with boys, girls demonstrated lower sexual self-adaptability, and their overall sexual adaptability was more susceptible to the family environment.

**Keywords:** sexual adaptability; family environment; personality; adolescents

Citation: Zhao, R.; Lv, J.; Gao, Y.; Li, Y.; Shi, H.; Zhang, J.; Wu, J.; Wang, L. Association between Family Environment and Adolescents' Sexual Adaptability: Based on the Latent Profile Analysis of Personality Traits. *Children* **2023**, *10*, 191. https://doi.org/10.3390/children10020191

Academic Editor: Brian Littlechild

Received: 9 December 2022
Revised: 9 January 2023
Accepted: 17 January 2023
Published: 19 January 2023

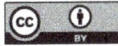

**Copyright:** © 2023 by the authors. Licensee MDPI, Basel, Switzerland. This article is an open access article distributed under the terms and conditions of the Creative Commons Attribution (CC BY) license (https://creativecommons.org/licenses/by/4.0/).

## 1. Introduction

There is an increasing consensus that sexual issues are not a unique topic confined to the adult world [1]. In puberty, children develop rapidly in sexual aspects, and their accompanying mental state also changes, both of which are more likely to produce health hazards and adverse behaviors [2,3]. Psychosexual health is closely related to human sexual activities [4]. The essence of psychosexual health is a good state of individual internal sexual psychological coordination and external sexual behavior adaptation. It mainly refers to good sexual cognition, correct sexual attitude and healthy sexual behavior. Of these, sexual adaptation is an important part. In a study of Chinese adolescents, sexual adaptation meant that they could happily accept their sexual changes and consciously constrain and adjust their sexual desires and behaviors according to the requirements of social and cultural norms. Sexual adaptation includes the identification of their own gender, the adaptation to social, moral and cultural norms and regulating and controlling sexual behavior and sexual activities [5]. Studies have shown that gender disapproval and maladaptation are related to adolescent mental distress and sexual injury [6,7], and a lack of sexual control and effective sex education have been associated with risky behaviors such as adolescent dating and sexual violence [8,9], as well as an increased risk of early pregnancy [10]. Maladaptation to social norms can lead to self-doubt and self-denial, and some people cannot generally interact with the opposite sex in adulthood.

It is necessary and fundamental to investigate the current status of adolescent sexual adaptation. Several studies have found that personality, gradually formed and developed through the interaction of heredity and environment, is closely related to sexual behavior and sexual health [11,12]. Human beings, particularly adolescents, are "social animals", and, therefore, naturally impacted by the social environments surrounding them, especially the family environment. A large number of studies have proved that there exists a significant association between the family environment and adolescent sexual development [13,14]. For example, parent–child communication is a protective factor of adolescent sexual behavior and sexual health. In addition, the more effective family monitoring is, the lower the proportion of teenagers with risky sexual behaviors [15,16].

Currently, research on sexual problems of Chinese adolescents focuses on sexual behavior, but little research has been found to study the psychosexual aspects of adolescent sexuality. In addition, few studies have addressed the critical questions regarding how the family environment affects the sexual and psychological status of adolescents, not to mention what role personality factors may play. To fill this research gap, we conducted a cross-sectional study to assess the relationship between the family environment and psychosexual health in adolescents with different personality characteristics, including the relationship with sexual adaptation.

We aim to determine whether the family environment affects sexual adaptability and whether this association is consistent among various personality traits in adolescents. Additionally, we intend to identify whether there exist different trends between the two genders previously defined regarding these associations. Therefore, more precise health interventions could be carried out in the future.

## 2. Materials and Methods

*Study Design and Participants*

In November 2019, we conducted a cross-sectional study in Putuo district, Shanghai and Datong City, Shanxi province. Middle and high school students aged 12–18 were surveyed. Classes were chosen as the sampling unit, and the sampling method comprised multistage, stratified and cluster sampling. Three stages in the sampling process were as follows: (i) for each city, three middle schools, including one senior high school and two junior schools, were selected (six schools in total); (ii) for each school, 4 classes were randomly selected (24 classes in total); (iii) all the students in the selected classes were surveyed. Before the survey, we sent out passive consent letters to the parents or guardians of all subjects via their schools. The parents or guardians were required to return a signed form if they did not want their child to participate in the survey. Then, we obtained active consent from the subjects, including asking whether they agreed to participate voluntarily at the very beginning. A total of 1331 people was surveyed, 25 of whom declined to participate, leading to a response rate of 98.12%. We also conducted data quality control. For instance, 200 of the 1306 people surveyed failed to pass the lie detection questions in the later stage. In the adolescent psychosexual health scale, there are 4 pairs of polygraph questions in the design. If three pairs or more responses were inconsistent, we excluded them when analyzing the data. Thus, the final analysis ended up with 1106 subjects with a passing rate of 84.68%. As shown in Figure 1.

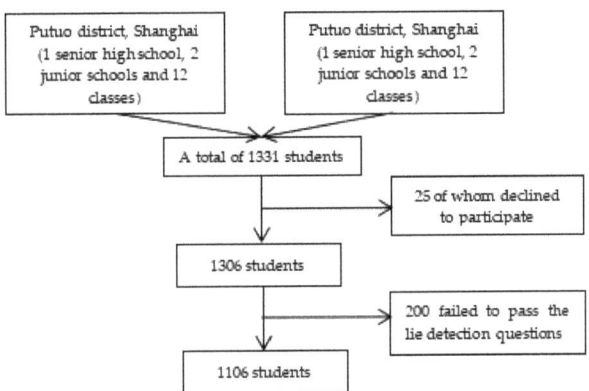

**Figure 1.** Sampling frame.

## 3. Measures

The *sexual adaptation subscale* from the widely accepted *adolescent psychosexual health scale* in China was employed to measure sexual adaptation (Cronbach's α = 0.818), which included the following dimensions: sexual control (measured with six items), sexual self-adaptation (measured with five items) and sexual social adaptation (measured with nine items). The answer options of all items were "very inconsistent = 1 point", "moderately inconsistent = 2 points", "uncertain = 3 points", "moderately consistent = 4 points" and "very consistent = 5 points". Some answers were reversely scored based on the question.

The *family environment scale* (FES) [17], which is a common international scale, was employed to measure the family environment status of adolescents (Cronbach's α = 0.826). Seven subscales with high reliability and validity in China were used in this study, including cohesion, expressiveness, conflict, intellectual–cultural orientation, active–recreational orientation, organization and a control subscale, each containing ten relevant items.

Personality was measured by using the *NEO five-factor inventory* (NEO-FFI) [18], and we used the version with 60 items (Cronbach's α = 0.712). The scale contains five subscales: neuroticism, extroversion, openness, agreeableness and conscientiousness, each containing 12 entries.

Other demographic characteristics were measured by using a self-administered questionnaire, including demographic characteristics and knowledge, attitudes and behaviors related to psychosexual health.

## 4. Statistical Analysis

Summary tables with frequencies were provided for all the categorical variables. Chi-squared tests were used to compare the differences in demographic characteristics between sexes. For all the continuous variables, the mean and standard deviations were presented. T-tests were used to compare the differences in sexual control, sexual self-adaptability and sexual and social adaptation subscale scores of different sex and geographical characteristics.

Furthermore, a potential profile analysis was employed to classify adolescents with different personality traits, with a score of five dimensions on the personality scale as a manifest variable for the latent profile analysis of adolescent personality characteristics.

In the end, the mixed regression model (MRM) was used to analyze the relationship between the family environment and adolescent sexual adaptability. In addition, the latent category variables obtained from the above analysis were used as moderators to establish the mixture regression model.

All statistical tests were considered statistically significant based on the two-sided 0.05 level of significance (i.e., $p < 0.05$). All analyses were performed using SAS® 9.4 and Mplus7.4.

## 5. Results

Descriptive statistics for all demographic characteristics are shown in Table 1. Among the 1106 participants aged 14–19 (SD = 2.49), 51.63% came from Shanghai and 48.37% from Shanxi. The grade levels were 58.68% in junior high school and 41.32% in senior high school. Of the participants, 82.46% reported living with their parents, 3.89% with their grandparents and 11.03% in school dormitories. In total, 86.06% reported their father's education level to be senior high school or higher, 53.62% of whom were aged 42 years or less. Additionally, 83.54% reported their mother's education level to be senior high school or higher, 67.73% of whom were aged 42 years or less. The per capita monthly income of 42.40% of the target families was more than CNY 6000.

**Table 1.** Demographic characteristics of all respondents based on sex.

| | Total (n = 1106) | Boys (n = 519) | Girls (n = 587) | $\chi^2$ p-Value |
|---|---|---|---|---|
| **Region** | | | | 0.995 |
| Shanghai | 51.63 | 51.64 | 51.62 | |
| Shanxi | 48.37 | 48.36 | 48.38 | |
| **Grade** | | | | 0.240 |
| Junior high school | 58.68 | 59.54 | 57.92 | |
| Senior high school | 41.32 | 40.46 | 42.08 | |
| **Main mode of residence** | | | | 0.643 |
| Live with parents | 82.46 | 81.50 | 83.30 | |
| Live with grandparents | 3.89 | 4.43 | 3.41 | |
| Board in school | 11.03 | 11.75 | 10.39 | |
| **Father's education attainment** | | | | 0.056 |
| Junior high school or below | 13.92 | 15.03 | 12.95 | |
| High school, technical secondary school or vocational school | 29.66 | 26.59 | 32.37 | |
| Junior college | 22.42 | 21.19 | 23.51 | |
| Bachelor's degree or above | 34.00 | 37.19 | 31.18 | |
| **Mother's education attainment** | | | | 0.155 |
| Junior high school or below | 16.46 | 15.22 | 17.55 | |
| High school, technical secondary school or vocational school | 30.38 | 28.71 | 31.86 | |
| Junior college | 22.69 | 22.35 | 23.00 | |
| Bachelor's degree or above | 30.47 | 33.72 | 27.60 | |
| **Father's age** | | | | 0.021 |
| <35 | 1.72 | 2.89 | 0.68 | |
| 35~ | 51.90 | 52.41 | 51.45 | |
| 43~ | 35.71 | 35.45 | 35.95 | |
| 50~ | 10.67 | 9.25 | 11.93 | |
| **Mother's age** | | | | 0.381 |
| <35 | 3.35 | 4.05 | 2.73 | |
| 35~ | 64.38 | 64.93 | 63.88 | |
| 43~ | 28.21 | 27.75 | 28.62 | |
| 50~ | 4.06 | 3.28 | 4.77 | |
| **Per capita monthly income (CNY)** | | | | 0.544 |
| <3000 | 35.08 | 35.07 | 35.09 | |
| 3000~ | 22.51 | 20.81 | 24.02 | |
| 6000~ | 20.07 | 20.42 | 19.76 | |
| 10,000~ | 22.33 | 23.70 | 21.12 | |

The average scores for adolescent sexual adaptation are shown in Table 2. The average scores of sexual control for boys and girls were 3.54 ± 0.50 and 3.56 ± 0.44, respectively. The difference was not statistically significant ($p = 0.329$). The average social adaptation score of boys was 3.77 ± 0.68. The girls' score for this factor was 3.76 ± 0.67. There was no statistical significance ($p = 0.779$). However, in terms of sexual self-adaptation, the boys' average score of 4.32 ± 0.64 was significantly higher than the girls' average score of 4.01 ± 0.77 ($p < 0.001$). Therefore, the difference between the boys' and girls' overall average sexual adaptation scores was significant ($p = 0.007$).

Table 2. Average score for each factor of sexual adaptation based on sex and region.

| Subscale Score | Sex | | | Region | | |
|---|---|---|---|---|---|---|
| | Boys ($n = 519$) | Girls ($n = 587$) | $p$ | Shanghai ($n = 571$) | Shanxi ($n = 535$) | $p$ |
| Sexual control | 3.54 ± 0.50 | 3.56 ± 0.44 | 0.329 | 3.60 ± 0.48 | 3.50 ± 0.45 | <0.001 |
| Sexual self-adaptation | 4.32 ± 0.64 | 4.01 ± 0.77 | <0.001 | 4.16 ± 0.68 | 4.15 ± 0.78 | 0.946 |
| Social adaptation | 3.77 ± 0.68 | 3.76 ± 0.67 | 0.779 | 3.84 ± 0.70 | 3.68 ± 0.64 | <0.001 |
| Overall average score | 3.84 ± 0.46 | 3.76 ± 0.46 | 0.007 | 3.85 ± 0.47 | 3.74 ± 0.45 | <0.001 |

The analysis of students from different regions revealed that the average scores of students for sexual control and social adaptation were different ($p < 0.001$), and the average scores of the two factors in Shanghai students were higher than those of Shanxi students. No statistical significance was found in terms of sexual self-adaptation ($p = 0.946$).

As shown in Table 3, we selected scores on the NEO five-factor inventory as explicit variables to analyze adolescent personality characteristics based on the latent profile analysis and fitted models 1–4. The smaller the fitting index AIC (Akaike information criteria) and BIC (Bayesian information criteria) values were, the better the model fit. In this study, it was found that the AIC, BIC and aBIC decreased monotonically with increasing categories. Model entropy reached the maximum at the third classification, with 0.732 for the male model and 0.812 for the female model. Moreover, the LMR value was no longer significant in the fourth classification. Therefore, the models with three potential categories were selected as the best models.

Table 3. Model comparison of latent profile analysis (personality variables).

| No. of Classes | AIC | BIC | aBIC | Entropy | LMR | BLRT | The Most Likely Number of Class Members |
|---|---|---|---|---|---|---|---|
| Boys | | | | | - | - | |
| 1C | 17,878.351 | 17,920.870 | 17,889.128 | 1.000 | | | 519 |
| 2C | 17,392.947 | 17,460.977 | 17,410.190 | 0.721 | 0.000 | 0.000 | 241/278 |
| 3C | 17,264.324 | 17,357.866 | 17,288.033 | 0.732 | 0.003 | 0.000 | 116/281/122 |
| 4C | 17,235.073 | 17,354.126 | 17,265.248 | 0.732 | 0.325 | 0.000 | 148/25/234/103 |
| Girls | | | | | | | |
| 1C | 20,118.511 | 20,162.261 | 20,130.515 | 1.000 | - | - | 587 |
| 2C | 19,557.426 | 19,627.427 | 19,576.632 | 0.785 | 0.000 | 0.000 | 392/195 |
| 3C | 19,393.933 | 19,490.183 | 19,420.341 | 0.812 | 0.004 | 0.000 | 355/66/166 |
| 4C | 19,355.279 | 19,477.780 | 19,388.890 | 0.797 | 0.107 | 0.000 | 17/162/84/324 |

Note: aBIC is BIC for sample correction; entropy is classification accuracy index, the value range is 0–1, the closer the Entropy is to 1, the more accurate the model classification is; LMR is likelihood ratio test index; BLRT is likelihood based on bootstrap ratio test.

Based on the results of the latent profile analysis, students of both male and female genders were divided into three categories according to their personality characteristics. The results of boys and girls were similar. As shown in Figures 2 and 3, the first category was relatively balanced in neuroticism, extroversion, openness, agreeableness and conscientiousness, and was named the balanced group. The second category of subjects had higher neuroticism scores than the other groups, and was called the high-neuroticism group. The third category of subjects had lower neuroticism scores, but the other features were higher;

we named this the low-neuroticism and high-others group. Among boys, there were 116 (22.35%) in the first category, 281 (54.14%) in the second category and 122 (23.51%) in the third category. There were 355 (60.48%) girls in the first category, 66 girls (11.24%) in the second category and 166 (28.28%) girls in the third category.

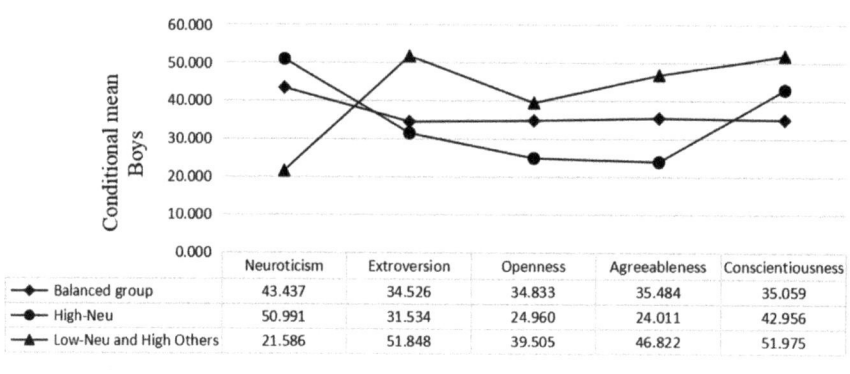

Figure 2. Plot of the conditional mean distribution for the latent categories (boys).

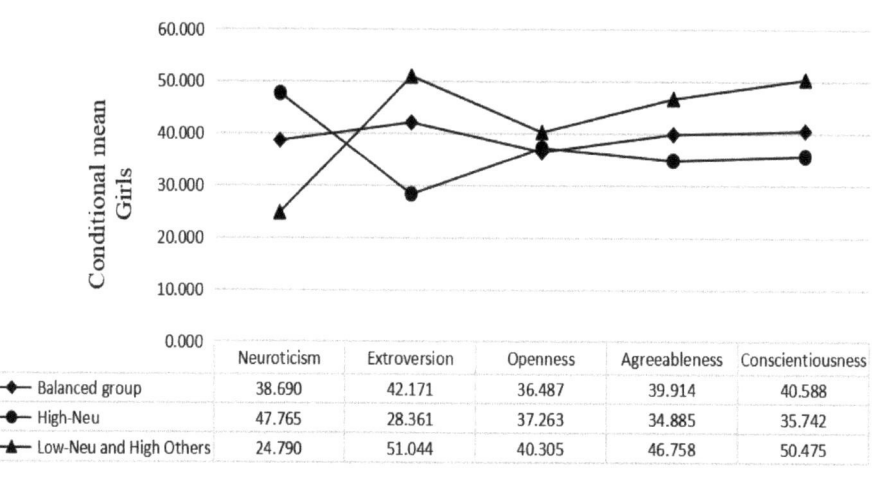

Figure 3. Plot of the conditional mean distribution for the latent categories (girls).

The 519 boys and 587 girls were divided into three latent categories. Possible influencing factors were included in the model, with the latent category variable "personality characteristics" as the moderator, the scores of different factors in the family environment scale as the predictor variable and the scores of adolescent sexual control, sexual self-adaptability and sexual social adaptability classified as the dependent variables. Thus, the mixed regression model of the relationship between the family environment and adolescent sexual adaptability was constructed.

The results showed that for boys with different personality traits, no family environmental factors influenced their sexual control ability, sexual self-adaptability and sexual social adaptability. As shown in Table 4, for girls in the first category, the balanced group, expressiveness factors in the family environment improved their sexual adaptability ($p < 0.05$), intellectual–cultural orientation and organization promoted their social adaptability ($p < 0.05$) and active–recreational orientation and control decreased their social adaptability ($p < 0.05$). For girls in the second category, the high-neuroticism group, cohesion in the family environment facilitated their sexual control ($p < 0.05$), while conflict and organization reduced their sexual control ability and active–recreational orientation decreased their sexual adaptation ($p < 0.05$). For girls in the third category, the low-neuroticism and high-others group, no family-environment-related factors were found to influence their sexual adaptability.

Table 4. Mixture regression model of family environment and adolescent's sexual adaptability (personality latent category variables as the moderator).

| Sexual Adaptation | Family Environment Variables (Based on Personality) | Estimate | S.E. | Est./S.E | p |
|---|---|---|---|---|---|
| Sexual Control | | | | | |
| | Girl-High-Neu Group | | | | |
| | Cohesion | 0.116 | 0.040 | 2.900 | 0.004 |
| | Conflict | −0.112 | 0.041 | −2.759 | 0.006 |
| | Organization | −0.100 | 0.051 | −1.967 | 0.049 |
| Sexual Self-Adaptation | | | | | |
| | Girl-Balanced Group | | | | |
| | Expressiveness | 0.108 | 0.025 | 4.425 | 0.000 |
| Social Adaptation | | | | | |
| | Girl-Balanced Group | | | | |
| | Intellectual–cultural orientation | 0.043 | 0.020 | 2.088 | 0.037 |
| | Active–recreational orientation | −0.048 | 0.020 | −2.433 | 0.015 |
| | Organization | 0.055 | 0.027 | 2.062 | 0.039 |
| | Control | −0.052 | 0.022 | −2.386 | 0.017 |
| | Girl-High-Neu Group | | | | |
| | Active–recreational orientation | −0.270 | 0.132 | −2.052 | 0.040 |

Note: *The model controls the demographic characteristics and only displays the significance variables ($p < 0.05$).*

## 6. Discussion

To the best of our knowledge, there have been few studies on the relationship between the family environment and psychosexual health in China, and most studies focused on the parent–child communication [19] and parenting style [20]. Studies showing the impact of the family environment from various dimensions on the psychosexual health of adolescents are relatively rare. In addition, a large number of studies found that the formation of personality is related to the family environment [21,22], and there is a certain relationship between personality and sexual activities [23], so it is necessary to stratify personality when analyzing the impact of the family environment on adolescent psychosexual health. However, thus far, we have not found papers published on this subject. Our research results also confirmed that for adolescents with different personality traits, the influence of the family environment on their sexual adaptability was different.

Among girls, the subjects in the first group of personality traits (the group with balanced scores) had the most dimensions affected by the family environment, and a total of five dimensions affected their sexual self-adaptation and sexual social adaptation. For girls of this type, the intellectual–cultural orientation, organization, active–recreational orientation and control factors in the family environment all influenced their sexual social adaptability, among which intellectual–cultural orientation and organization had positive effects, while active–recreational orientation and control had negative effects. Family knowledge helped to develop a much healthier lifestyle, overcome difficulties and handle stress, and family intellectual–cultural orientation was the supportive basis of building a good interpersonal relationship. Studies have found that the less knowledgeable family members are, the more mental health problems teenagers have [24]. This study also showed that family knowledge of female adolescents had a positive correlation with their sexual social adaptability. Organization in the family environment is a manifestation of achieving unified action easily within a family, and girls in highly organized families in this study had better social adaptability. Adolescence is a critical period for gender identity, peer relationships and self-identity. Different teenagers of different genders express their emotions in different ways. Men often express their emotions through behavior, while women often do so through verbal communication [25]. This study showed that family expressiveness has a protective effect on female sexual self-adaptation, suggesting that positive emotional expression in the family of female adolescents is conducive to improving sexual self-adaptation.

For girls with personality traits in the second group (in which the neuroticism score was higher than the other groups), the influence of the family environment mainly focused on sexual control. Family cohesion exerts a positive influence on sexual control, and it is an important embodiment of the quality of family relationships. Other studies also show that a poor quality of family relationships is significantly related to the occurrence of teenagers browsing pornographic information and looking at pornographic pictures [26]. Conflict and organization had a negative influence on sexual control. Conflict means a disharmony of the family environment, and organization refers to a scheduled, demanding and planned mode of action in the family. Some studies show that conflict and too much emphasis on rules in the family environment cause psychological pressure on adolescents [27]. Adolescents in this family environment may be more inclined to relieve their pressure through sexual release. At the same time, research has found that active–recreational orientation can have a negative impact on teenagers' sexual social adaptation, which may be related to the inner conflict caused by the fact that excessive emphasis on entertainment may deviate from social norms.

However, research on male students shows that the influence of the family environment on their psychosexual health is relatively low. In our study, no matter what kind of personality traits the boys had, we did not find any family environment factors that had an impact on their sexual control, sexual self-adaptability and sexual social adaptability. From the above results, we can see that, compared to the girls, the psychosexual development of male adolescents was less affected by the family environment. Other existing studies have also shown that there are gender differences between boys and girls in terms of many psychological issues [28], and that girls are more susceptible to the family environment [29]. A study on adolescents in eastern China found that the family environment would cause a higher occurrence of hysteria tendency among girls than among men. [30]. In addition, gender differences existed in other aspects of our study. We found that girls had lower sexual self-adaptability than boys, and the difference was statistically significant, which was similar to research results from other countries [31,32]. The difference is likely related to the dual perception held for both genders. Our investigation of adolescents' sexual adaptation mainly started from the three aspects of accepting their own physical characteristics, their own gender identity and acceptance and harmony with the opposite sex. Some relevant studies have shown that a low level of self-acceptance is related to depression and anxiety [33], and also associated with low self-esteem and low life satisfaction [34]. Therefore, more attention should be paid to girls' sexual self-adaptability, as it is of greater realistic value. Although, in recent decades, international and Chinese scholars have committed to promoting gender equality, the physiological differences between men and women, the constraints of traditional ideas and the gender division of labor and power inequality in work and family are still influential in reality. Among Chinese adolescents, there still exist gender differences in the acceptance and identification of their own gender, which suggests that a gender-differentiated intervention strategy should be adopted in the family scheme to encourage adolescents to happily accept their sexual changes and consciously constrain and adjust their sexual desires and behaviors according to the requirements of social and cultural norms.

## 7. Conclusions

We found that girls' sexual self-adaptability was lower than boys; meanwhile, girls' overall sexual adaptability was more susceptible to various dimensions of the family environment. For female adolescents with different personality traits, the influence of the family environment on their sexual adaptability was different. This suggests that a gender-differentiated and personality-differentiated intervention strategy should be adopted in the family scheme to promote sexual adaptation.

## 8. Limitations

Our study had some limitations. First, at present, the definition of the family environment is very broad, and Chinese and international scholars hold different opinions. Although the family environment scale (FES) is a widely used measurement tool, its application in China also has limitations (this study removed the subscale that was obviously not suitable for China), and the subscale applied in this study was not inclusive enough to cover all aspects of the family environment. Second, this study was only a cross-sectional study of two research sites, suggesting that the research results may not directly represent the overall situation of the whole country, and that there was also some uncertainty in the causal inference. In the future, more regions should be included in our longitudinal studies. Third, we found that adolescents in Shanghai and Shanxi showed differences in the scores of sexual social adaptability and sexual control, but due to the limited length of the paper, we did not further analyze the geographical differences and the possible reasons.

## 9. Future Prospects

Based on the relevant evidence provided by this study, adolescent psychosexual health interventions with different gender and personality characteristics could be conducted, which could further improve the sexual mental health level of Chinese adolescents. At the same time, we hope that the whole of society pays attention to adolescents' psychosexual health, especially the problems related to girls' sexual adaptability.

**Author Contributions:** Conceptualization, J.L., HS., J.W. and L.W.; Methodology, R.Z., J.L., Y.G., Y.L., H.S., J.Z. and L.W.; Formal analysis, R.Z., Y.G. and J.Z.; Investigation, Y.L. and J.Z.; Data curation, Y.L.; Writing – original draft, R.Z.; Writing – review & editing, J.L., Y.G., H.S., J.W. and L.W.; Supervision, J.W. All authors have read and agreed to the published version of the manuscript.

**Funding:** The study was funded by the Youth Project of Shanghai Municipal Health Commission (20174Y0190), The National Social Science Fund of China (19BRK015), the Shanghai Institute for Biomedical and Pharmaceutical Technologies (ZC19-11-1) and The Fifth Round of the Three-Year Public Health Action Plan of Shanghai (GWV-10.1-XK08). The funders had no role in the study design, data collection, analysis, decision to publish or preparation of the manuscript.

**Institutional Review Board Statement:** The study was conducted in accordance with the Declaration of Helsinki and approved by the Institutional ethics committee of the Shanghai Institute of Planned Parenthood Research (PJ2017–25). Approval date: 10 May 2017.

**Informed Consent Statement:** Before the survey, we sent out passive consent letters to the parents or guardians of all subjects via their schools. The parents or guardians were required to return a signed form if they did not want their child to participate in the survey. We obtained active consent from the subjects by asking all subjects if they agreed to participate at the very beginning of the survey.

**Data Availability Statement:** The datasets used and/or analyzed during the current study are available from the corresponding author on reasonable request.

**Acknowledgments:** The authors thank the cooperation of the school and students involved.

**Conflicts of Interest:** The authors declare no conflict of interest.

# References

1. Fortenberry, J.D. Puberty and adolescent sexuality. *Horm. Behav.* **2013**, *64*, 280–287. [CrossRef] [PubMed]

2. Layland, E.K.; Ram, N.; Caldwell, L.L.; Smith, E.A.; Wegner, L. Leisure Boredom, Timing of Sexual Debut, and Co-Occurring Behaviors among South African Adolescents. *Arch. Sex. Behav.* **2021**, *50*, 2383–2394. [CrossRef] [PubMed]
3. Warner, T.D.; Warner, D.F. Precocious and Problematic? The Consequences of Youth Violent Victimization for Adolescent Sexual Behavior. *J. Dev. Life-Course Criminol.* **2019**, *5*, 554–586. [CrossRef] [PubMed]
4. Dosch, A.; Rochat, L.; Ghisletta, P.; Favez, N.; Van der Linden, M. Psychological Factors Involved in Sexual Desire, Sexual Activity, and Sexual Satisfaction: A Multi-factorial Perspective. *Arch. Sex. Behav.* **2016**, *45*, 2029–2045. [CrossRef]
5. Luo, Y.; Zheng, Y. Preliminary study of sexual mental health during adolescence. *Chin. J. Psychol. Sci.* **2006**, *29*, 661–664+657.
6. Lian, Q.; Zuo, X.; Yu, C.; Lou, C.; Tu, X.; Zhou, W. Associations of Gender Dissatisfaction with Adolescent Mental Distress and Sexual Victimization. *Children* **2022**, *9*, 1221. [CrossRef]
7. Milano, W.; Ambrosio, P.; Carizzone, F.; De Biasio, V.; Foggia, G.; Capasso, A. Gender Dysphoria, Eating Disorders and Body Image: An Overview. *Endocr. Metab. Immune Disord. Drug Targets* **2020**, *20*, 518–524. [CrossRef]
8. Miller, E.; Jones, K.A.; McCauley, H.L. Updates on adolescent dating and sexual violence prevention and intervention. *Curr. Opin. Pediatr.* **2018**, *30*, 466–471. [CrossRef]
9. Pokhrel, P.; Bennett, B.L.; Regmi, S.; Idrisov, B.; Galimov, A.; Akhmadeeva, L.; Sussman, S. Individualism-Collectivism, Social Self-Control and Adolescent Substance Use and Risky Sexual Behavior. *Subst. Use Misuse* **2018**, *53*, 1057–1067. [CrossRef]
10. Molina Cartes, R.; González Araya, E. Teenage pregnancy. *Endocr. Dev.* **2012**, *22*, 302–331. [CrossRef]
11. Song, Y.M.; Sung, J.; Lee, K. Associations Between Adiposity and Metabolic Syndrome Over Time: The Healthy Twin Study. *Metab. Syndr. Relat. Disord.* **2017**, *15*, 124–129. [CrossRef] [PubMed]
12. Ibabe, I. Adolescent-to-Parent Violence and Family Environment: The Perceptions of Same Reality? *Int. J. Environ. Res. Public Health* **2019**, *16*, 2215. [CrossRef] [PubMed]
13. Kaestle, C.E.; Allen, K.R.; Wesche, R.; Grafsky, E.L. Adolescent Sexual Development: A Family Perspective. *J. Sex Res.* **2021**, *58*, 874–890. [CrossRef] [PubMed]
14. Huang, J.P.; Xia, W.; Sun, C.H.; Zhang, H.Y.; Wu, L.J. Psychological distress and its correlates in Chinese adolescents. *Aust. New Zealand J. Psychiatr.* **2009**, *43*, 674–681. [CrossRef] [PubMed]
15. Dittus, P.J.; Michael, S.L.; Becasen, J.S.; Gloppen, K.M.; McCarthy, K.; Guilamo-Ramos, V. Parental Monitoring and Its Associations With Adolescent Sexual Risk Behavior: A Meta-analysis. *Pediatrics* **2015**, *136*, e1587–e1599. [CrossRef] [PubMed]
16. Rogers, A.A.; Ha, T.; Stormshak, E.A.; Dishion, T.J. Quality of Parent-Adolescent Conversations About Sex and Adolescent Sexual Behavior: An Observational Study. *J. Adolesc. Health Off. Publ. Soc. Adolesc. Med.* **2015**, *57*, 174–178. [CrossRef]
17. Moos, R.H. Conceptual and empirical approaches to developing family-based assessment procedures: Resolving the case of the Family Environment Scale. *Fam. Process* **1990**, *29*, 199–211. [CrossRef]
18. McCrae, R.R.; Costa, P.T.A. contemplated revision of the NEO Five-Factor Inventory. *Personal. Individ. Differ.* **2004**, *36*, 587–596. [CrossRef]
19. Xie, Q.H.; Yang, Y.P.; Ou, W.; He, J.; Wang, Z. Parent-child communication and their relationship with sexual mental health among left-behind middle school students in northern Guizhou province. *Chin. J. Sch. Health* **2014**, *6*, 898–900. [CrossRef]
20. Li, X.; Xiao, T.; Liu, Y.; Liu, Q.; Jiang, H.; Wang, H.J.; Wang, H.D. Correlations among adolescent sexual knowledge, sexual attitude, family-rearing style and self-protection consciousness. *Chin. J. Health Educ.* **2018**, *4*, 317–320+324. [CrossRef]
21. Krauss, S.; Orth, U.; Robins, R.W. Family environment and self-esteem development: A longitudinal study from age 10 to 16. *J. Personal. Soc. Psychol.* **2020**, *119*, 457–478. [CrossRef] [PubMed]
22. Persson, B. Genotype-Environment Correlation and Its Relation to Personality—A Twin and Family Study. *Twin Res. Hum. Genet. Off. J. Int. Soc. Twin Stud.* **2020**, *4*, 228–234. [CrossRef] [PubMed]
23. Allen, M.S.; Walter, E.E. Linking big five personality traits to sexuality and sexual health: A meta-analytic review. *Psychol. Bull.* **2018**, *144*, 1081–1110. [CrossRef] [PubMed]
24. Cong, E.Z.; Wu, Y.; Cai, Y.Y.; Chen, H.Y.; Xu, Y.F. Association of suicidal ideation with family environment and psychological resilience in adolescents. *Chin. J. Contemp. Pediatr.* **2019**, *5*, 479–484. [CrossRef]
25. Lowry, R.; Johns, M.M.; Gordon, A.R.; Austin, S.B.; Robin, L.E.; Kann, L.K. Nonconforming Gender Expression and Associated Mental Distress and Substance Use Among High School Students. *JAMA Pediatr.* **2018**, *172*, 1020–1028. [CrossRef]
26. Ybarra, M.L.; Mitchell, K.J. Exposure to internet pornography among children and adolescents: A national survey. *Cyberpsychology Behav.* **2005**, *8*, 473–486. [CrossRef]
27. Lucas-Thompson, R.G.; Goldberg, W.A. Family relationships and children's stress responses. *Adv. Child Dev. Behav.* **2011**, *40*, 243–299. [CrossRef]
28. Marjoribanks, K. Family contexts, individual characteristics, proximal settings, and adolescents' aspirations. *Psychol. Rep.* **2002**, *91*, 769–779. [CrossRef]
29. Fuligni, A.J.; Zhang, W. Attitudes toward family obligation among adolescents in contemporary urban and rural China. *Child Dev.* **2004**, *75*, 180–192. [CrossRef]
30. Zhao, G.; Xie, L.; Xu, Y.; Cheng, Q. A Multicenter Cross-sectional Study on the Prevalence and Impact Factors of Hysteria Tendency in the Eastern Chinese Adolescents. *Iran. J. Public Health* **2018**, *47*, 1854–1864.
31. Matud, M.P.; López-Curbelo, M.; Fortes, D. Gender and Psychological Well-Being. *Int. J. Environ. Res. Public Health* **2019**, *16*, 3531. [CrossRef] [PubMed]

32. Brederecke, J.; Scott, J.L.; de Zwaan, M.; Brähler, E.; Neuner, F.; Quinn, M.; Zimmermann, T. Psychometric properties of the German version of the Self-Image Scale (SIS-D). *PLoS ONE* **2020**, *15*, e0230331. [CrossRef] [PubMed]
33. Kaltiala-Heino, R.; Bergman, H.; Työläjärvi, M.; Frisén, L. Gender dysphoria in adolescence: Current perspectives. *Adolesc. Health Med. Ther.* **2018**, *9*, 31–41. [CrossRef] [PubMed]
34. MacInnes, D.L. Self-esteem and self-acceptance: An examination into their relationship and their effect on psychological health. *J. Psychiatr. Ment. Health Nurs.* **2006**, *13*, 483–489. [CrossRef]

**Disclaimer/Publisher's Note:** The statements, opinions and data contained in all publications are solely those of the individual author(s) and contributor(s) and not of MDPI and/or the editor(s). MDPI and/or the editor(s) disclaim responsibility for any injury to people or property resulting from any ideas, methods, instructions or products referred to in the content.

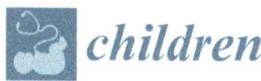 

Article

# The Influence of Parent's Cardiovascular Morbidity on Child Mental Health: Results from the National Health Interview Survey

Biplab Kumar Datta [1,2], Ashwini Tiwari [1,*], Elinita Pollard [3] and Havilah Ravula [3]

[1] Institute of Public and Preventive Health, Augusta University, Augusta, GA 30912, USA
[2] Department of Population Health Sciences, Medical College of Georgia, Augusta University, Augusta, GA 30912, USA
[3] Department of Psychological Sciences, Augusta University, Augusta, GA 30912, USA
* Correspondence: atiwari@augusta.edu

**Abstract:** Background: This study assessed the association between cardiovascular disease (CVD), the leading cause of death in the United States, among parents and child mental health. Methods: Our sample included 9076 children aged 6 to 17 years. Data were pooled from the 2016–2018 waves of the National Health Interview Survey. We fitted a logistic regression to obtain the odds ratios in favor of child mental health problems for parental CVD. We also fitted a multinomial logistic regression to obtain the odds in favor of the severity of mental health problems (i.e., minor, definite, and severe). Results: The adjusted odds of facing difficulties for a child of a parent with CVD were 1.64 (95% CI: 1.28–2.11) times that of their peers whose parents did not have CVD. The adjusted relative risk of facing minor and definite difficulties for a child of a parent with CVD were 1.48 (95% CI: 1.13–1.94) and 2.25 (95% CI: 1.47–3.46) times that of their peers of parents without CVD. Conclusions: The results suggest a strong association between child mental health and parental cardiovascular morbidity, demonstrating the need for the development or adaptation of existing public health interventions to facilitate mental health support for children of parents with CVD.

**Keywords:** cardiovascular disease; child mental health; parents; chronic disease

Citation: Datta, B.K.; Tiwari, A.; Pollard, E.; Ravula, H. The Influence of Parent's Cardiovascular Morbidity on Child Mental Health: Results from the National Health Interview Survey. Children 2023, 10, 138. https://doi.org/10.3390/children10010138

Academic Editor: Tingzhong Yang

Received: 14 December 2022
Revised: 3 January 2023
Accepted: 6 January 2023
Published: 11 January 2023

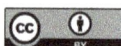

Copyright: © 2023 by the authors. Licensee MDPI, Basel, Switzerland. This article is an open access article distributed under the terms and conditions of the Creative Commons Attribution (CC BY) license (https://creativecommons.org/licenses/by/4.0/).

## 1. Introduction

Cardiovascular diseases (CVD) are the leading causes of morbidity and mortality worldwide [1]. In general, CVD risk is associated with prevalent risk factors such as childhood obesity, adulthood obesity, hypertension, consumption of low-quality foods, diabetes, and smoking [2–5]. Further, several studies offer evidence on independent links between CVD development and non-traditional predictors such as psychosocial stress, low socioeconomic status, negative affective reactions and emotions, sleep deprivation, and a lack of social support [6–10].

It is projected that by 2030, 40.5% of people in the United States will have some form of CVD [11]. Further, a growing concern has been the rising incidence of premature CVD, or CVD occurring among males aged ≤55 years and females aged ≤65 years [12], who are likely caregivers for children and adolescent populations. As such, it is critical to consider that the adverse effects of CVD may not only have implications for the individual with CVD, but downstream effects on child functioning and wellbeing.

To date, however, no studies have examined the direct or indirect impact of parental CVD on child health outcomes. Related literature on chronic pain, which may also be observed in CVD cases [13], could provide relevant insight on the plausible relationship between parental CVD and child mental health and behaviors. For example, recent evidence and a systematic review suggest that parental chronic pain and illness increase the risk of child psychological dysfunction, including increased internalizing symptoms for depression and anxiety [14,15]. Parental illness may also potentially affect child mental health through financial strain as well, which can increase parenting stress [16]. It is conceivable that in the case of CVD, reciprocal consequences of psychological distress may exacerbate CVD symptoms. In turn, these cyclical effects may extend the chronicity and severity of the disease, which are associated with exacerbating mental health symptoms among children [17]. As such, the investigation of the relationship between parental CVD conditions and children's mental health may indeed be warranted.

CVD research in general is limited in its exploration of related household effects among children. Extant literature instead focuses on associations between CVD and factors known to increase the risk for poor child outcomes. For example, the risk of CVD morbidity and mortality among adults is linked to the development of chronic stress, depression, and anxiety [18–20]. While unexplored in the context of CVD, such poor parental mental health is a known risk factor for behavioral and mental health outcomes among children. Further, several empirical studies among younger and adolescent aged children of parents with mental health symptoms indicate that children may experience difficulties in social interactions and emotion regulation, as well as internalizing disorder symptoms such has depression and anxiety [21–24]. Yet, the potentially meaningful association between parental CVD and child outcomes has remained unexplored.

Addressing this gap is critical to help identify resources and relevant public health strategies to reduce the risk of mental health adversity among children. As such, the primary objective of the current study was to use nationally representative data to examine whether parental CVD diagnosis is associated with negative mental health among children under 18 years of age.

## 2. Materials and Methods

### 2.1. Data

We used data from the 2016, 2017, and 2018 waves of the National Health Interview Survey (NHIS). The NHIS data include a "Sample Child file" that provides information on children aged 17 and under; and a "Sample Adult file" that provides information on individuals aged 18 and over. Both files include unique identifiers for families within a household and persons within a family. Further, the "Sample Child file" includes information on a sample child's relationship with a sample adult in the family. This allowed us to match children from the "Sample Child file" with their parents in the "Sample Adult file". Our study sample included 9080 children aged 6 to 17 years, for whom we were able to match children and parents in both data files.

### 2.2. Measures

In the "Sample Child" survey, under the "Child Mental Health Brief Questionnaire" module, adult respondents were asked if the respondent thought that the child had difficulties in any of the following areas: (i) emotions; (ii) concentration; (iii) behavior; or (iv) being able to get along with other people. The response options were as follows: (i) no; (ii) yes—minor difficulties; (iii) yes—definite difficulties; and (iv) yes—severe difficulties. A child was deemed to have mental health problems if they reported having minor, definite, or severe difficulties in any of the aforementioned areas. We later checked sensitivity by defining mental health problems as having definite or severe difficulties. For the general analysis, the binary outcome variable took the value 1 if minor, definite, or severe difficulties were reported, and 0 if otherwise. For the sensitivity analysis, the binary outcome variable took the value 1 if definite or severe difficulties were reported, and 0 if otherwise.

As a robustness check, we considered four mental health indicators as follows: (i) the child has many worries or often seemed worried; (ii) the child is often unhappy, depressed, or tearful; (iii) the child is generally well behaved and usually does what adults request; and (iv) the child has good attention span. Adult respondents were asked whether in the past six months preceding the survey, these conditions were not, somewhat, or certainly true for the child. A child was deemed to have the condition if it was reported somewhat or certainly true.

In the "Sample Adult" module, respondents were asked if they were ever told by a doctor or other health professionals that they had (i) coronary heart disease; (ii) angina pectoris; (iii) myocardial infarction; and (iv) any other heart condition or heart disease. A respondent was determined to have cardiovascular morbidity if they reported having any of these conditions.

*2.3. Statistical Analysis*

We first assessed the frequency of children having no, minor, definite, and severe problems by parent's CVD condition. We performed adjusted Wald tests to examine whether the differences were statistically significant. Level of significance was set at 5% level.

Next, we estimated a binomial logistic regression to obtain the odds ratios in favor of mental health problem for parent's CVD condition indicator. Our outcome variable was a binary variable indicating whether the child had a mental health problem or not. Our explanatory variable was another binary variable indicating whether the parent of the child had CVD or not.

We then estimated a multivariable specification where we controlled for several sociodemographic characteristics of children and their parents. Correlates related to children include age, sex, and race. Correlates related to parents include age, sex, marital status, educational attainment, employment status, and self-reported health conditions. We also accounted for household income (as share of federal poverty level threshold) and U.S. Census Bureau region fixed effects. Of note, these covariates were not included in the model to assess their relationship with the outcome variable, but to examine whether the relationship between child mental health problems and parent's CVD condition persisted after taking these sociodemographic attributes into account.

As a sensitivity check, both univariate and multivariable specifications were also estimated for child mental health problems, defined as having "definite or severe" difficulties instead of "minor, definite, or severe" difficulties. Next, separate logistic regressions were estimated for the four mental health conditions to check the robustness of the original results. The outcome variable for each condition was a binary variable indicating whether that condition was true for the child.

Lastly, we estimated a multinomial logistic regression to assess the degree of severity of the problem. We obtained unadjusted and adjusted relative risk ratios in favor of having (i) minor difficulties; (ii) definite difficulties; and (iii) severe difficulties, relative to the base outcome of "no difficulty" for the parent's CVD indicator. All estimates were obtained using complex survey weight of the NHIS and using Stata 17.0 software.

## 3. Results

Around 6% of the children in our sample had parents with CVD. Table 1 presents the descriptive statistics of the study participants by parent's CVD condition. For the majority of the children (~70%), data on the mother's information was included. Approximately 60% of parents were married in child households. While the children's and their parents' sex and race, in general, were comparable across the exposure (i.e., parent had CVD) and the control (i.e., parent did not have CVD) groups, the percent of parents with marital dissolution/disruption (i.e., widowhood, divorce, or separation) was higher (29% vs. 19%) among those who had CVD. Parents with CVD had lower (66% vs. 74%) employment and poorer self-reported health (Table 1).

**Table 1.** Descriptive statistics.

| | Percentage of Children | | |
|---|---|---|---|
| | All | Parent Did Not Have CVD | Parent Had CVD |
| Child's sex | | | |
| Male | 51.21 | 51.33 | 49.35 |
| Female | 48.79 | 48.67 | 50.65 |
| Race | | | |
| White | 52.48 | 52.16 | 57.41 |
| Black | 14.27 | 14.31 | 13.76 |
| Hispanic | 23.89 | 24.2 | 19.18 |
| Other | 9.36 | 9.34 | 9.66 |
| Parent's sex | | | |
| Male | 29.43 | 29.26 | 31.98 |
| Female | 70.57 | 70.74 | 68.02 |
| Parent's marital status | | | |
| Married | 61.27 | 61.54 | 57.25 |
| Never married | 12.8 | 13.01 | 9.55 |
| Living with partner | 6.35 | 6.48 | 4.27 |
| Widowed/divorced/separated | 19.58 | 18.97 | 28.93 |
| Parent's education | | | |
| College graduate | 36.26 | 36.29 | 35.83 |
| <High school diploma | 12.85 | 13 | 10.59 |
| High school graduate | 19.01 | 19.21 | 16.03 |
| Some college | 31.87 | 31.5 | 37.56 |
| Parent's employment | | | |
| Not employed | 26.27 | 25.75 | 34.26 |
| Employed | 73.73 | 74.25 | 65.74 |
| Parent's self-reported health | | | |
| Excellent | 30.6 | 31.63 | 14.86 |
| Very good | 34.62 | 35.22 | 25.41 |
| Good | 25.74 | 25.25 | 33.14 |
| Fair | 7.43 | 6.67 | 19.07 |
| Poor | 1.62 | 1.23 | 7.51 |
| Household income | | | |
| ≥400% of FPL | 30.39 | 30.53 | 28.29 |
| <100% of FPL | 19.8 | 19.48 | 24.67 |
| 100% to <200% of FPL | 22.8 | 22.96 | 20.35 |
| 200% to <400% of FPL | 27.01 | 27.03 | 26.69 |
| Observations | 9076 | 8513 | 563 |

Note: Estimates were obtained using complex survey weights. Parent's marital status was not available for 5 observations. Parent's education was not available for 13 observations. Parent's employment status was not available for 4 observations. Parent's self-reported health status was not available for 1 observation. Household income was not available for 399 observations.

Among children whose parents did not have CVD, 77.0% reported no difficulties in in emotions, concentration, behavior, or being able to get along with other people. This proportion was 15.0 percentage-points (pp) lower among children whose parents had CVD. Though the difference between children with parents having and not having CVD was not statistically significant for the "severe" difficulties outcome, statistically significant differences were observed for both "minor" and "definite" difficulties outcomes (Table 2).

**Table 2.** Share of children having difficulties in emotions, concentration, behavior, or being able to get along with other people—by parent's cardiovascular diseases.

|  | No Difficulty | Difficulties | | |
|---|---|---|---|---|
|  |  | Minor | Definite | Severe |
| Parent's CVD |  |  |  |  |
| No | 77.03 | 16.88 | 4.61 | 1.48 |
|  | (75.89, 78.16) | (15.89, 17.87) | (4.05, 5.16) | (1.18, 1.79) |
| Yes | 62.00 | 23.89 | 11.39 | 2.73 |
|  | (56.92, 67.07) | (19.58, 28.19) | (8.02, 14.77) | (1.27, 4.19) |
| Difference |  |  |  |  |
| CVD—No CVD | −15.03 *** | 7.00 ** | 6.79 *** | 1.24 |
|  | (−20.22, −9.85) | (2.6, 11.41) | (3.37, 10.21) | (−0.24, 2.72) |
| Observations | 6832 | 1608 | 477 | 159 |

Note: Estimates were obtained using complex survey weights. *** $p < 0.001$, ** $p < 0.01$.

Table 3 presents the crude and adjusted odds of having mental health problems. The odds of having minor, definite, or severe difficulties for children whose parents had CVD were 2.1 times that of their counterparts whose parents did not have CVD. When the socioeconomic and demographic characteristics, along with parent's self-reported health status, were accounted for, the adjusted odds ratio slightly decreased to 1.6. Similar were the results for the odds of having definite, or severe difficulties. Children whose parents had CVD were 2.5 times more likely to have definite, or severe difficulties compared with children whose parents did not have CVD. Like the original specification, the adjusted odds ratio in the sensitivity analysis was also slightly smaller.

**Table 3.** Crude and adjusted odds ratios in favor of difficulties in emotions, concentration, behavior, or being able to get along with other people.

|  | Original Specification | | Sensitivity Analysis | |
|---|---|---|---|---|
|  | Crude Odds Ratio | Adjusted Odds Ratio | Crude Odds Ratio | Adjusted Odds Ratio |
| CVD | 2.056 *** | 1.641 *** | 2.535 *** | 1.862 *** |
|  | (1.643, 2.571) | (1.279, 2.105) | (1.843, 3.487) | (1.295, 2.677) |
| Child's age | 1.016 | 1.014 | 1.028 | 1.030 |
|  | (0.998, 1.033) | (0.993, 1.036) | (0.999, 1.059) | (0.997, 1.065) |
| Child's sex |  |  |  |  |
| Male | Ref. | Ref. | Ref. | Ref. |
| Female | 0.627 *** | 0.609 *** | 0.517 *** | 0.509 *** |
|  | (0.561, 0.701) | (0.541, 0.685) | (0.424, 0.630) | (0.412, 0.630) |
| Race |  |  |  |  |
| White | Ref. | Ref. | Ref. | Ref. |
| Black | 0.988 | 0.710 ** | 0.859 | 0.542 ** |
|  | (0.816, 1.196) | (0.565, 0.892) | (0.642, 1.151) | (0.369, 0.798) |
| Hispanic | 0.698 *** | 0.553 *** | 0.724 * | 0.493 *** |
|  | (0.596, 0.816) | (0.457, 0.669) | (0.561, 0.934) | (0.364, 0.667) |
| Other | 0.816 * | 0.758 * | 0.778 | 0.645 * |
|  | (0.666, 0.999) | (0.611, 0.941) | (0.547, 1.107) | (0.447, 0.933) |
| Parent's age | 0.992 | 0.992 | 0.989 | 0.988 |
|  | (0.984, 1.000) | (0.982, 1.002) | (0.975, 1.003) | (0.972, 1.005) |
| Parent's sex |  |  |  |  |
| Male | Ref. | Ref. | Ref. | Ref. |
| Female | 1.593 *** | 1.352 *** | 2.031 *** | 1.634 *** |
|  | (1.374, 1.846) | (1.147, 1.595) | (1.549, 2.662) | (1.222, 2.186) |

Table 3. Cont.

|  | Original Specification | | Sensitivity Analysis | |
| --- | --- | --- | --- | --- |
|  | Crude Odds Ratio | Adjusted Odds Ratio | Crude Odds Ratio | Adjusted Odds Ratio |
| Parent's marital status |  |  |  |  |
| Married | Ref. | Ref. | Ref. | Ref. |
| Never married | 1.748 *** | 1.550 *** | 1.931 *** | 1.438 |
|  | (1.466, 2.085) | (1.233, 1.949) | (1.465, 2.545) | (0.999, 2.070) |
| Living with partner | 1.796 *** | 1.658 *** | 2.655 *** | 2.352 *** |
|  | (1.418, 2.274) | (1.283, 2.142) | (1.867, 3.776) | (1.624, 3.406) |
| Widowed/divorced/separated | 1.709 *** | 1.471 *** | 2.277 *** | 1.676 *** |
|  | (1.477, 1.978) | (1.236, 1.750) | (1.796, 2.887) | (1.262, 2.226) |
| Parent's education |  |  |  |  |
| College graduate | Ref. | Ref. | Ref. | Ref. |
| < High school diploma | 1.211 | 0.957 | 1.374 | 0.755 |
|  | (0.983, 1.491) | (0.733, 1.248) | (0.960, 1.965) | (0.492, 1.156) |
| High school graduate | 1.182 | 0.903 | 1.446 * | 0.835 |
|  | (0.999, 1.398) | (0.732, 1.113) | (1.077, 1.941) | (0.598, 1.168) |
| Some college | 1.448 *** | 1.086 | 1.373 * | 0.774 |
|  | (1.254, 1.673) | (0.914, 1.292) | (1.073, 1.756) | (0.594, 1.009) |
| Parent's employment |  |  |  |  |
| Not employed | Ref. | Ref. | Ref. | Ref. |
| Employed | 0.676 *** | 0.812 ** | 0.672 *** | 0.996 |
|  | (0.598, 0.766) | (0.694, 0.951) | (0.548, 0.825) | (0.785, 1.263) |
| Parent's self-reported health |  |  |  |  |
| Excellent | Ref. | Ref. | Ref. | Ref. |
| Very good | 1.656 *** | 1.596 *** | 1.812 *** | 1.685 ** |
|  | (1.391, 1.971) | (1.326, 1.921) | (1.297, 2.530) | (1.190, 2.385) |
| Good | 2.526 *** | 2.455 *** | 3.376 *** | 3.137 *** |
|  | (2.114, 3.017) | (2.017, 2.988) | (2.423, 4.702) | (2.192, 4.490) |
| Fair | 3.679 *** | 3.305 *** | 5.480 *** | 4.694 *** |
|  | (2.913, 4.646) | (2.547, 4.288) | (3.798, 7.908) | (3.109, 7.086) |
| Poor | 7.088 *** | 4.856 *** | 11.865 *** | 7.873 *** |
|  | (4.702, 10.686) | (3.128, 7.539) | (7.085, 19.871) | (4.462, 13.891) |
| Household income |  |  |  |  |
| ≥400% of FPL | Ref. | Ref. | Ref. | Ref. |
| <100% of FPL | 1.752 *** | 1.073 | 2.416 *** | 1.570 * |
|  | (1.474, 2.082) | (0.832, 1.384) | (1.802, 3.241) | (1.031, 2.392) |
| 100% to <200% of FPL | 1.384 *** | 1.037 | 1.979 *** | 1.516 * |
|  | (1.172, 1.635) | (0.837, 1.284) | (1.499, 2.613) | (1.094, 2.100) |
| 200% to <400% of FPL | 1.176 | 0.970 | 1.073 | 0.886 |
|  | (0.997, 1.386) | (0.802, 1.172) | (0.789, 1.459) | (0.628, 1.249) |
| Observations | 9076 | 8663 | 9076 | 8663 |

Note: Estimates were obtained using complex survey weights. *** $p < 0.001$, ** $p < 0.01$, * $p < 0.05$. The multivariable specification controls for U.S. region fixed effects. In original specification, having mental health problem was defined as having minor-, definite-, or severe difficulties. In the sensitivity analysis, having mental health problem was defined as having definite, or severe difficulties.

Results of the robustness analyses for different mental health indicators are presented in Table 4. Compared with children whose parents did not have CVD, children whose parents had CVD were 1.3 times more likely to have many worries or often seemed worried. Children whose parents had CVD were also more likely to often be unhappy, depressed, or tearful. While no statistically significant difference in being well behaved or usually doing what adults request was observed between children with parents having and not-having CVD, children whose parents had CVD were 29.3% less likely to have a good attention span.

Table 4. Crude and adjusted odds ratios in favor of mental health indicators.

|  | Has Many Worries/Often Seemed Worried | Often Unhappy/ Depressed/ Tearful | Well Behaved/ Usually Does What Adults Request | Has Good Attention Span |
|---|---|---|---|---|
| A. Unadjusted |  |  |  |  |
| CVD | 1.754 *** | 1.866 *** | 0.617 | 0.604 ** |
|  | (1.406, 2.187) | (1.440, 2.419) | (0.349, 1.090) | (0.447, 0.818) |
| Observations | 9070 | 9070 | 9075 | 9072 |
| B. Adjusted |  |  |  |  |
| CVD | 1.307 * | 1.401 * | 0.764 | 0.717 * |
|  | (1.034, 1.653) | (1.060, 1.852) | (0.414, 1.411) | (0.516, 0.996) |
| Observations | 8658 | 8660 | 8663 | 8660 |

Note: Estimates were obtained using complex survey weights. *** $p < 0.001$, ** $p < 0.01$, * $p < 0.05$. The multivariable specification controls for child's age, sex, and race; parent's age, sex, marital status, educational attainment, employment status, and self-reported health status; household income and U.S. region fixed effects.

Lastly, the results of the multinomial specifications are presented in Table 5. Relative to the base outcome of no difficulty, children whose parents had CVD were 1.8, 3.1, and 2.3 times more likely to have minor-, definite-, and severe- difficulties, respectively, than those of their peers whose parents did not have CVD. The adjusted relative risk ratios were similar, though not statistically significant for the severe difficulties outcome.

Table 5. Relative risk ratios in favor of difficulties in emotions, concentration, behavior, or being able to get along with other people.

|  | Base Outcome: No Difficulty | Outcome I: Minor Difficulties | Outcome II: Definite Difficulties | Outcome III: Severe Difficulties |
|---|---|---|---|---|
| A. Unadjusted |  |  |  |  |
| CVD | Ref. | 1.758 *** | 3.073 *** | 2.282 ** |
|  |  | (1.363, 2.268) | (2.128, 4.439) | (1.265, 4.118) |
| B. Adjusted |  |  |  |  |
| CVD | Ref. | 1.480 ** | 2.250 *** | 1.605 |
|  |  | (1.129, 1.938) | (1.465, 3.455) | (0.890, 2.897) |

Note: Estimates were obtained using complex survey weights. *** $p < 0.001$, ** $p < 0.01$. The multivariable specification adjusted for the following covariates: child's age, child's sex, child's race, parent's age, parent's sex, parent's marital status, parent's educational attainment, parent's employment status, parent's self-reported health, household income as ratio of Federal Poverty Level, and U.S. region fixed effects.

## 4. Discussion

To the best of our knowledge, this is the first study to investigate associations between parental CVD with child mental health outcomes. Our findings indicate that children of parents with CVD may be more vulnerable to experiencing poor mental health outcomes compared to children whose parents do not have CVD. The findings of the current study are in concordance with the studies illustrating that parental illness may increase risk of mental health difficulties and psychosocial maladjustment among children and adolescents [25,26]. These results are also be in line with previous research that suggests parental illness can impact children's health-related quality of life, psychosomatic complaints, and life satisfaction [27–29].

Findings from the current study may be explained by several mechanisms. For example, some studies indicate that parental physical illness may increase existing, or create new caring demands placed on a child in a household [30,31]. For example, young caregivers under 18 years of age, referred to as 'young carers' [32], may be responsible for domestic, social, and emotional support responsibilities. The role-reversal and potential disruptions to routine functioning, may place them at risk of 'young carer penalty' [33], a term encompassing the new strains associated with caregiving across a youth's personal and external ecological systems. Drawing from evidence on youth carers, higher levels of caregiving among the youth of parents with chronic illness is associated with an increased likelihood of mental illness [34,35] and potential isolation [36]. However, we caution that more research is needed to understand the role of caregiving responsibilities among the youth of parents with CVD in predicting youth well-being.

Another explanation may be the effects of CVD on parent–child interactions. Although there is a dearth of literature in this area, and while beyond the scope of this paper, it is possible that the relationship between parent and child is negatively affected by the development or long-term burden of CVD in the household. As illustrated by McDowell and Parke's [37] tripartite model, parent–child interactions can have a significant influence over a child's development, including social competence. Relatedly, negative peer interactions, such as ostracization, are linked to poor mental health outcomes among children [38]. Taken together, child mental health outcomes among parents with CVD may be an indirect byproduct of a confluence of factors.

Notably, while this study could not examine parental mental health relative to CVD diagnosis or the temporality of these variables, pre-existing mental illness among parents may have a proximal effect on child mental health, as a family history of mental disorders, such as depression, is considered to be a strong predictor of developing disorders in adolescence [39]. It is also of importance to consider the role of other aforementioned psychosocial factors linked to CVD prognosis among adults. Recent findings suggest that perceptions of poor social support and a higher burden of stress among parents are likely to negatively impact parenting skills and child wellbeing [40]. The effects of psychosocial domains of influence on child health should be of rising interest to researchers studying at-risk parents for CVD following the COVID-19 pandemic, which heightened social isolation and mental illness for populations worldwide.

Our findings should be interpreted with some caution. First, in these cross-sectional data, we were not able to identify whether a parent's CV condition preceded a child's mental health condition and vice versa. As such, we cannot assume a causal interpretation. Second, due to the survey design, we were limited to data coming from one parent. Third, the CV conditions were self-reported; there was no information on the severity or frequency of the condition. Despite these limitations, our analyses using nationally representative data present a strong association between parental CVD condition and children's mental health outcomes.

## 5. Conclusions

This study provides an important contribution in understanding the association between parental cardiovascular morbidity and child mental health. Our findings suggest that children of parents with CVD may experience significant mental health adversity. While more longitudinal research is needed to understand how parental CVD relates to child mental illness, our findings suggest that children should be considered as an important target in therapeutic interventions for parents with CVD to prevent downstream adverse outcomes.

Of importance to note, the burden of CVD in the United States is substantial in magnitude and there are sizable disparities by socioeconomic status [41]. Children from lower SES groups may have a disproportionately higher risk of having mental health issues, channeled through their parents' cardiovascular health. This concern is particularly relevant to the pandemic, which has exacerbated the financial constraint across many households [42], and has had prognostic CVD implications for patients [43]. With an ever-growing population of adults who may be living with cardiovascular morbidity, future directions must recognize that child outcomes may be influenced by parental health. The promotion of existing cardiovascular prevention strategies may therefore not only have implications for improving CVD incidence, but for potentially preventing long-term child mental health illness.

**Author Contributions:** Conceptualization, B.K.D. and A.T.; Data curation, B.K.D.; Formal analysis, B.K.D.; Methodology, B.K.D.; Supervision, B.K.D.; Validation, B.K.D. and A.T.; Writing—original draft, B.K.D., A.T., H.R. and E.P.; Writing—review & editing, B.K.D., A.T., H.R. and E.P. All authors have read and agreed to the published version of the manuscript.

**Funding:** This research received no external funding.

**Institutional Review Board Statement:** This study used publicly available anonymized secondary data, and therefore, ethical approval was not required. The datasets for this study meet the definition of NIH Exempt Human Subjects Research under the following exemption criteria—"Exemption 4: involves the collection/study of data or specimens if publicly available, or recorded such that subjects can not be identified". The survey protocol of the NHIS (Protocol # 2015-08) was approved by the Research Ethics Review Board of the National Center for Health Statistics and the U.S. Office of Management and Budget.

**Informed Consent Statement:** Not applicable.

**Data Availability Statement:** We used Public Use version of the NHIS, which is publicly available to download from the National Center for Health Statistics, Centers for Disease Control and Prevention, by accessing the following URL: https://www.cdc.gov/nchs/nhis/data-questionnaires-documentation.htm, accessed on 5 January 2023.

**Conflicts of Interest:** The authors declare no conflict of interest.

## References

1. World Health Organization. *Cardiovascular Diseases (CVDs)*; World Health Organization: Geneva, Switzerland, 2021.
2. Esposito, K.; Giugliano, D. Diet and inflammation: A link to metabolic and cardiovascular diseases. *Eur. Heart J.* **2006**, *27*, 15–20. [CrossRef] [PubMed]
3. Virani, S.S.; Alonso, A.; Benjamin, E.J.; Bittencourt, M.S.; Callaway, C.W.; Carson, A.P.; Chamberlain, A.M.; Chang, A.R.; Cheng, S.; Delling, F.N.; et al. Heart Disease and Stroke Statistics—2020 Update: A Report From the American Heart Association. *Circulation* **2020**, *141*, e139–e596. [CrossRef] [PubMed]
4. Benjamin, E.J.; Virani, S.S.; Callaway, C.W.; Chamberlain, A.M.; Chang, A.R.; Cheng, S.; Chiuve, S.E.; Cushman, M.; Delling, F.N.; Deo, R.; et al. Heart Disease and Stroke Statistics—2018 Update: A Report From the American Heart Association. *Circulation* **2018**, *137*, e67–e492. [CrossRef] [PubMed]
5. Mozaffarian, D.; Benjamin, E.J.; Go, A.S.; Arnett, D.K.; Blaha, M.J.; Cushman, M.; Das, S.R.; de Ferranti, S.; Després, J.-P.; Fullerton, H.J.; et al. Heart Disease and Stroke Statistics—2016 Update. *Circulation* **2016**, *133*, e38–e360. [CrossRef]
6. Low, C.A.; Thurston, R.C.; Matthews, K.A. Psychosocial factors in the development of heart disease in women: Current research and future directions. *Psychosom. Med.* **2010**, *72*, 842–854. [CrossRef]
7. Everson-Rose, S.A.; Lewis, T.T. Psychosocial factors and cardiovascular diseases. *Annu. Rev. Public Health* **2004**, *26*, 469–500. [CrossRef]
8. Kivimäki, M.; Kawachi, I. Work Stress as a Risk Factor for Cardiovascular Disease. *Curr. Cardiol. Rep.* **2015**, *17*, 74. [CrossRef]
9. Nagai, M.; Hoshide, S.; Kario, K. Sleep duration as a risk factor for cardiovascular disease—A review of the recent literature. *Curr. Cardiol. Rev.* **2010**, *6*, 54–61. [CrossRef]
10. Dar, T.; Radfar, A.; Abohashem, S.; Pitman, R.K.; Tawakol, A.; Osborne, M.T. Psychosocial Stress and Cardiovascular Disease. *Curr. Treat. Options Cardiovasc. Med.* **2019**, *21*, 23. [CrossRef]
11. Heidenreich, P.A.; Trogdon, J.G.; Khavjou, O.A.; Butler, J.; Dracup, K.; Ezekowitz, M.D.; Finkelstein, E.A.; Hong, Y.; Johnston, S.C.; Khera, A.; et al. Forecasting the Future of Cardiovascular Disease in the United States. *Circulation* **2011**, *123*, 933–944. [CrossRef]
12. Rodgers, J.L.; Jones, J.; Bolleddu, S.I.; Vanthenapalli, S.; Rodgers, L.E.; Shah, K.; Karia, K.; Panguluri, S.K. Cardiovascular Risks Associated with Gender and Aging. *J. Cardiovasc. Dev. Dis.* **2019**, *6*, 19. [CrossRef] [PubMed]
13. Fayaz, A.; Ayis, S.; Panesar, S.S.; Langford, R.M.; Donaldson, L.J. Assessing the relationship between chronic pain and cardiovascular disease: A systematic review and meta-analysis. *Scand. J. Pain* **2016**, *13*, 76–90. [CrossRef] [PubMed]
14. Higgins, K.S.; Birnie, K.A.; Chambers, C.T.; Wilson, A.C.; Caes, L.; Clark, A.J.; Lynch, M.; Stinson, J.; Campbell-Yeo, M. Offspring of parents with chronic pain: A systematic review and meta-analysis of pain, health, psychological, and family outcomes. *Pain* **2015**, *156*, 2256–2266. [CrossRef] [PubMed]
15. Kaasbøll, J.; Lydersen, S.; Indredavik, M.S. Psychological symptoms in children of parents with chronic pain—The HUNT study. *Pain* **2012**, *153*, 1054–1062. [CrossRef] [PubMed]
16. Cozza, S.J.; Holmes, A.K.; Van Ost, S.L. Family-Centered Care for Military and Veteran Families Affected by Combat Injury. *Clin. Child Fam. Psychol. Rev.* **2013**, *16*, 311–321. [CrossRef] [PubMed]

17. Kaasbøll, J.; Skokauskas, N.; Lydersen, S.; Sund, A.M. Parental Chronic Illness, Internalizing Problems in Young Adulthood and the Mediating Role of Adolescent Attachment to Parents: A Prospective Cohort Study. *Front. Psychiatry* **2021**, *12*, 807563. [CrossRef]
18. Gan, Y.; Gong, Y.; Tong, X.; Sun, H.; Cong, Y.; Dong, X.; Wang, Y.; Xu, X.; Yin, X.; Deng, J.; et al. Depression and the risk of coronary heart disease: A meta-analysis of prospective cohort studies. *BMC Psychiatry* **2014**, *14*, 371. [CrossRef]
19. Havranek, E.P.; Mujahid, M.S.; Barr, D.A.; Blair, I.V.; Cohen, M.S.; Cruz-Flores, S.; Davey-Smith, G.; Dennison-Himmelfarb, C.R.; Lauer, M.S.; Lockwood, D.W.; et al. Social Determinants of Risk and Outcomes for Cardiovascular Disease. *Circulation* **2015**, *132*, 873–898. [CrossRef]
20. Levine, G.N.; Cohen, B.E.; Commodore-Mensah, Y.; Fleury, J.; Huffman, J.C.; Khalid, U.; Labarthe, D.R.; Lavretsky, H.; Michos, E.D.; Spatz, E.S.; et al. Psychological Health, Well-Being, and the Mind-Heart-Body Connection: A Scientific Statement From the American Heart Association. *Circulation* **2021**, *143*, e763–e783. [CrossRef]
21. Smith, M. Parental mental health: Disruptions to parenting and outcomes for children. *Child Fam. Soc. Work.* **2004**, *9*, 3–11. [CrossRef]
22. Amrock, S.M.; Weitzman, M. Parental Psychological Distress and Children's Mental Health: Results of a National Survey. *Acad. Pediatr.* **2014**, *14*, 375–381. [CrossRef] [PubMed]
23. Madigan, S.; Oatley, H.; Racine, N.; Fearon, R.P.; Schumacher, L.; Akbari, E.; Cooke, J.E.; Tarabulsy, G.M. A Meta-Analysis of Maternal Prenatal Depression and Anxiety on Child Socioemotional Development. *J. Am. Acad. Child Adolesc. Psychiatry* **2018**, *57*, 645–657.e8. [CrossRef] [PubMed]
24. Sieh, D.S.; Meijer, A.M.; Oort, F.J.; Visser-Meily, J.M.A.; Van der Leij, D.A.V. Problem Behavior in Children of Chronically Ill Parents: A Meta-Analysis. *Clin. Child Fam. Psychol. Rev.* **2010**, *13*, 384–397. [CrossRef] [PubMed]
25. Pakenham, K.I.; Cox, S. The Effects of Parental Illness and Other Ill Family Members on the Adjustment of Children. *Ann. Behav. Med.* **2014**, *48*, 424–437. [CrossRef] [PubMed]
26. Barkmann, C.; Romer, G.; Watson, M.; Schulte-Markwort, M. Parental Physical Illness as a Risk for Psychosocial Maladjustment in Children and Adolescents: Epidemiological Findings From a National Survey in Germany. *Psychosomatics* **2007**, *48*, 476–481. [CrossRef]
27. Pilato, J.; Dorard, G.; Chevrier, B.; Leu, A.; Untas, A. Quality of Life of Adolescents Facing a Parental Illness: A Person-Oriented Approach. *Int. J. Environ. Res. Public Health* **2022**, *19*, 7892. [CrossRef]
28. de Roos, S.A.; Iedema, J.; de Boer, A.H. Quality of Life of Schoolchildren Living with a Long-Term Sick Parent: The Role of Tasks at Home, Life Circumstances and Social Support. *Int. J. Environ. Res. Public Health* **2022**, *19*, 7043. [CrossRef]
29. Jørgensen, S.E.; Thygesen, L.C.; Andersen, A.; Due, P.; Michelsen, S.I. Parental Illness and Life Satisfaction among Young People: A Cross-Sectional Study of the Importance of School Factors. *Int. J. Environ. Res. Public Health* **2022**, *19*, 2719. [CrossRef]
30. Aldridge, J. Where are we now? Twenty-five years of research, policy and practice on young carers. *Crit. Soc. Policy* **2017**, *38*, 155–165. [CrossRef]
31. Kavanaugh, M.S.; Stamatopoulos, V.; Cohen, D.; Zhang, L. Unacknowledged Caregivers: A Scoping Review of Research on Caregiving Youth in the United States. *Adolesc. Res. Rev.* **2016**, *1*, 29–49. [CrossRef]
32. Cheesbrough, S.; Harding, C.; Webster, H.; Taylor, L.; Aldridge, J. *The Lives of Young Carers in England Omnibus Survey Report: Research Report*; Department for Education: London, UK, 2017.
33. Stamatopoulos, V. The young carer penalty: Exploring the costs of caregiving among a sample of Canadian youth. *Child Youth Serv.* **2018**, *39*, 180–205. [CrossRef]
34. Becker, S. Global Perspectives on Children's Unpaid Caregiving in the Family: Research and Policy on 'Young Carers' in the UK, Australia, the USA and Sub-Saharan Africa. *Glob. Soc. Policy* **2007**, *7*, 23–50. [CrossRef]
35. Levine, C.; Hunt, G.G.; Halper, D.; Hart, A.Y.; Lautz, J.; Gould, D.A. Young Adult Caregivers: A First Look at an Unstudied Population. *Am. J. Public Health* **2005**, *95*, 2071–2075. [CrossRef] [PubMed]
36. Bursnall, S.; Pakenham, K.I. Too Small for Your Boots! Understanding the experience of children when family members acquire a neurological condition. In *Health and Healing after Traumatic Brain Injury: Understanding the Power of Family, Friends, Community, and Other Support Systems: Understanding the Power of Family, Friends, Community, and Other Support Systems*; ABC-CLIO: Santa Barbara, CA, USA, 2013; pp. 87–100.
37. McDowell, D.J.; Parke, R.D. Parental correlates of children's peer relations: An empirical test of a tripartite model. *Dev. Psychol.* **2009**, *45*, 224. [CrossRef] [PubMed]
38. Williams, K.D. Ostracism. *Annu. Rev. Psychol.* **2006**, *58*, 425–452. [CrossRef]
39. Thapar, A.; Collishaw, S.; Pine, D.S.; Thapar, A.K. Depression in adolescence. *Lancet* **2012**, *379*, 1056–1067. [CrossRef]
40. Gaspar, T.; Gomez-Baya, D.; Trindade, J.S.; Botelho Guedes, F.; Cerqueira, A.; de Matos, M.G. Relationship Between Family Functioning, Parents' Psychosocial Factors, and Children's Well-Being. *J. Fam. Issues* **2022**, *43*, 2380–2397. [CrossRef]
41. Min, Y.I.; Anugu, P.; Butler, K.R.; Hartley, T.A.; Mwasongwe, S.; Norwood, A.F.; Sims, M.; Wang, W.; Winters, K.P.; Correa, A. Cardiovascular Disease Burden and Socioeconomic Correlates: Findings from the Jackson Heart Study. *J. Am. Heart Assoc.* **2017**, *6*, e004416. [CrossRef]

42. Andrade, C.; Gillen, M.; Molina, J.A.; Wilmarth, M.J. The Social and Economic Impact of Covid-19 on Family Functioning and Well-Being: Where do we go from here? *J. Fam. Econ. Issues* **2022**, *43*, 205–212. [CrossRef]
43. Madjid, M.; Safavi-Naeini, P.; Solomon, S.D.; Vardeny, O. Potential Effects of Coronaviruses on the Cardiovascular System: A Review. *JAMA Cardiol.* **2020**, *5*, 831–840. [CrossRef]

**Disclaimer/Publisher's Note:** The statements, opinions and data contained in all publications are solely those of the individual author(s) and contributor(s) and not of MDPI and/or the editor(s). MDPI and/or the editor(s) disclaim responsibility for any injury to people or property resulting from any ideas, methods, instructions or products referred to in the content.

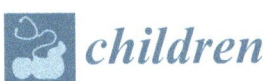

Article

# Psychometric Properties of the Chinese Version of the Brief Interpersonal Competence Questionnaire for Adolescents

Liuyue Huang [1,2], Junrun Huang [3], Zhichao Chen [3], Weiwei Jiang [3], Yi Zhu [4,*] and Xinli Chi [3,5,*]

1. Department of Psychology, Faculty of Social Sciences, University of Macau, Macao 999078, China
2. Center for Cognitive and Brain Sciences, Institute of Collaborative Innovation, University of Macau, Macao 999078, China
3. School of Psychology, Shenzhen University, Shenzhen 518060, China
4. School of Early-Childhood Education, Nanjing Xiaozhuang University, Nanjing 210017, China
5. The Shenzhen Humanities & Social Sciences Key Research Bases of the Center for Mental Health, Shenzhen 518060, China
* Correspondence: ryzhu@foxmail.com (Y.Z.); xinlichi@szu.edu.cn (X.C.)

**Abstract:** This study aimed to evaluate the psychometric properties of the Brief Interpersonal Competence Questionnaire (ICQ-15) administered to Chinese adolescents. A sample of 1705 adolescents (Mean age = 14.08, SD = 3.22, 46.5% male) completed a questionnaire including the Chinese version of the ICQ-15, as well as measurements of well-being, psychological resilience, and depression. To examine the psychometric properties of the ICQ-15, item analyses (item–total correlation and normality test), confirmatory factor analysis, concurrent validity analyses, multi-group analyses, and internal consistency analyses were performed. The results of the item analyses suggested a good item–total correlation, and the item scores were distributed approximately normally. The confirmatory factor analysis showed that the five-factor model had acceptable fit indices. The concurrent validity analyses indicated that the Chinese version of the ICQ-15 had a satisfactory concurrent validity. The multi-group analyses proved the measurement invariance across females and males, as well as participants in early, middle, and late adolescence. The ICQ-15 demonstrated satisfactory internal consistency reliability among Chinese adolescents. The ICQ-15 presents good psychometric properties and can be used to assess interpersonal competence in Chinese adolescents.

**Keywords:** social competence; measurement; adolescents; validity study

## 1. Introduction

Interpersonal relationships play an influential role in a person's life-span development and well-being [1]. A growing body of research indicates that individuals with good interpersonal relationships have a higher sense of well-being, greater academic resilience, more adaptive coping styles, and healthier physical conditions [2–4]. In contrast, poor interpersonal competence may result in interpersonal conflicts and even lead to the progression of internalizing and externalizing behaviors [5]. Notably, adolescents are in a critical period of transition from childhood to adulthood, with the pursuit of independence from their parents and the need for more social interactions with their peers. As such, interpersonal competence becomes particularly important at this stage [6]. A meta-analysis of 51 studies in China found that 24.3% of Chinese adolescents suffer from depression symptoms [7]. After the outbreak of COVID-19, adolescents' mental health problems have become a major concern in our society. A meta-analysis including 80,879 adolescents from around the world showed the pooled prevalence rate was 25.2% for depression and 20.5% for anxiety during the COVID-19 pandemic [8]. Local researchers are urged to pay special attention to adolescents' mental health and explore ways to improve it.

A key approach to promoting adolescents' mental well-being may be facilitating their interpersonal competence, whose lack has been shown to have a close negative association with mental health (e.g., depression) [9,10]. Similar to studies with adults, adolescents with deficient interpersonal competence were also found to be at a higher risk for loneliness, anxiety, and even suicidal behavior [11,12]. Conversely, adolescents with good interpersonal relationships are likely to experience fewer mental health problems and better school adaption and subjective well-being [13]. In this respect, interpersonal competence is particularly crucial for the healthy development of adolescents.

With the rise of research interest in adolescents' interpersonal competence, well-validated measures have become indispensable. In addition to providing scientific tools for assessing adolescents' interpersonal competence, scales with good reliability and validity can contribute to the evaluation of the effectiveness of related interventions. Indeed, interpersonal competence can be changed through interventions, particularly in the early years of life (i.e., childhood and adolescence) [14]. Existing studies have shown interventions targeted at social competence could improve adolescents' interpersonal efficacy and mental health status [15,16]. However, interpersonal competence improvement is a long-term, dynamic process that requires continuous evaluation [17]. There are times when studies are conducted under constrained settings (e.g., assessment time and cost). For example, there are large-scale investigations on the comprehensive development status of students or intensive clinical progress follow-up studies. A refined scale is required to reduce the response burden of the participants in these research contexts. As a result, both research and practice require short-form scales that are validated to measure interpersonal competence.

Regarding the current assessments of individuals' interpersonal relationships, there are two main categories. Most scales are disease-focused and based on the diagnosis systems of the International Classification of Diseases [18] or the Diagnostic and Statistical Manual of Mental Disorders [19]. The other category is from the perspective of positive aspects (e.g., strength and competence). To date, most existing scales for interpersonal relationships validated in the Chinese population were mainly designed to measure social problems, such as social anxiety and social phobia [20,21]. Notably, perspectives based on a "problem perspective" are prone to attach negative labels to the adolescents [22], which may have a negative influence on their self-identity.

In contrast, scales from the perspective of development are beneficial to reduce stigma. Several scales were developed to measure social competence from a positive perspective. For example, the 77-item Multidimensional Social Competence Scale showed acceptable psychometric properties among general young adults [23]. Nevertheless, too many questions may lead to burnout in large-scale testing and intensive evaluation. The Interpersonal Competence Questionnaire (ICQ), developed by Buhrmester and colleagues [24], is a widely used interpersonal competence measurement. The ICQ contains 40 items with five dimensions: initiation of a relationship, negative assertion, disclosure, emotional support, and conflict management. This questionnaire has been used in various countries and is now available in many different languages, including Chinese [25], German [26], Polish [27], Italian [28], and Korean [29], with good psychometric properties. However, the ICQ, with 40 items may be burdensome to administer in time- or cost-constrained conditions such as when performing comprehensive large-scale studies (e.g., adolescents development census) or intensive measurement studies (e.g., clinical progress follow-up) [17]. To increase the feasibility of the ICQ for routine assessments in research and clinical practice, Coroiu et al. [17] simplified and validated a 15-item version of the Interpersonal Competence Questionnaire (ICQ-15) on the basis of the ICQ. Consistent with the theoretical structure of the original scale, the ICQ-15 retained the five dimensions (three questions for each dimension). Not only the ICQ-15 showed good validity in the general adult population (age 18–90) but also facilitated the assessment of interpersonal competence under various environmental constraints.

The ICQ-15 has been validated in adolescent populations in Germany [17] and Spain [30], with the demonstration of good psychometric properties. However, the ICQ-15 has yet to be adapted to and validated in the Chinese adolescent population. As interpersonal competence is an essential part of the developmental process of adolescents, this study proposed to adapt the ICQ-15 and evaluate its reliability and validity among Chinese adolescents. To this end, the present study aimed to adapt the ICQ-15 to the Chinese context and to examine its validity in Chinese adolescents. We hypothesized that the Chinese version of IC1-15 has good psychometric properties.

## 2. Method

*2.1. Participants*

According to a recent proposition of the period of adolescence, adolescence spans the years between late childhood and early adulthood (ages 10 to 24 years, see [31]. The present study recruited participants aged 10 to 24 years. A total of 2100 questionnaires were distributed, and 1991 questionnaires were returned, with a response rate of 94.81%. The valid sample size was 1705 after excluding 291 invalid questionnaires, due, for example, to too short response times or invalid answers (e.g., all items were given the same answer or did not pass the attention check test). The control of the response time was performed after participants' submission according to the answering time recorded by the system. The online survey platform has the function of recording the participants' response time. According to the length of the survey, those participants who completed the whole questionnaire in less than 5 min were considered to be invalid cases. The mean age was 14.08 years (SD = 3.22). There were 793 (46.5%) male students and 912 (53.5%) female students. Regarding the school level, 271 (15.9%) were college students, 272 (16.0%) were high school students, 552 (32.3%) were middle school students, and 610 were elementary school students (35.8%).

*2.2. Procedure*

We used a convenience sampling method to collect data from May to June 2021 in five schools in Shenzhen, China, including one elementary school, one secondary school, two 12-year schools (primary to senior high school), and one university. Students from elementary, middle, and high schools were a cluster convenience sample. The research team collaborated with the school institutions and recruited most students in these sampling schools. The university participants were recruited by snowball sampling. The university student population was recruited by means of posters on university school web forums and social media platforms (e.g., WeChat, QQ). Moreover, no incentive was provided to the participants from primary to senior high school. Participants from the university were offered the opportunity to enter a draw for RMB 1~100, cash (equivalent to USD 0.14~14 at the time of the assessment). All participants could decide to withdraw from the study at any time. All participants included in the final analyses provided informed consent. All data were collected online via Sojump (https://www.wjx.cn/) (accessed on 8 December 2022), a widely used online questionnaire platform in China. There were no missing data in this study because all items needed to be completed before submission. This research project was approved by the Ethics Committee of Shenzhen University (No:2020005).

*2.3. Instruments*

2.3.1. Brief Form of Interpersonal Competence Questionnaire (ICQ-15)

ICQ-15 [17] is the short version of the widely used ICQ [24], with 15 items containing 5 dimensions: initiation of a relationship (items 2, 7, 9), negative assertion (items 10, 12, 13), disclosure (items 3, 5, 8), emotional support (items 4, 11, 14), and conflict management (items 1, 6, 15). The participants were invited to rate these items according to how challenging each social behavior was for them. The answers were scored on a 5-point Likert scale from 1 (= I am poor at this) to 5 (= I am extremely good at this). Higher scores indicate better interpersonal competence.

In the present study, after authorization from the author of the ICQ-15, three researchers who were proficient in both Chinese and English independently translated the scale to obtain a preliminary Chinese version. Two certified translators further ensured that the translated scale was accurate and conformed to Chinese language habits. Next, it was back-translated by an English-speaking professional, and then a native English speaker evaluated its semantic equivalence. Finally, through convenience sampling, thirteen students (five college students, two high school students, three middle school students, and three elementary school students) were recruited to assess the scale's readability. A developmental psychologist skilled in English was asked to review the final Chinese version of the scale. We provide the final Chinese version of the ICQ-15 for adolescents in the Appendix A (Table A1).

2.3.2. Five-Item World Health Organization Well-Being Index (WHO-5)

The WHO-5 was developed by the World Health Organization to test subjective well-being in adults [32] and was further validated as a measure of well-being assessment among adolescents [33]. The scale consists of five items, scored on a six-point Likert scale from 0 (= at no time) to 5 (= all of the time), with the total score being the sum of the five items' scores. Higher scores indicate higher levels of psychological well-being. The Cronbach's alpha coefficient for the scale in this study was 0.92.

2.3.3. Ten-Item Connor-Davidson Resilience Scale (CD-RISC-10)

This study used the 10-item Connor-Davidson Resilience Scale (CD-RISC-10) to assess the level of psychological resilience [34]. The CD-RISC-10 was validated in Chinese population [35]. It is a 5-point Likert scale ranging from 0 (= not true at all) to 4 (= true nearly all the time), with higher scores representing higher levels of psychological resilience. The Cronbach's alpha coefficient for this scale in this study was 0.93.

2.3.4. Patient Health Questionnaire-9 (PHQ-9)

The depressive symptoms were assessed by the Patient Health Questionnaire-9 (PHQ-9) in the preceding two weeks [36]. The PHQ-9 was validated in a Chinese adolescent population, demonstrating good psychometric properties [37]. The answers were scored on a 4-point scale from 0 (= not at all) to 3 (= nearly every day), with higher scores representing higher levels of depression. The Cronbach's alpha coefficient for the scale in this study was 0.90.

*2.4. Statistics and Analyses*

We first analyzed the data for item–total correlation. Second, a normality test was performed on the scores of the 15 items to examine whether the responses presented a normal distribution. There are sufficient research findings to support a five-factor correlated structure of the scale. Previous research has shown that confirmatory factor analysis (CFA) can be conducted on theoretically structured or mature scales without performing an exploratory factor analysis (EFA) [38]. The EFA can be applied if the CFA results are not acceptable. The full version of the ICQ was validated in Chinese adolescents [25,39], and the scores presented good structural validity as the original theoretical model proposed by Buhrmester et al. [24]. Thus, in this study, the data were analyzed by CFA to test their structural validity. For an acceptable model fit, the following goodness of fit measures were used: Comparative Fit Index (CFI) $\geq$ 0.90, Tucker–Lewis Index (TLI) $\geq$ 0.90, and root-mean-square error for approximation (RMSEA) $\leq$ 0.10. Fourth, as reviewed above, interpersonal competence plays an influential role in determining general well-being, psychological resilience, and depression. In this context, Pearson's correlation analyses were performed between the ICQ-15 and these criteria variables to assess the ICQ-15 concurrent validity. Fourth, measurement invariance is a prerequisite of a scale for comparison between different groups [40]. Hence, two multi-group analyses of the ICQ-15 were then conducted to examine the measurement invariance of this scale across genders and stages of adolescent development. Specifically, participants aged 10–13 years were grouped into early adolescence, participants aged 14–17 years were grouped into middle adolescence, and participants between the age of 18 years and early adulthood were grouped into late adolescence [31,41]. We examined configural invariance first, followed by metric invariance, scalar invariance, and strict variance. A configuration invariance test determines if the same factor structure applies to different groups. Metric invariance indicates whether the factor loadings are the same across groups. A scalar invariance indicates the presence of equal item intercepts across groups. Invariance of residual variance across groups is defined as strict invariance. The cutoff criteria for measurement invariance were 0.02 for the change of CFI and 0.03 for the change for RMSEA, as suggested by Rutkowski and Svetina for large-size samples [42]. The CFA and multi-group analyses were performed using a robust maximum likelihood (MLR) estimator. Finally, the internal consistency reliability of the ICQ-15 was examined. This study used SPSS 23.0 and Mplus 8.3 for data analyses.

## 3. Results

### 3.1. Item Analyses

The item–total correlation was analyzed by Pearson correlation. The results showed that the item–total correlation coefficients ranged from 0.57 to 0.77 ($ps < 0.001$). The normality test showed the kurtosis and skewness of the scores of the ICQ-15 items were from −1.01 to 0.08 (Table 1), i.e., within the cutoff score of ±1.50 [43]. The results suggested the items' scores followed an approximately normal distribution.

**Table 1.** Kurtosis and skewness of the scores of the ICQ-15 items ($n = 1705$).

| Item | 1 | 2 | 3 | 4 | 5 | 6 | 7 | 8 | 9 | 10 | 11 | 12 | 13 | 14 | 15 |
|---|---|---|---|---|---|---|---|---|---|---|---|---|---|---|---|
| Skewness | −0.16 | −0.42 | −0.20 | −0.47 | −0.20 | −0.38 | −0.17 | −0.43 | −0.22 | −0.13 | −0.69 | 0.08 | −0.03 | −0.52 | −0.47 |
| Kurtosis | −0.55 | −0.52 | −0.98 | −0.30 | −0.98 | −0.47 | −0.95 | −0.66 | −1.01 | −0.79 | −0.01 | −1.00 | −0.96 | −0.22 | −0.66 |

### 3.2. Structural Validity

The results of the CFA showed that the model fitted well, with the standard loading coefficients of the items on the factors ranging from 0.64 to 0.91 (see Table 2). The fit indices were $\chi^2 = 524.49$, $df = 80$, CFI = 0.95, TLI = 0.93, and RMSEA = 0.06, and all met the psychometric criteria.

**Table 2.** Standardized factor loadings for the five-factor model of the ICQ-15 ($n = 1705$).

| Initiation of Relationship | | Negative Assertion | | Disclosure | | Emotional Support | | Conflict Management | |
|---|---|---|---|---|---|---|---|---|---|
| Item | Loadings | Item | Loadings | Item | Loadings | Item | Loadings | Item | Loadings |
| 2 | 0.77 | 10 | 0.64 | 3 | 0.70 | 4 | 0.80 | 1 | 0.65 |
| 7 | 0.79 | 12 | 0.91 | 5 | 0.79 | 11 | 0.79 | 6 | 0.82 |
| 9 | 0.73 | 13 | 0.91 | 8 | 0.79 | 14 | 0.81 | 15 | 0.60 |

### 3.3. Concurrent Validity

The results of concurrent validity analyses showed that the scores of the total and five subscales of the ICQ-15 showed a moderate to strong correlation with the scores of the WHO-5 and the CD-RISC-10 ($r = 0.51$, $r = 0.53$; $ps < 0.001$) and a negative correlation with the scores of the PHQ-9 with moderate strength ($r = −0.32$; $p < 0.001$). Detailed data are presented in Table 3.

### 3.4. Multi-Group Analyses

Two multi-group analyses were conducted to test for measurement invariance among males and females, as well as in different age groups. After adding restrictions, the change of model fit indices (CFI and RMSEA) were less than the cutoff criteria of 0.020 between the male and the female groups (See Table 4) [42]. The results indicated that the ICQ-15 scale had good measurement invariance when comparing the male and the female groups. Details are shown in Table 4.

Table 3. Correlation coefficients between the ICQ-15 and other related measures and inter-factor correlations between ICQ-15 factors (n = 1705).

|        | WHO-5  | CD-RISC-10 | PHQ-9   | F1     | F2     | F3     | F4     | F5     |
|--------|--------|------------|---------|--------|--------|--------|--------|--------|
| F1     | 0.50 * | 0.47 *     | −0.33 * |        |        |        |        |        |
| F2     | 0.40 * | 0.39 *     | −0.24 * | 0.59 * |        |        |        |        |
| F3     | 0.44 * | 0.41 *     | −0.30 * | 0.74 * | 0.52 * |        |        |        |
| F4     | 0.39 * | 0.47 *     | −0.24 * | 0.68 * | 0.56 * | 0.64 * |        |        |
| F5     | 0.36 * | 0.46 *     | −0.22 * | 0.59 * | 0.48 * | 0.55 * | 0.71 * |        |
| ICQ-15 | 0.51 * | 0.53 *     | −0.32 * | 0.88 * | 0.77 * | 0.84 * | 0.86 * | 0.79 * |

Note. *: Significant at the 0.001 level (two-tailed); WHO-5: Well-Being Index Scale; CD-RISC-10: 10-item Connor–Davidson Resilience Scale; PHQ-9: Patient Health Questionnaire-9; ICQ-15: Brief form of the Interpersonal Competence Scale. F1: initiation of a relationship; F2: negative assertion; F3: disclosure; F4: emotional support; F5: conflict management.

Table 4. Results of the multi-group analysis between males and females (n = 1705).

|               | $\chi^2$ | df  | CFI   | TLI   | RMSEA | △CFI  | △RMSEA |
|---------------|----------|-----|-------|-------|-------|-------|--------|
| Configural MI | 651.354  | 160 | 0.944 | 0.927 | 0.060 | -     | -      |
| Weak MI       | 693.361  | 175 | 0.941 | 0.929 | 0.059 | 0.003 | −0.001 |
| Strong MI     | 764.039  | 190 | 0.935 | 0.928 | 0.060 | 0.006 | 0.001  |
| Strict MI     | 786.243  | 205 | 0.934 | 0.932 | 0.058 | 0.001 | −0.002 |

Note. CFI: Comparative Fit Index. TLI: Tucker–Lewis Index. RMSEA: Root-Mean-Square Error for Approximation. MI: Measurement Invariance.

As a result of the multi-group analysis, the change in the fit indexes of CFI, TLI, and RMSEA between the participants in early, middle, and late adolescence was less than the cutoff criteria of 0.020 [42], indicating that the ICQ-15 scale has acceptable measurement invariance across these development periods. Details are shown in Table 5.

Table 5. Results of the multi-group analysis between different stages of adolescent development.

|               | $\chi^2$ | df  | CFI   | TLI   | RMSEA | △CFI   | △RMSEA |
|---------------|----------|-----|-------|-------|-------|--------|--------|
| Configural MI | 768.704  | 240 | 0.944 | 0.926 | 0.062 | -      | -      |
| Weak MI       | 863.323  | 270 | 0.937 | 0.926 | 0.062 | −0.007 | 0.000  |
| Strong MI     | 1027.317 | 300 | 0.923 | 0.919 | 0.065 | −0.014 | −0.007 |
| Strict MI     | 1176.197 | 330 | 0.910 | 0.914 | 0.067 | −0.013 | −0.005 |

Note. CFI: Comparative Fit Index. TLI: Tucker–Lewis Index. RMSEA: Root-Mean-Square Error for Approximation. MI: Measurement Invariance.

### 3.5. Internal Consistency Reliability Analyses

The Cronbach's α coefficient for the scores of the ICQ-15 was 0.93. The Cronbach's α coefficients for the scores of the five subscales (i.e., initiation of a relationship, negative assertion, disclosure, emotional support, and conflict management) were 0.81, 0.85, 0.80, 0.84, and 0.73, respectively. The McDonald's ω coefficient for the scores of the ICQ-15 was 0.93, and that for the scores of the five subscales was 0.81, 0.87, 0.80, 0.84, and 0.73 in the same sequential as above, respectively.

## 4. Discussion

The purpose of this study was to examine the applicability of the ICQ-15 among Chinese adolescents and to enrich the measurement tools for improving interpersonal competence targeted at Chinese adolescents. The findings indicated the ICQ-15 has satisfactory item–total correlation and discrimination. The CFA showed an acceptable model fit index. The multi-group analyses showed that there was measurement invariance across males and females as well as across different stages of adolescence. The results supported our research hypothesis. Consistent with previous research [25–30], this study supports the interpersonal relationship competency scale consisting of five dimensions: initiation of a relationship, negative assertion, disclosure, emotional support, and conflict management.

The findings of the concurrent validity analysis showed that adolescents' interpersonal competence was positively correlated with subjective well-being and psychological resilience at a medium to high intensity, i.e., the stronger the interpersonal competence, the better the subjective well-being and psychological resilience, which is similar to the findings of previous studies [13,44]. This may be because adolescents are at a crucial transitional period in their development, where the influence of peer relationships becomes more prominent than in childhood. Adolescents with good interpersonal competence are likely to have higher levels of social support and benign emotional support. Therefore, they are more likely to feel connected with others, which will lead to a higher self-determination and more satisfaction in their lives [44]. In addition, when faced with distress situations, adolescents with high interpersonal competence can better regulate their emotions with the support of their families and peers, which will contribute to constructive stress coping strategies and better adaption. Thus, individuals with strong interpersonal competence may have a greater sense of well-being and psychological resilience in life. Interpersonal competence was also significantly and negatively associated with mental health problems, which is similar to the findings of previous studies [9,10]. The authors speculated that adolescents with poor interpersonal competence could face more negative interpersonal stress. Chronic negative stress can result in the impairment of adolescents' self-concept, endocrine system (e.g., cortisol dynamics), and nervous systems, ultimately affecting their psychological and even biological health [45].

The Cronbach's alpha coefficient for the ICQ-15 was 0.93, and the Cronbach's alpha coefficients of the five dimensions (initiation of a relationship, negative assertion, disclosure, emotional support, and conflict management) were 0.81, 0.85, 0.80, 0.84, and 0.73, respectively. Thus, the results indicated that the ICQ-15 has good internal consistency reliability, similar to the findings of a previous study [17]. Further, in the present study, after adding restrictions to the structural model of the ICQ-15, the subsequent change values of the fit indices all fell below 0.01, indicating that the Chinese version of the ICQ-15 scale has good measurement invariance across the male and female student groups and between the 10–24 age group.

There are some strengths of this study. First, the present study sample broadly covered all stages of adolescence, with good age representation. In addition, the Chinese version of the ICQ-15 validated in this study provides a concise and practical measurement for assessing adolescents' interpersonal competence. This is conducive to future interpersonal competence evaluation, behavioral experiments, or interventions. Third, this study found that adolescents with better interpersonal competence had higher subjective well-being and psychological resilience and fewer depressive symptoms, suggesting the importance of enhancing adolescents' interpersonal competence in education and clinical work. Cultivating the interpersonal competence of adolescents can promote their healthy development and enhance their adaptability. Overall, the ICQ-15 has good reliability and validity in the Chinese adolescent population and can be used as a scientific tool to measure the interpersonal skills of Chinese adolescents.

Several limitations to this study need to be noted. First, the subject group was mainly from Shenzhen City rather than a nation-wide sample. Future studies could increase the sample size including participants from other regions to minimize the geographical homogeneity of the participants. In addition, all assessments used in the present study were self-reported. Future studies could enrich the validity criteria by incorporating more assessment dimensions (other-rated scales, e.g., peer- or teacher-rated scales). Third, due to the constraints of the study sampling, the retest data could not be collected in this study. Thus, the test–retest reliability could not be obtained, which could be complemented in future studies.

## 5. Conclusions

This study assessed the reliability and validity of the ICQ-15 among Chinese adolescents. Item analyses, confirmatory factor analysis, concurrent validity analyses, multi-group analyses, and internal consistency analyses were performed on the scores of the ICQ-15 among 1705 Chinese adolescents. The results suggested good psychometric features of the Chinese version of the ICQ-15 which can be used as a tool for assessing interpersonal competence among Chinese adolescents.

**Author Contributions:** Conceptualization, L.H.; methodology, L.H. and J.H.; software, L.H. and J.H.; validation, L.H., Z.C. and W.J.; formal analysis, L.H. and J.H.; investigation, L.H.; resources, X.C. and Y.Z.; data curation, L.H., W.J. and X.C.; writing—original draft preparation, J.H. and L.H.; writing—review and editing, L.H., J.H., Z.C., W.J., X.C. and Y.Z.; supervision, X.C. and Y.Z.; project administration, X.C. and Y.Z.; funding acquisition, X.C. and Y.Z. All authors have read and agreed to the published version of the manuscript.

**Funding:** Y.Z. was funded by Shenzhen Basic Research Project (No. 20200814102701001). X.C. was supported by the Guangdong Basic and Applied Basic Research Foundation (Grant No. 2021A1515011330), Shenzhen Education Science Planning Project [grant number cgpy21001], and Shenzhen University-Lingnan University Joint Research Programme [grant number 202202001].

**Institutional Review Board Statement:** This research project was approved by the Ethics Committee of Shenzhen University (No: 2020005; Approved Date: 12 March 2020). All procedures performed in studies involving human participants were in accordance with the ethical standards of the institutional and/or national research committee and with the 1964 Helsinki Declaration and its later amendments or comparable ethical standards.

**Informed Consent Statement:** Informed consent was obtained from all subjects involved in the study.

**Data Availability Statement:** The data of this study are available in the open science framework (https://osf.io/27whc/ (accessed on 10 October 2022)).

**Acknowledgments:** The authors express their sincere gratitude to all the participants of the present study.

**Conflicts of Interest:** The authors declare no conflict of interest. The funders had no role in the design of the study; in the collection, analyses, or interpretation of data; in the writing of the manuscript, or in the decision to publish the results.

## Appendix A

**Table A1.** Chinese Version of the Brief form of Interpersonal Competence Questionnaire for Adolescents.

|  | 比较困难 1 | 勉强可以 2 | 基本可以 3 | 擅长 4 | 非常擅长 5 |
|---|---|---|---|---|---|
| 1. 当和好朋友的分歧快要发展成激烈争吵时，能够承认你可能是错的。 | | | | | |
| 2. 寻找一些事情，邀请你认为有趣和有吸引力的新朋友一起去做。 | | | | | |
| 3. 信任你的新朋友或者交往对象，让他/她看到你更柔软、敏感的一面。 | | | | | |
| 4. 帮助一个好朋友认识到他/她正在经历的问题的关键。 | | | | | |
| 5. 让一个新朋友了解"真实的"你。 | | | | | |
| 6. 在争吵中能够站在朋友的角度思考，真正理解他/她的观点。 | | | | | |
| 7. 向你可能想认识或交往的人介绍你自己。 | | | | | |
| 8. 卸下防御的"铠甲"，信任你的好朋友。 | | | | | |
| 9. 主动联系新朋友/熟人，约个时间聚一起做一些事。 | | | | | |

Table A1. Cont.

|  | 比较困难 1 | 勉强可以 2 | 基本可以 3 | 擅长 4 | 非常擅长 5 |
|---|---|---|---|---|---|
| 10. 当你的好朋友违背承诺时，能够与他/她直面矛盾。 | | | | | |
| 11. 当好朋友情绪低落时，能够说一些话或者做一些事情来支持他/她。 | | | | | |
| 12. 当朋友做了伤害你感情的事，能告诉他/她。 | | | | | |
| 13. 当同伴/熟人做了让你生气的事，能告诉他/她。 | | | | | |
| 14. 当你的好朋友需要帮助和支持时，能够以容易被对方接受的方式给到建议。 | | | | | |
| 15. 为了避免破坏关系的冲突，不对好朋友大发脾气(即使你更占理)。 | | | | | |

## References

1. Antonucci, T.C.; Ajrouch, K.J.; Webster, N.J.; Zahodne, L.B. Social Relations Across the Life Span: Scientific Advances, Emerging Issues, and Future Challenges. *Annu. Rev. Dev. Psychol.* **2019**, *1*, 313–336. [CrossRef]
2. Frisby, B.N.; Hosek, A.M.; Beck, A.C. The role of classroom relationships as sources of academic resilience and hope. *Commun. Q.* **2020**, *68*, 289–305. [CrossRef]
3. Kothari, B.H.; Blakeslee, J.; Miller, R. Individual and interpersonal factors associated with psychosocial functioning among adolescents in foster care: A scoping review. *Child Youth Serv. Rev.* **2020**, *118*, 105454. [CrossRef]
4. Nowicka, P.; Ek, A.; Grafström, E.; Johansson, T.; Nordin, K.; Neuman, N.; Reijs Richards, H.; Eli, K. How do interpersonal relationships affect children's weight management? A qualitative analysis of parents' long-term perceptions after obesity treatment. *Child Obes.* **2022**, *18*, 274–280. [CrossRef]
5. Prino, L.E.; Longobardi, C.; Fabris, M.A.; Parada, R.H.; Settanni, M. Effects of bullying victimization on internalizing and externalizing symptoms: The mediating role of alexithymia. *J. Child Fam. Stud.* **2019**, *28*, 2586–2593. [CrossRef]
6. Kiuru, N.; Wang, M.; Salmela-Aro, K.; Kannas, L.; Ahonen, T.; Hirvonen, R. Associations between Adolescents' Interpersonal Relationships, School Well-being, and Academic Achievement during Educational Transitions. *J. Youth Adolesc.* **2020**, *49*, 1057–1072. [CrossRef]
7. Tang, X.; Tang, S.; Ren, Z.; Wong, D. Prevalence of depressive symptoms among adolescents in secondary school in mainland China: A systematic review and meta-analysis. *J. Affect. Disord.* **2019**, *245*, 498–507. [CrossRef]
8. Racine, N.; McArthur, B.A.; Cooke, J.E.; Eirich, R.; Zhu, J.; Madigan, S. Global Prevalence of Depressive and Anxiety Symptoms in Children and Adolescents During COVID-19. *JAMA Pediatr.* **2021**, *175*, 1142. [CrossRef]
9. Bird, T.; Tarsia, M.; Schwannauer, M. Interpersonal styles in major and chronic depression: A systematic review and meta-analysis. *J. Affect. Disord.* **2018**, *239*, 93–101. [CrossRef]
10. Elsina, I.; Martinsone, B. Interpersonal Relationship Aspects as Perceived Risk and Social Support Factors in a Clinical Sample of Adolescents With Depression. *J. Relatsh. Res.* **2020**, *11*, E1. [CrossRef]
11. Moeller, R.W.; Seehuus, M. Loneliness as a mediator for college students' social skills and experiences of depression and anxiety. *J. Adolesc.* **2019**, *73*, 1–13. [CrossRef]
12. Dutton, C.E.; Rojas, S.M.; Badour, C.L.; Wanklyn, S.G.; Feldner, M.T. Posttraumatic Stress Disorder and Suicidal Behavior: Indirect Effects of Impaired Social Functioning. *Arch. Suicide Res.* **2016**, *20*, 567–579. [CrossRef]
13. Huber, L.; Plötner, M.; Schmitz, J. Social competence and psychopathology in early childhood: A systematic review. *Eur. Child Adoles. Psychiatry* **2019**, *28*, 443–459. [CrossRef]
14. Durlak, J.A.A.; Weissberg, R.P.A.; Pachan, M.A. A Meta-Analysis of After-School Programs That Seek to Promote Personal and Social Skills in Children and Adolescents. *Am. J. Commun. Psychol.* **2010**, *45*, 294–309. [CrossRef]
15. Ghelbash, Z.; Zarshenas, L.; Dehghan Manshadi, Z. A trial of an emotional intelligence intervention in an Iranian residential institution for adolescents. *Clin. Child Psychol. P* **2021**, *26*, 993–1002. [CrossRef]
16. Turner, D.T.; McGlanaghy, E.; Cuijpers, P.; van der Gaag, M.; Karyotaki, E.; MacBeth, A. A Meta-Analysis of Social Skills Training and Related Interventions for Psychosis. *Schizophr. Bull.* **2018**, *44*, 475–491. [CrossRef]
17. Coroiu, A.; Meyer, A.; Gomez-Garibello, C.; Brähler, E.; Hessel, A.; Körner, A. Brief Form of the Interpersonal Competence Questionnaire (ICQ-15) Development and Preliminary Validation with a German Population Sample. *Eur. J. Psychol. Assess.* **2015**, *31*, 272–279. [CrossRef]
18. Kogan, C.S.; Stein, D.J.; Maj, M.; First, M.B.; Emmelkamp, P.M.G.; Reed, G.M. The Classification of Anxiety and Fear-Related Disorders in the ICD-11. *Depress. Anxiety* **2016**, *33*, 1141–1154. [CrossRef]
19. Bögels, S.M.; Alden, L.; Beidel, D.C.; Clark, L.A.; Pine, D.S.; Stein, M.B.; Voncken, M. Social anxiety disorder: Questions and answers for the DSM-V. *Depress. Anxiety* **2010**, *27*, 168–189. [CrossRef]
20. Zhong, J.; Liu, J.; Xu, G.; Zheng, H.; Bowker, J.; Coplan, R.J. Measurement Invariance of Two Different Short Forms of Social Interaction Anxiety Scale (SIAS) and Social Phobia Scale (SPS) in Chinese and US Samples. *Eur. J. Psychol. Assess.* **2021**. [CrossRef]

21. Chen, B.; Zhang, R.; Zhang, Q.; Zheng, X. Reliability and Validity of the Social Anxiety Scale for Social Media Users (SAS-SMU) in Chinese University Students. *Chin. J. Clin. Psychol.* **2020**, *28*, 1190–1193, 1198.
22. Shek, D.T.; Dou, D.; Zhu, X.; Chai, W. Positive youth development: Current perspectives. *Adolesc. Health Med. Ther.* **2019**, *10*, 131–141. [CrossRef]
23. Trevisan, D.A.; Tafreshi, D.; Slaney, K.L.; Yager, J.; Iarocci, G. A psychometric evaluation of the Multidimensional Social Competence Scale (MSCS) for young adults. *PLoS ONE* **2018**, *13*, e206800. [CrossRef]
24. Buhrmester, D.; Furman, W.; Wittenberg, M.T.; Reis, H.T. Five domains of interpersonal competence in peer relationships. *J. Pers. Soc. Psychol.* **1988**, *55*, 991–1008. [CrossRef]
25. Wang, Y.; Zou, H.; Qu, Z. A Preliminary Revision of Interpersonal Competence Questionnaire (ICQ) for Chinese Junior Middle School Students. *Chin. J. Ment. Health* **2006**, *05*, 306–308.
26. Kanning, U.P. Development and Validation of a German-Language Version of the Interpersonal Competence Questionnaire (ICQ). *Eur. J. Psychol. Assess.* **2006**, *22*, 43. [CrossRef]
27. Górska, M. Psychometric Properties of the Polish Version of the Interpersonal Competence Questionnaire (ICQ-R). *Eur. J. Psychol. Assess.* **2011**, *27*, 186–192. [CrossRef]
28. Giromini, L.; De Campora, G.; Brusadelli, E.; D'Onofrio, E.; Zennaro, A.; Zavattini, G.C.; Lang, M. Validity and Reliability of the Interpersonal Competence Questionnaire: Empirical Evidence from an Italian Study. *J. Psychopathol. Behav. Assess.* **2016**, *38*, 113–123. [CrossRef]
29. Han, N.R.; Lee, D.G. Validation of the Korean Version of the Interpersonal Competence Questionnaire in Korean College Students. *Korean J. Couns. Psychother.* **2010**, *22*, 137–156.
30. Salavera, C.; Usán, P. Adaptación del cuestionario de competencia interpersonal ICQ-15 con población adolescente hispanohablante. *Rev. Iberoam. Diagnóstico Evaluación* **2018**, *3*, 29–39. [CrossRef]
31. Sawyer, S.M.; Azzopardi, P.S.; Wickremarathne, D.; Patton, G.C. The age of adolescence. *Lancet Child Adolesc. Health* **2018**, *2*, 223–228. [CrossRef]
32. Topp, C.W.; Ostergaard, S.D.; Sondergaard, S.; Bech, P. The WHO-5 Well-Being Index: A systematic review of the literature. *Psychother. Psychosom.* **2015**, *84*, 167–176. [CrossRef]
33. Wang, Z.; Bian, Q. Reliability and validity of the World Health Organization Five-item Well-Being Index for detecting depressive disorders in senior middle school students. *Chin. Ment. Health J.* **2011**, *25*, 279–283.
34. Campbell-Sills, L.; Stein, M.B. Psychometric analysis and refinement of the Connor-Davidson Resilience Scale (CD-RISC): Validation of a 10-item measure of resilience. *J. Trauma Stress* **2007**, *20*, 1019–1028. [CrossRef]
35. Wang, L.; Shi, Z.; Zhang, Y.; Zhang, Z. Psychometric properties of the 10-item Connor-Davidson Resilience Scale in Chinese earthquake victims. *Psychiat. Clin. Neuros.* **2010**, *64*, 499–504. [CrossRef]
36. Kroenke, K.; Spitzer, R.L.; Williams, J.B. The PHQ-9: Validity of a brief depression severity measure. *J. Gen. Intern. Med.* **2001**, *16*, 606–613. [CrossRef]
37. Hu, X.; Zhang, Y.; Liang, W.; Zhang, H.; Yang, S. Reliability and validity of Patient Health Questionnaire-9 (PHQ-9) in Chinese adolescents. *Sichuan Ment. Health* **2014**, *27*, 357–360.
38. Hurley, A.E.; Scandura, T.A.; Schriesheim, C.A.; Brannick, M.T.; Seers, A.; Vandenberg, R.J.; Williams, L.J. Exploratory and confirmatory factor analysis: Guidelines, issues, and alternatives. *J. Organ Behav.* **1997**, *18*, 667–683. [CrossRef]
39. Wei, Y. The Reliability and Validity of Interpersonal Competence Questionnaire in College Students. *Sch. Health China* **2005**, *26*, 1046–1048. [CrossRef]
40. Van de Schoot, R.; Lugtig, P.; Hox, J. A checklist for testing measurement invariance. *Eur. J. Dev. Psychol.* **2012**, *9*, 486–492. [CrossRef]
41. Smetana, J.G.; Campione-Barr, N.; Metzger, A. Adolescent Development in Interpersonal and Societal Contexts. *Annu. Rev. Psychol.* **2006**, *57*, 255–284. [CrossRef]
42. Rutkowski, L.; Svetina, D. Assessing the Hypothesis of Measurement Invariance in the Context of Large-Scale International Surveys. *Educ. Psychol. Meas.* **2014**, *74*, 31–57. [CrossRef]
43. Muthén, B.; Kaplan, D. A comparison of some methodologies for the factor analysis of non-normal Likert variables. *Br. Psychol. Soc.* **1985**, *38*, 171–189. [CrossRef]
44. Patrick, H.; Knee, C.R.; Canevello, A.; Lonsbary, C. The role of need fulfillment in relationship functioning and well-being: A self-determination theory perspective. *J. Pers. Soc. Psychol.* **2007**, *92*, 434–457. [CrossRef]
45. O'Connor, D.B.; Thayer, J.F.; Vedhara, K. Stress and health: A review of psychobiological processes. *Annu. Rev. Psychol.* **2021**, *72*, 663–688. [CrossRef]

**Disclaimer/Publisher's Note:** The statements, opinions and data contained in all publications are solely those of the individual author(s) and contributor(s) and not of MDPI and/or the editor(s). MDPI and/or the editor(s) disclaim responsibility for any injury to people or property resulting from any ideas, methods, instructions or products referred to in the content.

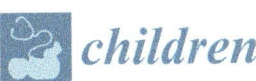

Article

# Psychological Resilience among Left-Behind Children in a Rural Area of Eastern China

Binyan Wang [1], Lihong Ye [1,2], Linshuoshuo Lv [1], Wei Liu [1], Fenfen Liu [1] and Yingying Mao [1,*]

1. School of Public Health, Zhejiang Chinese Medical University, Hangzhou 310053, China
2. School of Population Medicine and Public Health, Chinese Academy of Medical Sciences & Peking Union Medical College, Beijing 100730, China
* Correspondence: myy@zcmu.edu.cn

**Abstract:** Childhood is an important period for individuals' psychological development. Due to long-term separation from the parents, left-behind children (LBC) more easily develop deviation in cognition and abnormal personality. In this study, we aimed to explore the status of psychological resilience among LBC in a rural area of eastern China. We carried out a cross-sectional survey including middle and high school students from Qingyuan County of Zhejiang Province. Psychological resilience was measured using a modified scale developed for Chinese children. Data from a total of 1086 participants were collected, and the mean ± standard deviation score of psychological resilience was 4.11 ± 0.42. Multivariable linear regression analyses revealed that being a class leader ($p$ = 0.010) and having high self-evaluation of academic performance ($p$ < 0.001) were related with psychological resilience. Moreover, high contact frequency between parents and children ($p$ = 0.019) was associated with better psychological resilience among LBC. In conclusion, we found that being a class leader and having high self-evaluation of academic performance were associated with better psychological resilience among the children in this rural area and contact between parent and child was an essential factor associated with psychological resilience among LBC.

**Keywords:** left-behind children; parent–child communication; psychological resilience; child health

## 1. Introduction

Since the implementation of the reform and opening-up policy in China in the late 1970s, a great number of laborers from rural areas of China became urban city builders [1]. However, these migrant workers usually do not have equal treatments as citizens in terms of welfare, health care, as well as their children's accession to education in the cities they migrate to, and most of them are employed in low-paying jobs and living in poor conditions, which further discourages them from bringing their children with them [2]. Therefore, a majority of the migrant workers leave their children at home to be cared for by their relatives, friends, local community, or child institutions to reduce the living costs in the cities. As reported by the National Children's Fund (UNCIEF), the left-behind children (LBC) refer to the specific group of children who have been left-behind by adult migrants responsible for them, especially one or both parents [3]. The number of the so-called LBC is prominently high in the low- or middle-income countries worldwide. For example, approximately 27 percent of children in Philippine, 36 percent in Ecuador, and more than 40 percent in rural South Africa were estimated to be left behind [4]. In China, there were about 61 million rural children that were left behind by their migrant parents in 2010–2014, and the number has been proliferating [1]. Such labor migration seriously affected the physical and mental health of LBC, who were left uncared for [5].

In recent years, psychological problems of LBC have attracted increasing attention and concerns of the public both at home and abroad. Since long-term separation from their parents, most LBC could not receive adequate care and guidance from their parents and, thus, were at risk for developing psychological and behavioral problems, such as anxiety and depression. For example, it has been reported that the prevalence of psychological and behavioral problems, including loneliness, anxiety, depression, weak interpersonal relationships, and obsessive-compulsive symptoms, was high among LBC [6–13]. Moreover, a cross-sectional study of university students in Jiangsu province in China reported that left-behind experience in childhood was associated with worse mental health of late adolescence [14].

Recent studies related to LBC have placed much emphasis on mental health and its associated factors, while only a few studies have focused on the psychology of mental health from a positive perspective, aiming at investigating its protective factors. Psychological resilience refers to the effective response and adaptation in the face of difficulties or adversity [15]. It is a "rebound ability" with self-protection when life changes pose a challenge or a threat. The historical roots of resilience can be found in two bodies of literature: the psychological aspects of coping and the physiological aspects of stress [16]. Individual-level resilience requires positive experience and good personal relationships and perception of social support to confer resilience. Environmental factors can be imposed on an individual by external resources, such as living environment, school resource, and social assistance [17]. Observational studies have suggested that LBC had lower scores in psychological resilience, which may have more negative symptoms in adverse environments [18,19]. However, most previous studies on LBC's psychological resilience have not considered the dynamism and complex nature of family relationships, as well as students' performance at school. For instance, some of LBC's parents may return to their hometown after migrating for work for an extended period, but previous reports were limited with respect to the differences between current and previous LBC [20]. Furthermore, less attention has been paid to the contact between parents and children, which is an important family process of parent–child communication.

Therefore, in the present study, we aimed to understand the current situation of LBC's psychological resilience and its associated factors. We conducted a cross-sectional survey of middle school and high school students in Qingyuan County of Zhejiang Province, because Zhejiang Province is a relatively affluent province located in eastern China but there are a great number of LBC in remote mountainous and economically underdeveloped areas, such as Qingyuan county. Moreover, there is no relevant research on psychological resilience of LBC in rural areas of Zhejiang province to date.

## 2. Materials and Methods

### 2.1. Study Participants and Data Collection

The present study was carried out in Qingyuan County in Zhejiang Province, located in eastern China, from August to September in 2017. The protocol of this study was approved by Zhejiang Chinese Medical University Ethical Committee. Stratified random cluster sampling was used to include study participants. Briefly, the middle schools and high schools in Qingyuan county were first stratified into two groups based on their distances to the central town. Then one middle school and one high school were randomly selected from each stratum. All of the students in the selected schools were surveyed using a structured paper questionnaire ($n = 1086$). The survey was performed by School of Public Health at Zhejiang Chinese Medical University in co-operation with local health and educational authorities. We did not provide any incentives to the students.

Socio-demographic characteristics of the participants, including age, sex, ethnicity, location, household income, having siblings or not, type of school, being a class leader or not, self-evaluation of academic performance, as well as left-behind status, were collected using questionnaires by trained investigators. LBC were defined as children under 18 years old who have been left behind at their original residence for at least six months while one or both parents migrated to cities for work and were classified into "father migrated", "mother migrated", "both migrated", "past migrated", and a reference group of children (non-LBC). For LBC, parental migration status, type of caregivers, contact frequency between parent(s) and child, and frequency of parent(s) visiting the child were further collected.

The study participants' psychological resilience was assessed using a modified scale compiled by Hu et al. [21] from the Department of Psychology at Peking University in 2008, which included 27 items from two dimensions, personal strength and support. Personal strength included three factors: goal focus, emotion control, and positive cognition, and support included two factors: family support and interpersonal assistance. Participants were asked to indicate the extent to which they agreed with each item on a 5-point Likert rating scale (1 = strongly disagree; 5 = strongly agree). The scale was validated among children in China, and the internal consistency of the initial survey ($n$ = 283) was 0.85 and the reliability of the retest ($n$ = 420) was 0.83 [21].

## 2.2. Quality Control

The questionnaire used in the present study was developed after pre-survey and revision, and the investigators were trained before the survey. Before the survey, all participants were informed of the purpose of this study and the guidelines of the questionnaire. Participants were encouraged to answer the questions truthfully. The questionnaires were collected on site within a specified time. After the survey, on the same day, the investigators checked the quality of the questionnaire. If problems were found, a timely return visit was made. EpiData 3.02 software (EpiData Association, Denmark) was used to input the questionnaire data independently by two investigators, and the database was established after cross-validation.

## 2.3. Statistical Analysis

Statistical analysis was performed using R 3.3.0 (R core team). The scores of each item of psychological resilience were expressed in mean ± standard deviation (SD). The differences between groups were compared using two-sample t-test and one-way analyses of variance (ANOVA) for continuous variables, and chi-square test for categorical variables. Associated factors for psychological resilience were further analyzed using multivariable linear regression models. Two-sided $p$-values less than 0.05 were considered statistically significant.

## 3. Results

### 3.1. The Basic Characteristics of Study Participants

This study included a total of 1086 children aged 12–18 years from middle and high schools (Table 1). The percentage of females was 54.42%, and 97.42% of them were of Han ethnicity. Among them, 365 (33.6%) children were left behind, with 162 (44.4%) classified as both parents migrated, 142 (38.9%) as father migrated, 14 (3.8%) as mother migrated, and 47 (12.9%) as past migrated. In terms of caregivers, 162 (44.4%) were cared by single parent, 123 (33.7%) by grandparents, 49 (13.4%) by uncles and aunts, 12 (3.3%) by brothers/sisters, and 19 (5.2%) by themselves.

Compared with non-LBC, there were more LBC with parents who were divorced or passed away ($p$ = 0.002). There were no differences in the distributions of gender, ethnicity, household income, having sibling(s), being a class leader, and self-evaluation of academic performances were found between LBC and non-LBC ($p$ > 0.05).

Table 1. Psychological resilience among the study participants.

| Variables | | n | % | Psychological Resilience | | | Personal Strength | | | Support | | |
|---|---|---|---|---|---|---|---|---|---|---|---|---|
| | | | | M | SD | p | M | SD | p | M | SD | p |
| Sex | Female * | 591 | 54.42 | 4.12 | 0.42 | 0.396 | 4.02 | 0.57 | 0.025 | 4.25 | 0.42 | <0.001 |
| | Male | 495 | 45.58 | 4.10 | 0.43 | | 4.10 | 0.59 | | 4.10 | 0.43 | |
| Ethnicity | Han * | 1058 | 97.42 | 4.11 | 0.42 | 0.870 | 4.05 | 0.58 | 0.944 | 4.18 | 0.44 | 0.553 |
| | Others | 28 | 2.58 | 4.12 | 0.46 | | 4.05 | 0.65 | | 4.22 | 0.38 | |
| Location | Village * | 346 | 31.86 | 4.07 | 0.41 | 0.019 | 4.02 | 0.54 | 0.171 | 4.13 | 0.44 | 0.005 |
| | Town | 740 | 68.14 | 4.13 | 0.43 | | 4.07 | 0.60 | | 4.21 | 0.43 | |
| [1] Type of school | Middle school * student | 479 | 44.11 | 4.12 | 0.44 | 0.403 | 4.14 | 0.59 | <0.001 | 4.11 | 0.44 | <0.001 |
| | High school student | 607 | 55.89 | 4.10 | 0.41 | | 3.99 | 0.56 | | 4.24 | 0.42 | |
| Having sibling(s) | No * | 830 | 71.14 | 4.12 | 0.41 | 0.458 | 4.06 | 0.57 | 0.816 | 4.19 | 0.43 | 0.194 |
| | Yes | 256 | 23.57 | 4.09 | 0.45 | | 4.05 | 0.62 | | 4.15 | 0.44 | |
| Left-behind | No * | 721 | 66.39 | 4.11 | 0.41 | 0.652 | 4.05 | 0.58 | 0.959 | 4.19 | 0.43 | 0.360 |
| | Yes | 365 | 33.61 | 4.10 | 0.44 | | 4.05 | 0.59 | | 4.16 | 0.45 | |
| [2] Household income | Low * | 188 | 17.31 | 4.03 | 0.45 | 0.003 | 3.96 | 0.60 | <0.001 | 4.12 | 0.47 | 0.361 |
| | Moderate | 849 | 78.18 | 4.12 | 0.41 | | 4.06 | 0.56 | | 4.20 | 0.42 | |
| | High | 49 | 4.51 | 4.18 | 0.54 | | 4.27 | 0.70 | | 4.07 | 0.45 | |
| [3] Class leader | No * | 685 | 63.08 | 4.08 | 0.42 | <0.001 | 4.01 | 0.57 | <0.001 | 4.16 | 0.44 | 0.039 |
| | Yes | 401 | 36.92 | 4.17 | 0.43 | | 4.13 | 0.59 | | 4.22 | 0.43 | |
| Self-evaluation of academic performances | Bad * | 198 | 18.23 | 3.94 | 0.44 | <0.001 | 3.80 | 0.56 | <0.001 | 4.12 | 0.48 | 0.006 |
| | Below average | 174 | 16.02 | 4.05 | 0.39 | | 3.97 | 1.52 | | 4.15 | 0.44 | |
| | Average | 386 | 35.54 | 4.14 | 0.38 | | 4.11 | 0.54 | | 4.19 | 0.41 | |
| | Above average | 270 | 24.86 | 4.20 | 0.42 | | 4.18 | 0.59 | | 4.22 | 0.42 | |
| | Good | 58 | 5.34 | 4.25 | 0.54 | | 4.25 | 0.72 | | 4.25 | 0.50 | |

[1] Students in Grade 3 to 6 and Grade 7 to 8 were classified into middle school students and high school students, respectively. [2] The household income was self-rated as low, moderate, or high by the study participants. [3] The class leader was the students who help teachers to manage the class affairs. * Reference group. The bold indicated $p < 0.05$. Abbreviations: M, mean; SD, standard deviation.

### 3.2. The Psychological Resilience and Its Associated Factors among the Study Participants

As shown in Table 1, the average score of psychological resilience was higher in students from the town than those from the village ($p = 0.019$), and in class leaders than non-class leaders ($p < 0.001$). Higher household income and high self-evaluation of academic performances were associated with higher scores of psychological resilience, respectively ($p = 0.003$ and $p < 0.001$).

For the dimension of personal strength, the average score was higher in boys ($p = 0.025$), middle school students ($p < 0.001$), class leaders ($p < 0.001$), and those with higher household income ($p < 0.001$) and better self-evaluation of academic performances ($p < 0.001$). For the dimension of support, girls ($p < 0.001$), high school students ($p < 0.001$), those living in the town ($p = 0.005$), being a class leader ($p = 0.039$), and having better self-evaluation of academic performances scored better ($p = 0.006$).

In the multivariable linear regression models, statistically significant associations were observed for being a class leader ($\beta = 0.067$, $p = 0.010$) and better self-evaluation of academic performances ($\beta = 0.074$, $p < 0.001$) with higher scores of psychological resilience. For its two dimensions, higher household income ($\beta = 0.083$, $p = 0.032$), being a class leader ($\beta = 0.085$, $p = 0.017$) and better self-evaluation of academic performances ($\beta = 0.110$, $p < 0.001$) were associated with higher scores of personal strengths, while living in a village or town ($\beta = 0.078$, $p = 0.006$) and better self-evaluation of academic performances ($\beta = 0.029$, $p = 0.013$) were related with higher scores in support (Table 2).

**Table 2.** Multivariable linear regression analysis of factors associated with psychological resilience.

| Variables | Psychological Resilience | | | | Personal Strength | | | | Support | | | |
|---|---|---|---|---|---|---|---|---|---|---|---|---|
| | β | se | t | p | β | se | t | p | β | se | t | p |
| Location | 0.052 | 0.027 | 1.927 | 0.054 | 0.032 | 0.037 | 0.864 | 0.388 | 0.078 | 0.029 | 2.729 | **0.006** |
| [1] Household income | 0.047 | 0.028 | 1.663 | 0.097 | 0.083 | 0.039 | 2.148 | **0.032** | 0.002 | 0.030 | 0.056 | 0.956 |
| [2] Class leader | 0.067 | 0.026 | 2.584 | **0.010** | 0.085 | 0.036 | 2.399 | **0.017** | 0.045 | 0.027 | 1.641 | 0.101 |
| Self-evaluation of academic performances | 0.074 | 0.011 | 6.706 | **<0.001** | 0.110 | 0.015 | 7.317 | **<0.001** | 0.029 | 0.012 | 2.494 | **0.013** |

[1] The household income was self-rated as low, moderate, or high by the study participants. [2] The class leader was the students who help teachers to manage the class affairs. The variables that reach the statistically significant association for psychological resilience ($p < 0.05$) in the univariable analysis were included in the multivariable linear regression models. The bold indicated $p < 0.05$. Abbreviations: se, standard error.

### 3.3. The Psychological Resilience and Associated Factors in Left-Behind Children

However, the univariable and multivariable analysis did not show statistically significant differences in psychological resilience between LBC and non-LBC, nor in its two dimensions. Among LBC, in the univariable analysis, being a class leader ($p = 0.006$), higher self-evaluation of academic performances ($p < 0.001$), frequent contact between parent and child ($p = 0.004$), and frequent parental visit to children ($p = 0.028$) were associated with higher scores of psychological resilience (Table 3). Type of school ($p = 0.009$), being a class leader ($p = 0.029$), and higher self-evaluation of academic performances ($p < 0.001$) were associated with higher scores of personal strength, while sex ($p = 0.027$), high school students ($p = 0.001$), being a class leader ($p = 0.017$), and higher self-evaluation of academic performances ($p = 0.003$) were associated with higher scores of support. Moreover, psychological resilience among LBC was associated with the contact frequency between parents and children, with those contacting daily scoring the highest ($4.20 \pm 0.46$) and those contacting once per 30 days or more scoring the lowest ($3.96 \pm 0.48$) ($p = 0.004$). Similar scores and trends were found for both personal strength ($p = 0.019$) and support ($p = 0.012$).

Table 3. Psychological resilience among left-behind children.

| Variables | | No | % | Psychological Resilience | | | Personal Strength | | | Support | | |
|---|---|---|---|---|---|---|---|---|---|---|---|---|
| | | | | M | SD | p | M | SD | p | M | SD | p |
| Sex | Female * | 179 | 49.04 | 4.11 | 0.43 | 0.731 | 4.03 | 0.57 | 0.373 | 4.22 | 0.46 | 0.027 |
| | Male | 186 | 50.96 | 4.09 | 0.46 | | 4.08 | 0.61 | | 4.11 | 0.44 | |
| Ethnicity | Han * | 358 | 98.08 | 4.10 | 0.44 | 0.546 | 4.05 | 0.59 | 0.867 | 4.17 | 0.46 | 0.129 |
| | Others | 7 | 1.92 | 3.99 | 0.47 | | 4.01 | 0.66 | | 3.96 | 0.30 | |
| Location | Village * | 123 | 33.70 | 4.07 | 0.43 | 0.297 | 4.02 | 0.55 | 0.438 | 4.13 | 0.45 | 0.306 |
| | Town | 242 | 66.30 | 4.12 | 0.45 | | 4.07 | 0.61 | | 4.18 | 0.46 | |
| [1] Type of school | Middle school * | 181 | 49.59 | 4.11 | 0.45 | 0.651 | 4.13 | 0.61 | 0.009 | 4.09 | 0.45 | 0.001 |
| | High school | 184 | 50.41 | 4.09 | 0.43 | | 3.97 | 0.56 | | 4.24 | 0.45 | |
| Having sibling(s) | No * | 92 | 25.21 | 4.12 | 0.43 | 0.115 | 4.07 | 0.58 | 0.267 | 4.19 | 0.45 | 0.081 |
| | Yes | 273 | 74.79 | 4.04 | 0.47 | | 3.99 | 0.61 | | 4.09 | 0.45 | |
| [2] Household income | Low * | 69 | 18.90 | 4.03 | 0.47 | 0.109 | 3.97 | 0.60 | 0.052 | 4.10 | 0.47 | 0.716 |
| | Moderate | 275 | 75.34 | 4.12 | 0.43 | | 4.06 | 0.57 | | 4.19 | 0.45 | |
| | High | 21 | 5.75 | 4.16 | 0.54 | | 4.27 | 0.74 | | 4.02 | 0.43 | |
| [3] Class leader | No * | 127 | 34.79 | 4.06 | 0.45 | 0.006 | 4.00 | 0.58 | 0.029 | 4.12 | 0.47 | 0.017 |
| | Yes | 238 | 65.21 | 4.19 | 0.42 | | 4.15 | 0.60 | | 4.24 | 0.42 | |
| Self-evaluation of academic performances | Bad * | 74 | 20.27 | 3.91 | 0.48 | <0.001 | 3.77 | 0.58 | <0.001 | 4.08 | 0.50 | 0.003 |
| | Below average | 55 | 15.07 | 3.94 | 0.45 | | 3.86 | 0.53 | | 4.05 | 0.50 | |
| | Average | 126 | 34.52 | 4.16 | 0.38 | | 4.14 | 0.54 | | 4.19 | 0.41 | |
| | Above average | 94 | 25.75 | 4.24 | 0.41 | | 4.25 | 0.59 | | 4.22 | 0.40 | |
| | Good | 16 | 4.38 | 4.26 | 0.50 | | 4.18 | 0.60 | | 4.36 | 0.56 | |
| Parental migration status | Father-migrated * | 142 | 38.90 | 4.08 | 0.43 | 0.291 | 4.05 | 0.56 | 0.610 | 4.13 | 0.46 | 0.131 |
| | Mother-migrated | 14 | 3.84 | 3.98 | 0.52 | | 3.84 | 0.60 | | 4.15 | 0.56 | |
| | Both-migrated | 162 | 44.38 | 4.11 | 0.44 | | 4.05 | 0.59 | | 4.18 | 0.46 | |
| | Past migrated | 47 | 12.88 | 4.17 | 0.47 | | 4.12 | 0.67 | | 4.24 | 0.40 | |
| Type of caregivers | Single-parent * | 162 | 44.38 | 4.13 | 0.42 | 0.413 | 4.10 | 0.54 | 0.259 | 4.16 | 0.45 | 0.961 |
| | Grandparents | 123 | 33.70 | 4.05 | 0.45 | | 4.00 | 0.59 | | 4.12 | 0.46 | |
| | Uncles/aunts | 49 | 13.42 | 4.19 | 0.42 | | 4.09 | 0.61 | | 4.31 | 0.41 | |
| | Brothers/sisters | 12 | 3.29 | 4.17 | 0.46 | | 4.06 | 0.68 | | 4.31 | 0.43 | |
| | By oneself | 19 | 5.21 | 3.94 | 0.56 | | 3.91 | 0.81 | | 3.98 | 0.52 | |

**Table 3.** Cont.

| Variables | | No | % | Psychological Resilience | | | Personal Strength | | | Support | | |
|---|---|---|---|---|---|---|---|---|---|---|---|---|
| | | | | M | SD | p | M | SD | p | M | SD | p |
| Contact frequency with parents | 1 per 30 days or more * | 43 | 11.78 | 3.96 | 0.48 | **0.004** | 3.98 | 0.63 | **0.019** | 3.94 | 0.50 | **0.012** |
| | 1 per 15–30 days | 71 | 19.45 | 4.07 | 0.38 | | 3.97 | 0.50 | | 4.19 | 0.38 | |
| | 1 per 4–7 days | 107 | 29.32 | 4.09 | 0.45 | | 4.02 | 0.60 | | 4.17 | 0.46 | |
| | 1 per 2–3 days | 69 | 18.90 | 4.14 | 0.43 | | 4.09 | 0.58 | | 4.21 | 0.47 | |
| | Daily | 75 | 20.55 | 4.20 | 0.46 | | 4.18 | 0.62 | | 4.22 | 0.43 | |
| Frequency of parents visiting children | More than 1 year * | 32 | 8.77 | 4.05 | 0.48 | **0.028** | 4.04 | 0.68 | 0.052 | 4.07 | 0.52 | 0.113 |
| | Every 6 months to 1 year | 69 | 18.90 | 4.09 | 0.46 | | 4.01 | 0.60 | | 4.19 | 0.46 | |
| | Every 1–6 months | 153 | 41.92 | 4.05 | 0.40 | | 3.94 | 0.54 | | 4.12 | 0.43 | |
| | Every month | 111 | 30.41 | 4.20 | 0.46 | | 4.18 | 0.61 | | 4.23 | 0.45 | |

[1] Students in Grade 3 to 6 and Grade 7 to 8 were classified into middle school students and high school students, respectively. [2] The household income was self-rated as low, moderate, or high by the study participants. [3] The class leader was the students who help teachers to manage the class affairs. * Reference group. The bold indicated $p < 0.05$. Abbreviations: M, mean; SD, standard deviation.

As shown in the Tables 4 and 5, in the multivariable regression analysis, being a class leader (β = 0.121, $p$ = 0.010 in Table 4; β = 0.106, $p$ = 0.023 in Table 5) and higher self-evaluation of academic performance (β = 0.100 in Table 4, β = 0.108 in Table 5, both $p$ < 0.001) and high contact frequency between parents and children (β = 0.041, $p$ = 0.019 in Table 4) were associated with psychological resilience. For its two dimensions, higher self-evaluation of academic performance (β = 0.140 in Table 4, β = 0.147 in Table 5, both $p$ < 0.001) was associated with personal strength, and being a class leader (β = 0.116, $p$ = 0.020 in Table 4, β = 0.101, $p$ = 0.043 in Table 5), self-evaluation of academic performance (β = 0.049, $p$ = 0.019 in Table 4, β = 0.058, $p$ = 0.005 in Table 5), and contact frequency between parents and children (β = 0.045, $p$ = 0.017 in Table 4) were associated with support.

**Table 4.** Multivariable linear regression analysis of factors associated with psychological resilience among left-behind children.

| Variables | Psychological Resilience | | | | Personal Strength | | | | Support | | | |
|---|---|---|---|---|---|---|---|---|---|---|---|---|
| | β | se | t | $p$ | β | se | t | $p$ | β | se | t | $p$ |
| [1] Class leader | 0.121 | 0.047 | 2.585 | **0.010** | 0.114 | 0.062 | 1.842 | 0.066 | 0.116 | 0.050 | 2.333 | **0.020** |
| Self-evaluation of academic performances | 0.100 | 0.019 | 5.131 | **<0.001** | 0.140 | 0.026 | 5.472 | **<0.001** | 0.049 | 0.021 | 2.364 | **0.019** |
| Contact frequency with parents | 0.041 | 0.018 | 2.348 | **0.019** | 0.034 | 0.023 | 1.481 | 0.140 | 0.045 | 0.019 | 2.403 | **0.017** |

[1] The class leader was the students who help teachers to manage the class affairs. The variables that reach the statistically significant association for psychological resilience ($p$ < 0.05) in the univariable analysis were included in the multivariable linear regression models. To avoid collinearity, "Contact frequency with parents" and "Frequency of parents visiting children" were added to the linear regression model, respectively. The bold indicated $p$ < 0.05. Abbreviations: se, standard error.

**Table 5.** Multivariable linear regression analysis of factors associated with psychological resilience among left-behind children.

| Variables | Psychological Resilience | | | | Personal Strength | | | | Support | | | |
|---|---|---|---|---|---|---|---|---|---|---|---|---|
| | β | se | t | $p$ | β | se | t | $p$ | β | Se | t | $p$ |
| [1] Class leader | 0.106 | 0.047 | 2.278 | **0.023** | 0.101 | 0.061 | 1.642 | 0.101 | 0.101 | 0.050 | 2.028 | **0.043** |
| Self-evaluation of academic performances | 0.108 | 0.019 | 5.631 | **<0.001** | 0.147 | 0.025 | 5.833 | **<0.001** | 0.058 | 0.020 | 2.832 | **0.005** |
| Frequency of parents visiting children | 0.047 | 0.024 | 1.954 | 0.051 | 0.054 | 0.032 | 1.711 | 0.088 | 0.037 | 0.026 | 1.427 | 0.154 |

[1] The class leader was the students who help teachers to manage the class affairs. The variables that reach the statistically significant association for psychological resilience ($p$ < 0.05) in the univariable analysis were included in the multivariable linear regression models. To avoid collinearity, "Contact frequency with parents" and "Frequency of parents visiting children" were added to the linear regression model, respectively. The bold indicated $p$ < 0.05. Abbreviations: se, standard error.

Among non-LBC, univariable linear regression analysis showed that living in the town area ($p$ = 0.033), higher household income ($p$ = 0.012), being a class leader ($p$ = 0.023), and self-evaluation of academic performance ($p$ < 0.001) were associated with higher scores of psychological resilience (Table 6). Sex ($p$ = 0.033), higher household income ($p$ = 0.007), type of school ($p$ = 0.009), being a class leader ($p$ = 0.013) and higher self-evaluation of academic performances ($p$ < 0.001) were associated with higher scores of personal strength, while sex ($p$ < 0.001), living in the town ($p$ = 0.006), and type of school ($p$ = 0.001) were associated with higher scores of support. However, we did not observe the potential association between being a class leader ($p$ = 0.420), self-evaluation of academic performance ($p$ = 0.269) and support. In the multivariable linear regression analysis, being a class leader (β = 0.106, $p$ = 0.024) and higher self-evaluation of academic performance (β = 0.106, $p$ < 0.001) were associated with psychological resilience. In its two dimensions, higher self-evaluation of academic performance (β = 0.144, $p$ < 0.001) was associated with personal strength. Being a class leader (β = 0.100, $p$ = 0.045) and higher self-evaluation of academic performance (β = 0.058, $p$ = 0.005) were associated with support (Table 7).

Table 6. Psychological resilience among non-left-behind children.

| Variables | | No | % | Psychological Resilience | | | Personal Strength | | | Support | | |
|---|---|---|---|---|---|---|---|---|---|---|---|---|
| | | | | M | SD | p | M | SD | p | M | SD | p |
| Sex | Female * | 405 | 37.29 | 4.13 | 0.41 | 0.436 | 4.01 | 0.570 | **0.033** | 4.26 | 0.407 | **<0.001** |
| | Male | 316 | 29.10 | 4.10 | 0.42 | | 4.11 | 0.58 | | 4.09 | 0.43 | |
| Ethnicity | Han * | 700 | 64.46 | 4.11 | 0.41 | 0.583 | 4.05 | 0.57 | 0.986 | 4.19 | 0.43 | 0.147 |
| | Others | 21 | 1.93 | 4.17 | 0.46 | | 4.06 | 0.66 | | 4.31 | 0.66 | |
| Location | Village * | 223 | 20.53 | 4.07 | 0.40 | **0.033** | 4.02 | 0.43 | 0.261 | 4.12 | 0.43 | **0.006** |
| | Town | 498 | 45.86 | 4.14 | 0.42 | | 4.07 | 0.59 | | 4.22 | 0.42 | |
| [1] Type of school | Middle school * | 181 | 49.59 | 4.13 | 0.43 | 0.451 | 4.14 | 0.58 | **0.009** | 4.12 | 0.44 | **0.001** |
| | High school | 184 | 50.41 | 4.10 | 0.40 | | 4.00 | 0.56 | | 4.24 | 0.41 | |
| Having sibling(s) | No * | 557 | 51.29 | 4.11 | 0.40 | 0.757 | 4.05 | 0.56 | 0.595 | 4.19 | 0.43 | 0.809 |
| | Yes | 164 | 15.10 | 4.12 | 0.44 | | 4.08 | 4.08 | | 4.18 | 0.42 | |
| [2] Household income | Low * | 69 | 18.90 | 4.03 | 0.60 | **0.012** | 3.95 | 3.95 | **0.007** | 3.95 | 0.47 | 0.382 |
| | Moderate | 275 | 75.34 | 4.24 | 0.56 | | 0.77 | 0.77 | | 4.20 | 0.41 | |
| | High | 21 | 5.75 | 4.19 | 0.55 | | 4.26 | 0.69 | | 4.11 | 0.47 | |
| [3] Class leader | No * | 447 | 41.16 | 4.09 | 0.40 | **0.023** | 4.01 | 0.57 | **0.013** | 4.18 | 0.42 | 0.420 |
| | Yes | 274 | 25.23 | 4.16 | 0.43 | | 4.12 | 0.58 | | 4.21 | 0.43 | |
| Self-evaluation of academic performances | Bad * | 124 | 11.42 | 3.96 | 0.42 | **<0.001** | 3.82 | 0.55 | **<0.001** | 4.15 | 0.47 | 0.269 |
| | Below average | 119 | 10.96 | 4.10 | 0.36 | | 4.03 | 0.50 | | 4.20 | 0.40 | |
| | Average | 260 | 23.94 | 4.13 | 0.38 | | 4.09 | 0.54 | | 4.19 | 0.41 | |
| | Above average | 176 | 16.21 | 4.17 | 0.43 | | 4.14 | 0.59 | | 4.22 | 0.43 | |
| | Good | 42 | 3.87 | 4.24 | 0.56 | | 4.27 | 0.77 | | 4.20 | 0.47 | |

[1] Students in Grade 3 to 6 and Grade 7 to 8 were classified into middle school students and high school students, respectively. [2] The household income was self-rated as low, moderate, or high by the study participants. [3] The class leader was the students who help teachers to manage the class affairs. * Reference group. The bold indicated $p < 0.05$. Abbreviations: M, mean; SD, standard deviation.

**Table 7.** Multivariable linear regression analysis of factors associated with psychological resilience among non-left-behind children.

| Variables | Psychological Resilience | | | | Personal Strength | | | | Support | | | |
|---|---|---|---|---|---|---|---|---|---|---|---|---|
| | β | se | t | p | β | se | t | p | β | se | t | p |
| Location | 0.037 | 0.048 | 0.783 | 0.434 | 0.028 | 0.064 | 0.438 | 0.662 | 0.048 | 0.050 | 0.954 | 0.341 |
| [1] Household income | 0.028 | 0.048 | 0.590 | 0.556 | 0.062 | 0.064 | 0.966 | 0.335 | −0.013 | 0.051 | −0.260 | 0.795 |
| [2] Class leader | 0.106 | 0.047 | 2.272 | **0.024** | 0.112 | 0.060 | 1.8 | 0.073 | 0.100 | 0.049 | 2.014 | **0.045** |
| Self-evaluation of academic performances | 0.106 | 0.019 | 5.445 | **<0.001** | 0.144 | 0.026 | 5.562 | **<0.001** | 0.058 | 0.021 | 2.820 | **0.005** |

[1] The household income was self-rated as low, moderate, or high by the study participants. [2] The class leader was the students who help teachers to manage the class affairs. The variables that reach the statistically significant association for psychological resilience ($p < 0.05$) in the univariable analysis were included in the multivariable linear regression models. The bold indicated $p < 0.05$. Abbreviations: se, standard error.

## 4. Discussion

To the best of our knowledge, this is the first study to examine psychological resilience of children living in the rural areas of Zhejiang province in eastern China. In the present study, we found that being a class leader and self-evaluation of academic performance were associated with psychological resilience in this rural area of eastern China, and parent–child contact is an essential factor for psychological resilience among LBC.

There are several theories of resilience: (i) resilience is a positive psychological outcome among high-risk individuals [22]; (ii) resilience is a dynamic, interactive process that involves stress, pressure, and other adverse life events [23]; and (iii) resilience is the ability of an individual to cope with stress, frustration, trauma, and other adverse life events [24]. Compared to the first and the second theories, the theory of resilience as ability is largely measurable and is most directly amenable to therapeutic interventions. In the past few decades, studies have suggested the negative impact of parental migration on children's psychological resilience [19]. However, in the present study, we did not observe differences in scores of psychological resilience between LBC and non-LBC, which was not similar with results from previous studies [25]. This may be because the study participants in our study from Qingyuan County encountered various environmental diversities and LBC accounted for only one third of the study population. Moreover, studies showed that economic conditions were closely related to children's physical and mental health [26,27], since Zhejiang province is relatively affluent, the average levels of psychological resilience of children in the present study are relatively high. The students in this special area may have similar coping capacities with their general rural adversities or socio-economic challenges, despite their parental migration status. It is also possible that, due to the limited sample size, this study did not have enough statistical power. However, the results from our study are in consistency with the findings of another cross-sectional survey conducted in Yunyang County of Three Gorges Areas in the middle of China, which reported no differences in the resilience between LBC and non-LBC in middle school students [28].

As for the factors associated with psychological resilience among children living in the mountainous areas, we found that being class leader and self-evaluation of academic performances were potential determinants of psychological resilience. Results from the study by Wang et al. also showed that LBC with learning disabilities had statistically significantly lower scores of psychological resilience than those with excellent and median learning abilities [29]. Because children have learning pressure at school, their academic performance directly determines their psychological toughness. Therefore, our study suggested that teachers and parents should actively encourage students to help improve their academic performances. Moreover, our study also suggested that the scores of psychological resilience of the class leader students were higher than those of non-class leaders. The possible reasons may be that students who serve as class leaders have higher self-social value, and their self-esteem is easier to be satisfied, which is positively correlated with children's mental health. Therefore, it is suggested that schools pay more attention to cultivating the students' self-social value and self-esteem, especially for LBC.

Moreover, we also found that among LBC, parental–child contact was associated with psychological resilience. It is in consistency with findings from Zhou et al. that better parent–child communication was associated with better development of their mental health among LBC [19]. Results from the study by Wang et al. also showed that contact frequency with parents was closely related to LBC's mental health [30]. It could be seen that maintaining a high contact frequency was very important for the parents of migrant workers to timely and comprehensively grasp the living and school life of their children and maintain an intimate parent–child relationship. In addition, as the study conducted by Clarke et al. suggested, children who suffered from insecure parent relationships were more difficult in building resilience [31]. Therefore, communication between parents and children is necessary for the development of psychological resilience of LBC, leading to our suggestions that the parents of LBC should communicate with their children as much as possible and pick up their children for a reunion as much as possible. The study by Liu et al.

evaluated the impact of parental migration and parent–child relation types on psychological resilience of LBC and found that mother's remote migration had a significantly negative impact on psychological resilience of LBC [18]. In this study, though we did not detect statistically significant differences in psychological resilience among LBC with different migration statuses, our results showed that the scores of psychological resilience of LBC with mother out for work was the lowest. A study conducted in Ghana and Nigeria found similar results [32]. Since migrant mothers cannot take good care of their children's daily life, they also have difficulty in giving appropriate care and support emotionally; it is suggested that mothers stay at home to take care of LBC as much as possible.

This study has several limitations. First, this survey only included middle and high school students in Qingyuan, a rural area of Zhejiang province in eastern China. Further studies should broaden the research objectives and include students from other grades and from nonrural areas. Second, the data in the present study were collected by self-reported questionnaires with limited variables from the children, so further studies are warranted to collect further information on mental health and trauma exposure, which may also influence psychological resilience. In addition, this is a cross-sectional study with limited capacity in causal inference; therefore, we could not rule out the possibility that psychological resilience might contribute to children's academic performance or their contact with their parents. Further longitudinal studies are needed to investigate the causal associations between identified factors and psychological resilience and its potential underlying mechanisms.

## 5. Conclusions

In summary, this study suggested that being a class leader and self-evaluation of academic performance were related with psychological resilience in children in this rural area of eastern China, and parent–child contact is an important factor for psychological resilience among LBC. Targeted intervention programs, such as strengthening parental–child communications should be delivered to improve the psychological resilience among LBC in China.

**Author Contributions:** B.W. and Y.M., conceived the study; F.L., L.Y., L.L. and W.L. conducted survey; L.L. and L.Y. analyzed data; B.W. wrote the draft; and all of the authors revised and proofed the final draft. All authors have read and agreed to the published version of the manuscript.

**Funding:** The study was supported by Zhejiang Province Civil Policy Theory Research Plan under grant (ZMYB201652).

**Institutional Review Board Statement:** The study was reviewed and approved by the Ethical Committee of Zhejiang Chinese Medical University (No.170520-1) with approval date on 20 May 2017.

**Informed Consent Statement:** Not applicable.

**Data Availability Statement:** The datasets analyzed in this study are available from the corresponding author on reasonable request.

**Acknowledgments:** The authors sincerely thank all the participants and researchers involved in the present study.

**Conflicts of Interest:** The authors declare that the research was conducted in the absence of any commercial or financial relationships that could be construed as a potential conflict of interest.

## References

1. Yuan, P.; Wang, L. Migrant workers: China boom leaves children behind. *Nature* **2016**, *529*, 25. [CrossRef] [PubMed]
2. Chen, X.; Wang, L.; Wang, Z. Shyness-sensitivity and social, school, and psychological adjustment in rural migrant and urban children in China. *Child Dev.* **2009**, *80*, 1499–1513. [CrossRef] [PubMed]
3. UNICEF Welcomes State Council Guideline on the Protection of Left Behind Children. Available online: https://www.unicef.cn/en/press-releases/unicef-welcomes-state-council-guideline-protection-left-behind-children (accessed on 10 November 2022).

4. Fellmeth, G.; Rose-Clarke, K.; Zhao, C.; Busert, L.K.; Zheng, Y.; Massazza, A.; Sonmez, H.; Eder, B.; Blewitt, A.; Lertgrai, W.; et al. Health impacts of parental migration on left-behind children and adolescents: A systematic review and meta-analysis. *Lancet* **2018**, *392*, 2567–2582. [CrossRef] [PubMed]
5. Samson, M.; Fajth, G.; Francois, D. Cognitive capital, equity and child-sensitive social protection in Asia and the Pacific. *BMJ Glob. Health* **2016**, *1*, i19–i26. [CrossRef] [PubMed]
6. Gao, Y.; Li, L.; Chan, E.Y.; Lau, J.; Griffiths, S.M. Parental migration, self-efficacy and cigarette smoking among rural adolescents in south China. *PLoS ONE* **2013**, *8*, e57369. [CrossRef]
7. Gao, Y.; Li, L.P.; Kim, J.H.; Congdon, N.; Lau, J.; Griffiths, S. The impact of parental migration on health status and health behaviours among left behind adolescent school children in China. *BMC Public Health* **2010**, *10*, 56. [CrossRef]
8. He, B.; Fan, J.; Liu, N.; Li, H.; Wang, Y.; Williams, J.; Wong, K. Depression risk of 'left-behind children' in rural China. *Psychiatry Res.* **2012**, *200*, 306–312. [CrossRef]
9. Liu, H.; Zhou, Z.; Fan, X.; Wang, J.; Sun, H.; Shen, C.; Zhai, X. The influence of left-behind experience on college students' mental health: A cross-sectional comparative study. *Int. J. Environ. Res. Public Health* **2020**, *17*, 1511. [CrossRef] [PubMed]
10. Liu, W.; Li, J.; Huang, Y.; Yu, B.; Qin, R.; Cao, X. The relationship between left-behind experience and obsessive-compulsive symptoms in college students in China: The mediation effect of self-esteem. *Psychol. Health Med.* **2021**, *26*, 644–655. [CrossRef] [PubMed]
11. Qu, G.B.; Wu, W.; Wang, L.L.; Tang, X.; Sun, Y.H.; Li, J.; Wang, J. Systematic review and meta-analysis found higher levels of behavioural problems in male left-behind children aged 6–11 years. *Acta Paediatr.* **2018**, *107*, 1327–1334. [CrossRef]
12. Tang, W.; Wang, G.; Hu, T.; Dai, Q.; Xu, J.; Yang, Y.; Xu, J. Mental health and psychosocial problems among Chinese left-behind children: A cross-sectional comparative study. *J. Affect. Disord.* **2018**, *241*, 133–141. [CrossRef] [PubMed]
13. Zhou, Y.M.; Zhao, C.X.; Qi, Y.J.; Fan, H.; Huang, X.N.; Tian, X.B.; Sun, J.; Yi, Z. Emotional and behavioral problems of left-behind children in impoverished rural China: A comparative cross-sectional study of fourth-grade Children. *J. Adolesc. Health* **2020**, *67*, S48–S54. [CrossRef] [PubMed]
14. Wu, H.; Cai, Z.; Yan, Q.; Yu, Y.; Yu, N.N. The Impact of childhood left-behind experience on the mental health of late adolescents: Evidence from Chinese college freshmen. *Int. J. Environ. Res. Public Health* **2021**, *18*, 2778. [CrossRef] [PubMed]
15. Bonanno, G.A. Loss, trauma, and human resilience: Have we underestimated the human capacity to thrive after extremely aversive events? *Am. Psychol.* **2004**, *59*, 20–28. [CrossRef] [PubMed]
16. Tusaie, K.; Dyer, J. Resilience: A historical review of the construct. *Holist. Nurs. Pract.* **2004**, *18*, 3–8. [CrossRef] [PubMed]
17. Davydov, D.M.; Stewart, R.; Ritchie, K.; Chaudieu, I. Resilience and mental health. *Clin. Psychol. Rev.* **2010**, *30*, 479–495. [CrossRef] [PubMed]
18. Liu, H.; Liu, L.; Jin, X. The impact of parental remote migration and parent-child relation types on the psychological resilience of rural left-behind children in China. *Int. J. Environ. Res. Public Health* **2020**, *17*, 5388. [CrossRef]
19. Zhou, C.; Lv, Q.; Yang, N.; Wang, F. Left-behind children, parent-child communication and psychological resilience: A structural equation modeling analysis. *Int. J. Environ. Res. Public Health* **2021**, *18*, 5123. [CrossRef]
20. Zhang, H.; Zhou, H.; Cao, R. Bullying victimization among left-behind children in rural China: Prevalence and associated risk factors. *J. Interpers. Violence* **2021**, *36*, NP8414–NP8430. [CrossRef]
21. Hu, Y.; Gan, Y. Development and psychometric validity of the resilience scale for Chinese adolescents. *Acta Psychol. Sin.* **2008**, *40*, 902–912. [CrossRef]
22. Hopwood, M.; Treloar, C. Resilient coping: Applying adaptive responses to prior adversity during treatment for hepatitis C infection. *J. Health Psychol.* **2008**, *13*, 17–27. [CrossRef] [PubMed]
23. Luthar, S.S.; Cicchetti, D.; Becker, B. The construct of resilience: A critical evaluation and guidelines for future work. *Child Dev.* **2000**, *71*, 543–562. [CrossRef] [PubMed]
24. Bonanno, G.A.; Brewin, C.R.; Kaniasty, K.; Greca, A.M. Weighing the costs of disaster: Consequences, risks, and resilience in individuals, families, and communities. *Psychol. Sci. Public Interest* **2010**, *11*, 1–49. [CrossRef] [PubMed]
25. HQ, Z. Mental resilience and its influence factors in rural left-behind students. *Chin. J. Sch. Health* **2011**, *32*, 613–614. (In Chinese)
26. Wang, A.N.; Zhang, W.; Zhang, J.P.; Huang, F.F.; Ye, M.; Yao, S.Y.; Luo, Y.H.; Li, Z.H.; Zhang, J.; Su, P. Latent classes of resilience and psychological response among only-child loss parents in China. *Stress Health* **2017**, *33*, 397–404. [CrossRef] [PubMed]
27. Hostinar, C.E.; Miller, G.E. Protective factors for youth confronting economic hardship: Current challenges and future avenues in resilience research. *Am. Psychol.* **2019**, *74*, 641–652. [CrossRef]
28. Guo, X.; Liu, Q.; Wang, H.; Huang, K.; Lei, X.; Zhang, F.; Wang, Y. Resilience and its influential factors in left-behind middle school students in Yunyang County of Rural Three Gorges Areas in China: A cross-sectional survey. *Public Health* **2015**, *129*, 1479–1487. [CrossRef] [PubMed]
29. Wang, D.Q.; Shang, G.H.; Chen, X.B. Study on resilience and general self-efficacy with group psychological counseling among rural left-behind children. *Chin. J. Sch. Dr* **2016**, *30*, 801–803.
30. Wang, F.; Lin, L.; Xu, M.; Li, L.; Lu, J.; Zhou, X. Mental health among left-behind children in rural China in relation to parent-child communication. *Int. J. Environ. Res. Public Health* **2019**, *16*, 1855. [CrossRef]

31. Rose-Clarke, K.; Nambutr, W.; Kongkamud, A.; Lertgrai, W.; Prost, A.; Benyakorn, S.; Albakri, M.; Devries, K.; Salisbury, T.; Jampaklay, A. Psychosocial resilience among left-behind adolescents in rural Thailand: A qualitative exploration. *Sociol. Health Illn.* **2021**, *44*, 147–168. [CrossRef]
32. Cebotari, V.; Mazzucato, V.; Siegel, M. Child development and migrant transnationalism: The health of children who stay behind in Ghana and Nigeria. *J. Dev. Stud.* **2016**, *53*, 444–459. [CrossRef]

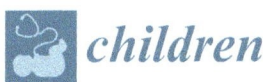 

*Review*

# Psychosis Caused by a Somatic Condition: How to Make the Diagnosis? A Systematic Literature Review

Nolwenn Dissaux [1,2,*], Pierre Neyme [3], Deok-Hee Kim-Dufor [1], Nathalie Lavenne-Collot [1,4], Jonathan J. Marsh [5], Sofian Berrouiguet [1,2], Michel Walter [1,2] and Christophe Lemey [1,2]

[1] Centre Hospitalier Régional et Universitaire de Brest, 2 Avenue Foch, 29200 Brest, France
[2] Unité de Recherche EA 7479 SPURBO, Université de Bretagne Occidentale, 29200 Brest, France
[3] Fondation du Bon Sauveur d'Alby, 30 Avenue du Colonel Teyssier, 81000 Albi, France
[4] Laboratoire du Traitement de l'Information Médicale, Inserm U1101, 29200 Brest, France
[5] Graduate School of Social Service, Fordham University, 113 West 60th Street, New York, NY 10023, USA
* Correspondence: nolwenn.dissaux@chu-brest.fr

**Abstract:** Background: First episode of psychosis (FEP) is a clinical condition that usually occurs during adolescence or early adulthood and is often a sign of a future psychiatric disease. However, these symptoms are not specific, and psychosis can be caused by a physical disease in at least 5% of cases. Timely detection of these diseases, the first signs of which may appear in childhood, is of particular importance, as a curable treatment exists in most cases. However, there is no consensus in academic societies to offer recommendations for a comprehensive medical assessment to eliminate somatic causes. Methods: We conducted a systematic literature search using a two-fold research strategy to: (1) identify physical diseases that can be differentially diagnosed for psychosis; and (2) determine the paraclinical exams allowing us to exclude these pathologies. Results: We identified 85 articles describing the autoimmune, metabolic, neurologic, infectious, and genetic differential diagnoses of psychosis. Clinical presentations are described, and a complete list of laboratory and imaging features required to identify and confirm these diseases is provided. Conclusion: This systematic review shows that most differential diagnoses of psychosis should be considered in the case of a FEP and could be identified by providing a systematic checkup with a laboratory test that includes ammonemia, antinuclear and anti-NMDA antibodies, and HIV testing; brain magnetic resonance imaging and lumbar puncture should be considered according to the clinical presentation. Genetic research could be of interest to patients presenting with physical or developmental symptoms associated with psychiatric manifestations.

**Keywords:** first-episode psychosis; differential diagnosis; initial work-up; systematic review

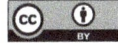

## 1. Introduction

First episode of psychosis (FEP) is a full-threshold clinical condition in which altered perceptions of reality, delusions, disorganized thoughts, and cognitive dysfunctions can be observed by others and are associated with functional decline [1]. FEP affects 3% of the population and typically manifests during adolescence or early adulthood. Additionally, FEP may pose severe consequences, such as suicidal behaviors. Following FEP, the clinical trajectory leads to a diagnosis of schizophrenia in 51% of cases and 32.5% for another non-affective psychotic disorder [2]. However, psychotic-like symptoms have been found to also reveal a somatic affection; for example, it is well-established that auditory hallucinations can be caused by temporal epilepsy [3]. Furthermore, several studies have found that psychotic-like experiences may be associated with physical disorders in ultra-high-risk patients [4] and that at least 5% of FEP could be caused by a physical disease [5,6]. It is thus essential to identify whether these somatic diseases potentially underlie FEP patients, especially since curative treatments for them exist in most cases. Moreover, over the past decade, studies have shown evidence that early detection of the first signs of psychosis and early intervention with a reduced duration of untreated psychosis (DUP) limit the negative impacts of the disorder [7,8].

Considering these results, guidelines focus on early intervention and treatment of FEP. However, the low specificity of FEP symptoms makes detection highly challenging, and even though guidelines propose a "general medical assessment" [1], no consensus of recommendation has been established for a comprehensive medical assessment to eliminate somatic causes. One of the main challenges in the case of FEP is to dual-diagnose co-occurring somatic diseases. Some pathologies may not be immediately clinically apparent, although a brief test can make the diagnosis. More commonly, there is no specific test, and the clinician will turn to a differential diagnosis based on unstructured clinical and paraclinical inferences. Furthermore, antipsychotics should be used with caution in some clinical conditions, such as encephalitis [9–11], indicating the sensitivity of FEP cases as well as the lethal risks that ill-informed treatment or medical mismanagement may pose. This systematic review aims to determine the physical diseases that can engender psychotic symptoms and the paraclinical exams that allow for the exclusion of these pathologies.

## 2. Materials and Methods

This review followed the Preferred Reporting Items for Systematic Reviews and Meta-Analyses (PRISMA) guidelines [12] to ensure comprehensive and transparent reporting of methods and results. The protocol was registered at the International Prospective Register of Systematic Reviews (PROSPERO) in June 2019 (registration number: CRD42020136243).

### 2.1. Search Strategy

Two independent authors searched the electronic database PubMed. A two-fold research strategy was used to ensure a complete search. The research terms used were as follows: "Schizophrenia/diagnosis"[MAJR] AND "Diagnosis, Differential"[MeSH Terms] AND review" and psychosis[Title/Abstract] AND diagnosis[Title/Abstract] AND neurologic[Title/Abstract] OR endocrinologic[Title/Abstract] OR metabolic[Title/Abstract] OR infectious[Title/Abstract] OR inflammatory[Title/Abstract] OR autoimmune[Title/Abstract] OR chromosomic[Title/Abstract] OR genetic[Title/Abstract] OR toxic[Title/Abstract].

In addition, a manual literature search was performed on the websites of academic societies to identify publications related to the subject.

Papers published until July 2021 were included.

### 2.2. Eligibility Criteria

Articles must have included the prerequisite topics, "first-episode psychosis differential diagnosis and/or related paraclinical features", with the language of the publication written in English.

Case reports were excluded to avoid non-relevant data or duplicates with reviews already reporting matching cases. The psychotic presentation of medical conditions such as brain tumors, traumatic brain disorders, substance abuse, and common thyroid disorders has been clearly established for several decades [1,13,14]. These somatic conditions are thus not detailed in this review, as they have not been the subject of active research within the last 15 years.

### 2.3. Data Collection

All potential studies were first exported into a reference citation manager (Zotero), and duplicates were removed. Two independent researchers separately performed the screening of titles and abstracts, full-text analysis, and selection of paraclinical exams. Disagreements were resolved through discussions until a consensus was reached and a third reviewer was available to resolve the rest of the disagreements.

Next, a narrative-descriptive summary was created for the selected studies.

As the selected studies use heterogeneous methods, we identified commonalities from them through a two-part analysis: (1) by study features (number of studies, theme, populations, bias, etc.); and (2) by studies' contributions to clinical psychiatry and implications for future research. Studies were classified according to the nosographic category they addressed (neurology, infectious diseases, etc.), the type of exam performed, and the type of study that was conducted (meta-analysis, literature review, etc.).

## 3. Results

### 3.1. Search Results

The electronic search returned 970 articles, and five recommendations were also identified through the hand-searched literature of publications in academic societies. A full-text evaluation was conducted for 130 articles, out of which 87 met the inclusion criteria and were included in the final synthesis (details in Appendix A). From these studies, autoimmune, metabolic, neurologic, infectious, and genetic differential diagnoses were identified for FEP, and the complete list of laboratory or imaging features required to confirm these diseases was drawn (detail in Appendix B).

Details of the search results are summarized in Figure 1.

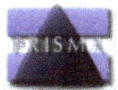

## PRISMA 2009 Flow Diagram

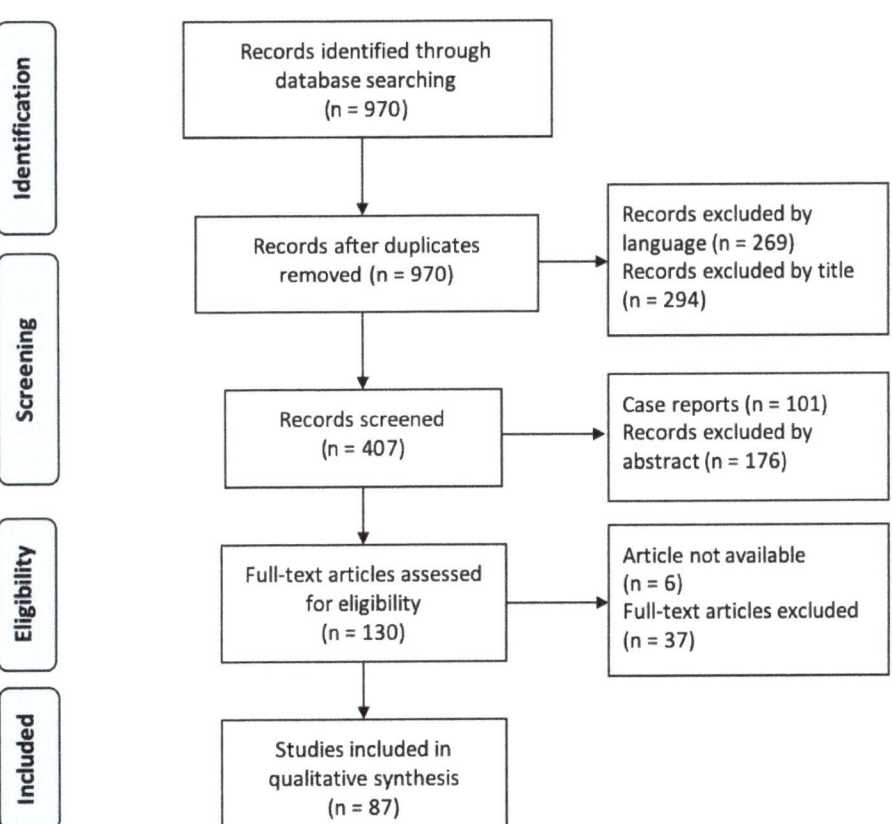

**Figure 1.** Prisma flow diagram for the literature search.

## 3.2. Autoimmune Diseases

Of the 87 articles, 38 concerned autoimmune diseases, of which systemic lupus erythematosus and limbic encephalitis were the most frequently described.

### 3.2.1. Limbic Encephalitis

Since the first description of limbic encephalitis in 1960, several antibodies responsible for these autoimmune brain inflammations have been discovered. The most frequent kind of limbic encephalitis is anti-N-Methyl-D-Aspartate (NMDA) receptor encephalitis, which predominantly affects children (35–40%) [9,15]. Other antibodies that are found in limbic encephalitis include anti-LG1, anti-GAD, anti-VGKC-Ab, anti-AMPA-r, and anti-GABA-r. Encephalitis with anti-NMDA-r, anti-AMPA-r, and anti-GABA-r antibodies has been strongly identified as being responsible for the manifestation of psychiatric symptoms [16–20]. It appears that psychotic symptoms are more frequent in limbic encephalitis with anti-NMDA-r antibodies in the form of drastic personality change [9], abnormal behavior (agitation, aggression, or catatonia), and delusions and hallucinations [15,21]. These symptoms can also be associated with irritability, insomnia, mood troubles [22,23], and a high level of anxiety [10,24]. Anti-NMDA receptor encephalitis is associated with cerebrospinal fluid (CSF) IgG antibodies against the GluN1 subunit of the NMDA receptor. Since antibody tests are not accessible in many institutions and it can take several weeks to obtain the results, most recent studies have aimed to improve knowledge of psychopathology and the clinical specificities of these diseases [25–30]. The clinical and paraclinical criteria have been defined to identify a probable anti-NMDA receptor encephalitis as soon as possible [31], but may not be sufficient in cases of autoimmune encephalitis without neurologic symptoms, and a systematic serum anti-NMDA-r antibodies test, electroencephalogram (EEG), and magnetic resonance imaging (MRI) of the brain are recommended [32]. For patients with psychotic symptoms presenting with clinical criteria or MRI or EEG signs, routine CSF should be mandatory [33,34].

### 3.2.2. Systemic Lupus Erythematosus

Systemic Lupus Erythematosus (SLE) is a prototype of a chronic, inflammatory, systemic autoimmune disease with unknown etiology, preferentially affecting females in their childbearing years [35,36], but two-thirds of pediatric patients develop neuropsychiatric symptoms [37]. Neuropsychiatric SLE (NPSLE) includes the neurologic syndromes of the central, peripheral, and autonomic nervous systems and psychiatric symptoms including depression, psychosis, and anxiety [37–39]. Delusions and hallucinations are the two main symptoms of SLE psychosis; however, they can also occur after administration of corticosteroids, and a differential diagnosis between NPSLE and cortico-induced neuropsychiatric disorders must further be considered [40]. The diagnosis of SLE is based on clinical and paraclinical criteria, but the lack of pathognomonic symptoms or test findings makes the diagnosis of NPSLE difficult to confirm. According to the last classification criteria for SLE, positive antinuclear antibodies are an obligatory criterion [41].

### 3.2.3. Hashimoto Encephalopathy

Two articles concerned Hashimoto encephalopathy (HE), a rare neuropsychiatric syndrome associated with Hashimoto thyroiditis, an autoimmune-mediated chronic inflammation of the thyroid. HE is more common in women and is associated with serologic evidence of antithyroid antibodies when other causes of encephalopathy are excluded [42]. In these cases, clinical manifestations include neurologic symptoms such as seizures or abnormal movements, impaired consciousness, and behavioral changes. Additionally, psychiatric symptoms including aggression, severe irritability, hallucinations, insomnia, and agitation have been described as dominant clinical features for all pediatric patients examined [43]. Brain MRI and EEG are recommended in all patients to account for the differential diagnosis of other possible encephalopathies, but the results are not specific to HE. The diagnosis is based on the identification of clinical manifestations that are associated with increased antithyroid antibodies, and all suspected patients presenting with acute or subacute encephalopathy or cognitive decline of unknown etiology should be tested for antithyroid antibodies in serum or CSF [44]. When the antibody titer is normal at presentation with persistent symptoms of HE and evidence for another diagnosis, follow-up determinations of antithyroid antibody titers can lead to a confirmed diagnosis [43].

3.2.4. Acute Disseminated Encephalomyelitis

Acute disseminated encephalomyelitis (ADEM) is an immune-mediated inflammatory process involving central nervous system white matter that mainly occurs in children [45]. ADEM typically follows a viral infection, but it can occasionally occur without any defined preceding trigger. The classical presentation is characterized by the acute onset of neurologic abnormalities. Several cases of initial presentation with acute psychosis have been reported. In these cases, fever and focal neurologic signs were absent on presentation [46]. Early MRI facilitates the diagnosis [47] and often reveals diffuse, symmetric white matter demyelinating lesions [45,48].

*3.3. Metabolic Diseases*

Inborn errors of metabolism (IEMs) are physiological defects or malfunctions due to full or partial loss of gene function, usually caused by autosomal recessively inherited enzyme defects [13]. Although metabolic diseases are not frequent, the number of articles concerning these pathologies has greatly increased over the last ten years. Their impact on the central nervous system can be responsible for psychiatric syndromes such as psychosis, depression, anxiety, or mania [49,50]. Niemann-Pick disease and Wilson's disease were the two main metabolic disorders described in the literature.

3.3.1. Niemann–Pick Disease

Niemann–Pick disease type C (NP–C) is a rare (<1/100,000 births) [51], autosomal recessive neurodegenerative disease caused by mutations in the NPC1 or NPC2 gene that lead to impaired intracellular lipid trafficking and excess storage of cholesterol and glycophospholids in the brain, liver, and other tissues [52]. Patients with NP–C show extreme clinical heterogeneity in their symptom profiles, ages at disease onset, and rates of disease progression [53]. Neurological disease onset typically occurs during childhood [53], and psychiatric manifestations are frequently reported with a high incidence of psychotic symptoms, comprising paranoid delusions, auditory hallucinations, and disorganized thoughts [54,55]. Psychiatric manifestations may remain isolated for several years, and most patients who initially present with psychotic symptoms do not have obvious abnormalities on neurological examination [56,57]. Although several biochemical markers have been evaluated to provide a low-invasive and inexpensive diagnostic method [58], the definite diagnosis of NP–C disease remains based on the demonstration of specific mutations in the genes NPC1 and NPC2 [59].

3.3.2. Wilson's Disease

Wilson's disease is an autosomal recessive disease that is more common than NP–C disease (6/100,000) [57] and commonly affects children or young adults [59,60]. It is caused by a mutation of a gene [ATP7B] encoding for a copper transportation protein, leading to copper accumulation in the liver, kidney, bones, and brain. Psychiatric symptoms appear early, and it has been estimated that one in two patients present psychiatric signs in the absence of other organic signs [61]. The most frequently reported psychiatric manifestations are mood disorders, including both depressive and manic elements [62–66], hallucinations [67–69], and personality changes with the emergence of irritability and aggressive behavior [70,71]. A meta-analysis found a 2.4% frequency of "frank psychosis" resembling schizophrenia [60]. Blood copper measurement and the existence of a conventional Kayser–Fleisher ophthalmic ring are important diagnostic indicators of Wilson's disease.

The current diagnosis is made through MRI findings indicating thalamic and lenticular nucleus hyper-signals [57].

### 3.3.3. Disorders of Homocysteine Metabolism

Homocysteine is an essential amino acid and is metabolized along pathways of remethylation or transsulfuration. Disorders of homocysteine metabolism (DHMs) are usually caused by the absence of an enzyme in one of these pathways. Two distinct enzymes are concerned: (1) methyltetrahydrofolate reductase deficiency in the remethylation pathway and (2) cystathionine beta synthase (CbS) deficiency in the transsulfuration pathway. These deficiencies lead to a functional deficiency of folate or B12 despite normal circulating levels [57,59]. DHMs are responsible for highly variable clinical features such as skeletal abnormalities, neurologic signs, and psychiatric problems that can essentially be characterized as psychotic symptoms [57,72]. Psychotic-like symptoms can be an isolated clinical feature [73] and often produce visual hallucinations [74]. Brain imaging sometimes shows demyelination but may also present as completely normal. An MRI scan of the spinal cord may show high signal intensity in the dorsal columns of the spinal cord, similar to that seen in pernicious anemia [59]. The diagnosis is based on amino acid chromatography and the determination of homocysteine [57].

### 3.3.4. Acute Intermittent Porphyria

Acute intermittent porphyria (AIP) is an autosomal dominant disease with variable penetrance that is linked to the deficiency of porphobilinogen deaminase, an enzyme that is involved in the biosynthesis of heme [59]. Clinical signs of AIP usually appear in adults, but cases of childhood onset have been reported [57,75,76]. The "classical triad" of symptoms consists of abdominal pains, psychiatric disturbances, and peripheral neuropathies. Psychiatric symptoms such as delusions, hallucinations, and the development of thought disorders [57] are frequent [75,77] and can be the single presenting feature [49,78]. Acute attacks are often triggered by porphyrinogenic treatments (contraceptives, barbiturates, sulfonamides, antiepileptics), sepsis, or alcohol ingestion [76]. The diagnosis of AIP should be considered in any psychiatric syndrome with unexplained cyclical pain [79]. This diagnosis is based on the measurement of delta-aminolevulinic acid in blood testing and porphibilinogene in urinalysis [57], which may be normal between attacks [59].

### 3.3.5. Cerebrotendinous Xanthomasis

Cerebrotendinous xanthomatosis (CTX) is a hereditary metabolic disorder characterized biochemically by sterol 27-hydroxylase deficiency, an enzyme involved in the degradation of cholesterol. This metabolic deficiency causes the formation of xanthomatous lesions (gradual buildup of cholestanol, a cholesterol metabolite) in various tissues, including the brain and tendons [59]. The estimated prevalence of CTX is <5 in 100,000, and it varies by country and ethnic group [80,81]. Clinically, patients usually have juvenile cataracts, tendinous xanthomata, and xanthomas (lipid accumulation in the superficial dermis) as visible signs [57]. Neurological signs and psychiatric disorders (psychotic manifestations, hallucinations) are often associated with CTX [82] and appear during adolescence. Acute psychotic-like episodes have been described, even though other behavioral disorders, especially attention-deficit hyperactivity disorders, are more frequent in childhood and adolescence [82]. In CTX cases, MRI shows a typical dendritic hyper-signal in the cerebellar nuclei regions. The diagnosis is confirmed by plasma cholestanol measurements and gene sequencing [57].

### 3.3.6. Arylsulfatase A Deficiency

Arylsulfatase A Deficiency, also known as metachromatic leukodystrophy (MLD), is an autosomal recessive disorder in which the partial or complete absence of arylsulfatase A leads to demyelination of the central and peripheral nervous systems [83]. The clinical presentation is heterogeneous with respect to the age of onset, the rate of progression, and the initial symptoms [84–86]. The neurological signs of MLD are often preceded by precursor symptoms in childhood, mainly behavioral disturbances and psychotic symptoms such as auditory hallucinations, bizarre delusions, and catatonic posturing [87]. The diagnosis should be suspected in individuals with progressive neurologic dysfunction, MRI evidence of leukodystrophy, or low arylsulfatase A activity in leukocytes [84]. The presence of sulfatides in urine is a useful indicator of the enzyme block [56]. The diagnosis of MLD can also be confirmed by molecular testing or after the identification of metachromatic lipid deposits in a nerve or brain biopsy [84].

3.3.7. Hereditary Transthyretin Amyloidosis

Hereditary transthyretin amyloidosis (ATTR) is a systemic disorder characterized by the extracellular deposition of misfolded transthyretin protein [88]. The clinical presentation is typically a slowly progressive sensorimotor and/or autonomic neuropathy [89] that is frequently accompanied by non-neuropathic features such as cardiomyopathy, nephropathy, vitreous opacities, and central nervous system (CNS) amyloidosis [90]. Individuals with leptomeningeal amyloidosis (LA) show CNS signs, including psychotic symptoms. The diagnosis of ATTR is established with the above clinical features, a biopsy showing amyloid deposits that bind to anti-TTR antibodies, and the identification of a heterozygous pathogenic variant in TTR by molecular testing [90]. In LA, the protein concentration in the CSF is usually high, and gadolinium-enhanced MRI typically shows an extensive increase in the surface of the brain, ventricles, and spinal cord [91].

3.3.8. Urea Cycle Disorders

Urea cycle disorders are caused by inherited enzyme deficiencies. Ornithine transcarbamylase enzyme deficiency is the most common of these diseases (1 in 8000 births) [92]. These disorders may evolve chronically during the neonatal period with mild symptoms until a first acute hyperammonemia episode appears. Patients present with symptoms related to the accumulation of ammonium in the body, including digestive, neurological, and psychotic symptoms [93]. These pathologies can easily be revealed by a measurement of plasma ammonemia.

3.3.9. Tay-Sachs Disease

Tay-Sachs disease (TSD) is an autosomal recessive lipid storage disorder caused by ß-hexosaminidase A deficiency. The prevalence of TSD is estimated to be 1 in 200,000 live births [94]. Three clinical variants of TSD, based on the age of onset, have been described in the literature [56]. Psychiatric signs may be the only manifestations of the chronic form, which usually presents in late childhood or adolescence; acute psychosis is reported in 30% to 50% of cases [95–97]. The presence of speech disturbances, gait abnormalities, movement disorders, and cognitive decline may indicate an underlying metabolic disorder. Most reports suggest that neuroleptic medications are rarely efficacious and may produce an unacceptably high risk/benefit ratio, whereas benzodiazepine may ameliorate the psychiatric and neurologic abnormalities in these patients [56,95,96].

*3.4. Neurologic Diseases*

3.4.1. Huntington's Disease

Huntington's disease (HD) is an incurable, autosomal dominant, neurodegenerative disease caused by an expanded CAG repeat in the huntingtin gene [98]. In HD, the production of a mutant protein leads to progressive motor impairment, psychiatric disorders, and cognitive decline [98,99]. The first manifestations begin around midlife. Neuropsychiatric symptoms, including psychosis, are highly prevalent and appear in the premotor phase [100]. According to the current criteria, the diagnosis is centered around the presence of involuntary choreiform movements and a positive genetic test for the CAG-expanded allele gene or a family history of HD [101].

### 3.4.2. Frontotemporal Dementia

Frontotemporal dementia (FTD) is a neurodegenerative disorder indicating a focal clinical syndrome; it is characterized by changes in one's personality and social conduct with circumscribed degeneration of the prefrontal and anterior temporal lobes [102]. Clinical and clinicopathological observations have found that people with younger-onset FTD frequently present with symptoms of schizophrenia, bipolar disorder, and affective disorders. When patients who are diagnosed with schizophrenia have an insidious and evolving cognitive deficiency, the probability of FTD is higher [103]. The characterization of FTD remains challenging, and, in the absence of definitive biomarkers, the diagnosis is based on clinical criteria including early behavioral disinhibition, apathy, perseverative behaviors, hyperorality, and executive deficits [104–106].

### 3.4.3. Wernicke Encephalopathy and Korsakoff's Psychosis

Wernicke encephalopathy (WE) is an acute neuropsychiatric condition caused by thiamine (vitamin B1) intracellular depletion in brain cells [107]. Alcohol misuse is the first cause of thiamine deficiency in industrialized countries but can also be seen in depleted teenage mothers in areas of poverty [108,109]. Korsakoff's psychosis results from inadequate treatment or a failure to diagnose WE in a timely manner and is characterized by severe short-term memory loss and hallucinations [110]. MRI investigations show thalamic, mamillary body, and frontal lobe atrophy, but the diagnosis remains based on clinical features and can be supported by a history of alcohol abuse [111,112].

### 3.4.4. Kleine–Levin Syndrome

Kleine–Levin syndrome (KLS) is a rare disease with an estimated prevalence of 1–2 per million people in France [113,114]. The triad of hypersomnia, megaphagia, and hypersexuality is classically reported in KLS cases, but the clinical presentation is rather hypersomnia with prolonged sleep times accompanied by a combination of cognitive, behavioral, and/or psychiatric disturbances. These symptoms also include depression, anxiety, and, rarely, suicidality [115]. Derealization, dissociation (feelings of mind-body disconnection), and altered perceptions are frequently described by patients with KLS [116]. The symptomatic periods alternate with intermitting periods of normalcy. Sleep monitoring and functional brain imaging during and between episodes are useful to support the diagnosis, which is based on clinical features [117,118].

### 3.4.5. Narcolepsy

Narcolepsy is a chronic sleep disorder that affects the regulation of sleep-wake cycles. It occurs in approximately 1 in 2000 individuals [119] and usually begins during adolescence. The classical symptoms of narcolepsy are excessive daytime sleepiness and sleep attacks, and the diagnosis is based on physiological testing, including nocturnal polysomnography and daytime EEG measurement of sleep latency. Hypnagogic/hypnopompic hallucinations are also reported, and the distinction between this presentation and the hallucinations of schizophrenia may be challenging in some clinical settings [119,120]. Most studies suggest that these psychotic symptoms are worsened by antipsychotic drugs; by contrast, they abate when narcolepsy is identified and treated with psychostimulants [119].

*3.5. Infectious Diseases*

A viral hypothesis for schizophrenia was seriously considered at the beginning of the 20th century [121]. More recent data show that some infectious agents, like toxoplasma gondii or CMV, could explain psychosis pathophysiology; however, a clear mechanism and a chronology are still difficult to establish. However, the human immunodeficiency virus appears to take a central role in these infectious etiologies [122], which are caused by well-known opportunistic agents [123].

### 3.5.1. Human Immunodeficiency Virus

Human Immunodeficiency Virus (HIV) is estimated to be associated with psychotic symptoms in 0.23% to 15% of cases [14]. These symptoms, characterized by persecutory, grandiose, and somatic delusions with hallucinations, present generally either in late-stage HIV or when patients have transitioned to acquired immunodeficiency syndrome (AIDS) [124,125]. One complicating factor in assessing this association is the fact that side effects of antiretrovirals include hallucinations [125]. HIV is diagnosed by the detection of antibodies (anti-HIV) in serum and confirmed by a Western blot test. In addition to a specific link between HIV and psychosis, some opportunistic infections related to HIV also trigger psychotic manifestations. Moreover, patients with HIV are at increased risk of developing extrapyramidal symptoms and tardive dyskinesia, particularly with the use of atypical antipsychotics [124,126]. Systematic testing (detection of anti-HIV antibodies in serum) is recommended in the case of FEP, but consent from each patient may be required, according to some state laws, before testing [127].

### 3.5.2. Toxoplasmosis

Toxoplasma gondii is an intracellular protozoan whose definitive host is the cat. Humans are infested by ingestion of contaminated food or water, or by congenital transmission to the fetus [128]. In immunocompetent hosts, primary infection typically remains asymptomatic. Toxoplasma is the most common infection in HIV-seropositive immunocompromised hosts, and in some cases, patients present with neurological or psychotic symptoms [129,130]. An MRI may show specific cerebral granuloma lesions, and the diagnosis is confirmed by serologic testing [129,131].

### 3.5.3. Cytomegalovirus

Cytomegalovirus (CMV) is a beta-herpesvirus that spreads by personal contact or congenital transmission. Most initial CMV infections are asymptomatic in immune-competent individuals, but reactivation may occur in cases of immunodeficiency (transplantation, HIV infection) and lead to psychiatric symptoms [130]. Clinical symptoms include deficits in concentration, memory, manipulation of knowledge, humor, and emotional expression [132]. A case of auditory hallucinations, delusions, and tangential thinking has also been described in the literature [133]. The diagnosis of CMV is confirmed by serologic testing.

### 3.5.4. Syphilis

Syphilis is a chronic, sexually transmitted disease caused by Treponema pallidum [134]. In the absence of adequate treatment, the disease follows several stages: primary, secondary, and tertiary syphilis. Neurosyphilis can occur at any stage of the disease but is classically associated with tertiary syphilis [134]. The clinical manifestations of neurosyphilis are not specific, and patients may present with psychotic symptoms mimicking psychiatric illness [14,135]. The diagnosis can be suspected based on clinical findings. The demonstration of T. pallidum in infected tissues or fluid confirms the diagnosis, but serologic testing remains the mainstay of laboratory diagnosis [135,136].

### 3.5.5. Lyme Borreliosis

Lyme borreliosis is a bacterial disease caused by a spirochete, Borrelia burgdoferi, which is transmitted by ticks. Its prevalence is correlated with the presence of forest areas [137]. If not treated at the initial stage, characterized by the apparition of erythema migrans, spirochetes spread in the organism and infect various organs, especially the nervous system. Neurological symptoms can occur several years after the initial infection, as spirochetes can remain quiescent for a long time [138]. The symptoms of Lyme neuroborreliosis (LNB) include encephalopathies and encephalomyelitis, but mood disturbances and psychotic symptoms are also described [139,140]. The CSF analysis is a key test for the diagnosis of LNB, which is based on several criteria defined in the article by Mygland et al. [141].

### 3.6. Genetic Diseases

The relationship between some genetic disorders and psychotic-like symptoms has been noted since the 1980s [142]. Because of the multiplicity of possible gene alterations and the low prevalence of these diseases, however, systematic genetic screening is not yet conceivable. However, genetic screening should be discussed in the case of a clinical presentation evocative of a genetic disorder. In most of these diseases, patients suffer from several physical disorders and may present with an intellectual disability, dysmorphia, or resistance to antipsychotic treatments. The genetic syndromes reported in the literature are 22q11 deletion syndrome, Prader–Willi syndrome, C9orf72 mutations, Fragile X premutation disorders [143,144], BSC1L mutation [145], 3q29 recurrent deletion [146], 15q duplication syndrome [147], and genetic mitochondrial disorders [148]. The syndromes that are most frequently found in cases of FEP are described below.

#### 3.6.1. 22q11 Deletion Syndrome

22q11 deletion syndrome is a common (1 in 4000 births) genetic disorder. Patients suffer from several physical disorders, such as congenital heart defects, palate defects, hypoparathyroidism, and immunologic abnormalities. This syndrome is also associated with psychiatric manifestations [149,150], and 23–32% of adults present with psychotic disorders [151,152]. This deletion is estimated to account for 1–2% of schizophrenia cases overall [153].

#### 3.6.2. Prader–Willi Syndrome

Prader–Willi syndrome (PWS) is a neurodevelopmental disorder resulting from a genetic anomaly on chromosome 15, with two main subtypes identified. The birth incidence is estimated at around 1 in 22,000 [154]. Patients with PWS usually present with an association of clinical features such as hypotonia, hypogonadism, hyperphagia, mild learning disabilities, and small hands and feet. A comorbid association of PWS with psychiatric disorders has been suggested in several studies [155,156]. In both genetic subtypes, psychiatric manifestations are mainly atypical affective disorders with or without psychotic symptoms [157,158].

#### 3.6.3. C9orf72 Mutations

C9orf72 mutations have been found in almost 12% of patients with FTD and are also associated with some forms of amyotrophic lateral sclerosis (ALS) [159]. In patients with FTD or ALS, late-onset psychotic disorders as the initial presentation have been reported to be more frequent when these diseases are secondary to the C9orf72 mutation [160–162].

## 4. Discussion

This systematic review reveals that many somatic illnesses, most of which may occur or begin during childhood or adolescence, can be responsible for psychotic symptoms. Determining the appropriate initial work-up implies that the prevalence of these pathologies and screening test features are to be taken into account [127].

### 4.1. Limitations

Studies published for the past fifteen years were selected to illustrate less-investigated, actual, and contemporary concerns about FEP. Well-known differential diagnoses (i.e., blood sugar troubles) do not require active academic research. As a consequence, these pathologies did not appear in this systematic review as they are systematically screened in current practice. As this literature review focused on clinical perspectives, the bibliographic search was restricted to medical databases. However, the probability that our pathology list will be representative of current research concerns is increased by the inclusion of the only review that has been published to date.

*4.2. Prevalence*

Diseases in which psychosis is a typical presentation (i.e., Wilson's disease, thyroid diseases, etc.) should be systematically screened for FEP [127]. Many of the diseases found in this review can potentially influence psychotic symptoms even if they are not the usual presentation, especially as some of these pathologies are very rare. It would be arduous, if not infeasible, to systematically screen every disease in which psychotic symptoms have been reported; however, it seems necessary to propose an initial work-up that will help physicians who suspect a somatic origin of a given disorder.

*4.3. Causality*

When a somatic disease is found in a patient with FEP, the question is whether this pathology is the cause of psychosis or a comorbidity. The stress-diathesis model of schizophrenia shows this distinction is difficult to make: a somatic disorder may act as an external stress factor in individuals with pre-existing vulnerability factors [163,164]. However, models have been proposed to assess whether an association can causally contribute to a pathological phenomenon [165,166], and three key principles (atypicality, temporality, and explicability) have been suggested to help establish a cause-and-effect relationship between a somatic condition and psychotic symptoms [14]. In an atypical presentation of FEP, psychotic symptoms that appear after the onset of a medical condition and the possibility of establishing a physiological link between a somatic lesion and psychotic symptoms may provide evidence of a secondary psychotic disorder.

*4.4. Exams*

4.4.1. Laboratory Tests

A consensus exists on the performance of laboratory screening, but opinions differ on how broad this screening should be [1,127,167,168]. Many diseases reported in this review may produce inflammation that can be detected with a C-reactive protein test.

An ammonemia measurement, which is a low-cost exam, should be systematically performed to eliminate hyperammonemia. Positive antinuclear and anti-NMDA antibodies associated with an inflammatory syndrome may reveal an autoimmune disorder such as SLE or limbic encephalitis. A negative syphilis serology allows for ruling out neurosyphilis. This serologic test may also show an underlying autoimmune disease in the case of false-positive results [169].

A TSH test is necessary to reveal thyroid dysfunction. It may also lend support in detecting HE [170]. Suspicion of Wilson's disease, which is the most frequent metabolic disorder responsible for psychotic symptoms, can be formally excluded with a negative result of the copper measurement in the blood.

All infectious diseases outlined in this review, except syphilis and LNB, appeared in cases of immunodeficiency in HIV-seropositive hosts. As the HIV-seropositive condition can itself be associated with psychotic manifestations, systematic detection is recommended in cases of FEP after recording consent from patients [14,129,130,171].

Additionally, this review highlights the role of genetic diseases, particularly the relationship between psychotic disorders and 22q11 deletion syndrome. Clinicians should systematically seek this genetic mutation when patients present with clinical manifestations such as a developmental delay or facial dysmorphology [149,172].

The main function of an electrocardiogram (ECG) is to identify a cardiac disease, which is of particular importance before introducing an antipsychotic treatment [1]. Conduction disorders detected in young patients should also lead clinicians to suspect lupus [173].

EEG is an inexpensive, easily available, and noninvasive exam that is helpful for the diagnosis of limbic encephalitis when specific signs are detected (extreme delta brush waves have been reported in 30% of cases) [16,31,174,175].

Most of the diseases reported in this review can be revealed by magnetic resonance imaging (MRI): signs of encephalitis [43,44], leukodystrophy [56], white matter lesions [173], diffuse cortical atrophy [162], or specific lesions of toxoplasmosis [129]. Even though cerebral computed tomography (CT) is considerably more feasible, this exam uses ionizing radiation. CT is also less sensitive than MRI in the diagnosis of cerebral lesions [3]. Moreover, studies report good patient compliance, and an economic analysis suggested that MRI could be cost-saving when the prevalence of organic causes is around 1%, while the prevalence of imaging findings that would influence clinical management is estimated at around 5% in the case of FEP [3,10,168,170,176].

### 4.4.2. Lumbar Puncture

This review emphasizes the increasing number of limbic encephalitis cases reported and the high probability of underdiagnosis of this pathology [10,177,178]. Considering these observations, lumbar puncture would be indicated in the FEP initial work-up [179,180]. The invasive aspect of this exam is highly counterbalanced by the opportunity to diagnose a curable disease and consider the risk of a paradoxical reaction to antipsychotics in the case of encephalopathy.

## 5. Conclusions

This review highlights that the timely diagnosis of a physical disease is fundamental when a patient presents with psychotic symptoms in order to (1) administer the appropriate therapy and (2) avoid paradoxical reactions to antipsychotics. This differential diagnosis is possible only if the appropriate exams are performed. The initial exams recommended are presented in Table 1. Specifically, our results indicate that laboratory tests, including the antinuclear antibody test, the test of anti-NMDA antibodies, and HIV testing, must be performed systematically. The benefit-risk ratio indicates that brain MRI should be considered in cases of FEP. Finally, lumbar puncture (which is an invasive exam) could be of interest for some patients, considering the clinical presentation. Future studies should provide additional data on the feasibility and acceptability of these exams, particularly lumbar punctures.

**Table 1.** Initial exams recommended in the case of a first episode of psychosis.

| | |
|---|---|
| Laboratory tests | C-reactive protein test<br>TSH<br>Ammonemia<br>Ceruloplasmin<br>FTA-ABS (fluorescent treponemal antibody absorbed)<br>HIV test (after obtaining consent from patients)<br>Antinuclear and anti-NMDA antibodies |
| Imaging | Brain MRI |
| Genetic tests | Karyotype and research of specific mutations, such as a 22q11 deletion, for patients presenting physical or developmental features associated with psychiatric manifestations |
| Others | ECG<br>EEG<br>Lumbar puncture in search of pleocytosis or oligoclonal bands in the CSF |

**Funding:** This research received no external funding.

**Institutional Review Board Statement:** Not applicable.

**Informed Consent Statement:** Not applicable.

**Data Availability Statement:** The data presented in this study are available in Appendix A.

**Acknowledgments:** This research was partially supported by Brest University and the Regional Hospital Center.

**Conflicts of Interest:** The authors declare that they have no known competing financial interest or personal relationships that could have appeared to influence the work reported in this paper.

## Appendix A

| Author/Date | Article Title | Article Characteristics | Type of Pathology | Disease |
|---|---|---|---|---|
| Ford B, McDonald A, Srinivasan S. 2019 [21] | Anti-NMDA receptor encephalitis: a case study and illness overview. | Case report (40-year-old female with first episode of psychotic symptoms) and review of anti-NMDA differential diagnoses. | Autoimmune | Limbic encephalitis |
| Wang HY, Li T, Li XL, Zhang XX, Yan ZR, Xu Y. 2019 [11] | Anti-N-methyl-D-aspartate receptor encephalitis mimics neuroleptic malignant syndrome: case report and literature review. | Case report (24-year-old male presenting with FEP and Neuroleptic Malignant Syndrome-like symptoms) and review of diagnosis criteria for anti-NMDAr encephalitis and NMS. | Autoimmune | Limbic encephalitis |
| Sarkis RA, Coffey MJ, Cooper JJ, Hassan I, Lennox B. 2019 [27] | Anti-N-Methyl-D-Aspartate Receptor Encephalitis: A Review of Psychiatric Phenotypes and Management Considerations: A Report of the American Neuropsychiatric Association Committee on Research. | Review of case reports and case series (283 articles included) with patients presenting with acute or subacute (<3 months) psychiatric symptoms and anti-NMDAr antibodies. 54% of the 544 case subjects had psychotic symptoms. | Autoimmune | Limbic encephalitis |
| Steiner J, Prüss H, Köhler S, Frodl T, Hasan A, Falkai P. 2018 [34] | Autoimmune encephalitis with psychosis: Warning signs, step-by-step diagnostics and treatment. | Overview of clinical signs of autoimmune encephalitis in patients with FEP. | Autoimmune | Limbic encephalitis |
| Endres D, Leypoldt F, Bechter K, Hasan A, Steiner J, Domschke K, Wandinger KP, Falkai P, Arolt V, Stich O, Rauer S, Prüss H, van Elst LT. 2020 [33] | Autoimmune encephalitis as a differential diagnosis of schizophreniform psychosis: clinical symptomatology, pathophysiology, diagnostic approach, and therapeutic considerations. | Overview of clinical signs and diagnostic strategy in autoimmune encephalitis as differential diagnoses of FEP. | Autoimmune | Limbic encephalitis |
| Guasp M, Giné-Servén E, Maudes E, Rosa-Justicia M, Martínez-Hernández E, Boix-Quintana E, Bioque M, Casado V, Módena-Ouarzi Y, Guanyabens N, Muriana D, Sugranyes G, Pacchiarotti I, Davi-Loscos E, Torres-Rivas C, Ríos J, Sabater L, Saiz A, Graus F, Castro-Fornieles J, Parellada E, Dalmau J. 2021 [32] | Clinical, Neuroimmunologic, and CSF Investigations in First Episode Psychosis. | Overview of clinical signs and diagnostic strategy in autoimmune encephalitis as differential diagnoses of FEP. | Autoimmune | Limbic encephalitis |
| Khajezadeh MA, Zamani G, Moazzami B, Nagahi Z, Mousavi-Torshizi M, Ziaee V. 2018 [37] | Neuropsychiatric Involvement in Juvenile-Onset Systemic Lupus Erythematosus. | Cross-sectional study including patients under 18 years old with a diagnosis of SLE. 3 of the 41 patients with neuropsychiatric signs had psychotic symptoms. | Autoimmune | Systemic lupus erythematosus |
| Honnorat J, Plazat LO. 2018 [15] | Autoimmune encephalitis and psychiatric disorders. | Review of psychiatric symptoms of autoimmune encephalitis. 4% of isolated psychotic symptoms in anti-NMDAR encephalitis. | Autoimmune | Limbic encephalitis |
| Lancaster E. 2015 [177] | Paraneoplastic Disorders. | Review of the clinical specificities of paraneoplastic disorders. | Autoimmune | Limbic encephalitis |
| Wang D, Hao Q, He L, He L, Wang Q. 2018 [181] | LGI1 antibody encephalitis—Detailed clinical, laboratory and radiological description of 13 cases in China. | Retrospective analysis of clinical presentation for 13 patients (ages 18–63) diagnosed with LGI1 antibody encephalitis. 46% had psychotic symptoms as an initial symptom. | Autoimmune | Limbic encephalitis |
| Bechter K, Deisenhammer F. 2017 [180] | Psychiatric syndromes other than dementia. | Overview of differential diagnostic issues in new-onset cases of severe mental illness, focusing on CSF abnormalities. | Autoimmune | Limbic encephalitis |

| Author/Date | Article Title | Article Characteristics | Type of Pathology | Disease |
|---|---|---|---|---|
| Hermans T, Santens P, Matton C, Oostra K, Heylens G, Herremans S, Lemmens. 2018 [182] | Anti-NMDA receptor encephalitis: still unknown and underdiagnosed by physicians and especially by psychiatrists? | Description of anti-NMDAR typical presentation and diagnostic criteria with a focus on the risk of delay in diagnosis illustrated by the case of a 25-year-old woman presenting with FEP. | Autoimmune | Limbic encephalitis |
| Lee J, Yu HJ, Lee J. 2018 [43] | Hashimoto encephalopathy in pediatric patients: Homogeneity in clinical presentation and heterogeneity in antibody titers. | Review of clinical manifestations, antibody titers, and treatment responses in 6 children (ages 10–17) diagnosed with Hashimoto encephalopathy. 66.7% presented with psychotic symptoms. | Autoimmune | Hashimoto encephalopathy |
| Voice J, Ponterio JM, Lakhi N. 2017 [183] | Psychosis secondary to an incidental teratoma: a "heads-up" for psychiatrists and gynecologists. | Pathophysiology overview of anti-NMDA encephalitis secondary to ovarian teratoma. Case report of a 17-year-old woman presenting with FEP. | Autoimmune | Limbic encephalitis |
| Chandra SR, Viswanathan LG, Sindhu DM, Pai AR. 2017 [29] | Subacute Noninfective Inflammatory Encephalopathy: Our Experience and Diagnostic Problems. | Clinical manifestation analysis for patients with immune-mediated encephalopathy. 70% of 42 patients (ages 11–75) presented with FEP. Delay to diagnosis could reach 2 years. | Autoimmune | Limbic encephalitis |
| Gable M, Glaser C. 2017 [17] | Anti-N-Methyl-d-Aspartate Receptor Encephalitis Appearing as a New-Onset Psychosis: Disease Course in Children and Adolescents Within the California Encephalitis Project. | Clinical characterization and laboratory findings in 24 patients aged <18 with anti-NMDAR encephalitis. 66% presented with FEP. Psychotic symptoms can persist for more than 3 weeks before other symptoms appear. | Autoimmune | Limbic encephalitis |
| Mantere O, Saarela M, Kieseppä T, Raij T, Mäntylä T, Lindgren M, Rikandi E, Stoecker W, Teegen B, Suvisaari J. 2018 [184] | Anti-neuronal anti-bodies in patients with early psychosis. | Investigation of antineuronal antibodies in blood samples from 70 patients with a FEP, 6 patients with a clinical high risk for psychosis, and 34 controls. One CHR patient had anti-NMDAR antibodies. All other tests were negative. | Autoimmune | Limbic encephalitis |
| Xiao X, Gui S, Bai P, Bai Y, Shan D, Hu Y, Bui-Nguyen TM, Zhou R. 2017 [185] | Anti-NMDA-receptor encephalitis during pregnancy: A case report and literature review. | Review of anti-NMDAR clinical manifestations during pregnancy. Case report of a 24-year-old pregnant woman presenting with FEP. | Autoimmune | Limbic encephalitis |
| Hao Q, Wang D, Guo L, Zhang B. 2017 [18] | Clinical characterization of autoimmune encephalitis and psychosis. | Retrospective study of clinical presentation and laboratory examinations for 70 patients (ages 12–75) diagnosed with autoimmune encephalitis. 44% had psychiatric symptoms as initial presentation. | Autoimmune | Limbic encephalitis |
| Singh RK, Bhoi SK, Kalita J, Misra UK. 2017 [186] | Cerebral Venous Sinus Thrombosis Presenting Feature of Systemic Lupus Erythematosus. | Overview of SLE complications. | Autoimmune | Systemic lupus erythematosus |
| Bost C, Pascual O, Honnorat J. 2016 [15] | Autoimmune encephalitis in psychiatric institutions: current perspectives. | Review of psychiatric and behavioral manifestations of autoimmune encephalitis. Psychotic symptoms are the first symptoms in >40% of patients. | Autoimmune | Limbic encephalitis |
| Schou M, Sæther SG, Borowski K, Teegen B, Kondziella D, Stoecker W, Vaaler A, Reitan SK. 2016 [187] | Prevalence of serum anti-neuronal autoantibodies in patients admitted to acute psychiatric care. | Investigation of serum prevalence of 6 anti-neuronal antibodies in 925 patients admitted to acute psychiatric inpatient care. | Autoimmune | Limbic encephalitis |
| Brenton JN, Goodkin HP. 2016 [30] | Antibody-Mediated Autoimmune Encephalitis in Childhood. | Review of autoimmune encephalitis occurring in childhood: clinical presentation and laboratory findings. | Autoimmune | Limbic encephalitis |
| Shimizu Y, Yasuda S, Kako Y, Nakagawa S, Kanda M, Hisada R, Ohmura K, Shimamura S, Shida H, Fujieda Y, Kato M, Oku K, Bohgaki T, Horita T, Kusumi I, Atsumi T. 2016 [40] | Post-steroid neuropsychiatric manifestations are significantly more frequent in SLE compared with other systemic autoimmune diseases and predict better prognosis compared with de novo neuropsychiatric SLE. | Analysis of psychiatric manifestations in 146 patients with SLE, 43 with NPSLE, and 162 with other systemic autoimmune diseases and comparison after administration of corticosteroids. | Autoimmune | Systemic lupus erythematosus |
| Lancaster, E. J Clin Neurol. 2016 [16] | The Diagnosis and Treatment of Autoimmune Encephalitis. | Overview of autoimmune encephalitis clinical presentation and ancillary test findings. | Autoimmune | Limbic encephalitis |

| Author/Date | Article Title | Article Characteristics | Type of Pathology | Disease |
|---|---|---|---|---|
| Lazar-Molnar E, Tebo AE. 2015 [23] | Autoimmune NMDA receptor encephalitis. | Review of NMDAR antibody encephalitis clinical manifestations and diagnostic strategies. | Autoimmune | Limbic encephalitis |
| Kruse JL, Jeffrey JK, Davis MC, Dearlove J, IsHak WW, Brooks JO 3rd. 2014 [19] | Anti-N-methyl-D-aspartate receptor encephalitis: a targeted review of clinical presentation, diagnosis, and approaches to psychopharmacologic management. | 2 case reports (16 and 19 year-old women with initial psychotic symptoms) and overview of the evaluation and treatment of anti-NMDAR encephalitis. | Autoimmune | Limbic encephalitis |
| Pollak TA, McCormack R, Peakman M, Nicholson TR, David AS. 2014 [188] | Prevalence of anti-N-methyl-D-aspartate (NMDA) receptor [corrected] antibodies in patients with schizophrenia and related psychoses: a systematic review and meta-analysis. | Systematic literature search, including 7 studies (1441 patients) to evaluate the prevalence of anti-NMDAR antibodies in patients with a primary psychiatric diagnosis without clinical signs of encephalitis. | Autoimmune | Limbic encephalitis |
| Armangue T, Petit-Pedrol M, Dalmau J. 2012 [24] | Autoimmune encephalitis in children. | Overview of autoimmune encephalitis clinical presentations in patients under 18 years old. | Autoimmune | Limbic encephalitis |
| de Holanda NC, de Lima DD, Cavalcanti TB, Lucena CS, Bandeira F. 2011 [44] | Hashimoto's encephalopathy: systematic review of the literature and an additional case. | Case report of a 23-year-old woman and systematic review of clinical features of Hashimoto encephalopathy (52 articles/130 patients). | Autoimmune | Hashimoto encephalopathy |
| Bertsias GK, Ioannidis JP, Aringer M, Bollen E, Bombardieri S, Bruce IN, Cervera R, Dalakas M, Doria A, Hanly JG, Huizinga TW, Isenberg D, Kallenberg C, Piette JC, Schneider M, Scolding N, Smolen J, Stara A, Tassiulas I, Tektonidou M, Tincani A, van Buchem MA, van Vollenhoven R, Ward M, Gordon C, Boumpas DT. 2010 [189] | EULAR recommendations for the management of systemic lupus erythematosus with neuropsychiatric manifestations: report of a task force of the EULAR standing committee for clinical affairs. | Recommendations. | Autoimmune | Systemic lupus erythematosus |
| Greenberg BM. 2009 [169] | The neurologic manifestations of systemic lupus erythematosus. | Overview of the neurologic and psychiatric clinical manifestations of SLE. | Autoimmune | Systemic lupus erythematosus |
| Hanly JG, Urowitz MB, Siannis F, Farewell V, Gordon C, Bae SC, Isenberg D, Dooley MA, Clarke A, Bernatsky S, Gladman D, Fortin PR, Manzi S, Steinsson K, Bruce IN, Ginzler E, Aranow C, Wallace DJ, Ramsey-Goldman R, van Vollenhoven R, Sturfelt G, Nived O, Sanchez-Guerrero J, Alarcón GS, Petri M, Khamashta M, Zoma A, Font J, Kalunian K, Douglas J, Qi Q, Thompson K, Merrill JT. 2008 [39] | Systemic Lupus International Collaborating Clinics. Autoantibodies and neuropsychiatric events at the time of systemic lupus erythematosus diagnosis: results from an international inception cohort study. | Analysis of the associations between autoantibodies and neuropsychiatric events in a cohort of 412 patients with a new diagnosis of SLE. | Autoimmune | Systemic lupus erythematosus |
| Steinlin MI, Blaser SI, Gilday DL, Eddy AA, Logan WJ, Laxer RM, Silverman ED. 1995 [190] | Neurologic manifestations of pediatric systemic lupus erythematosus. | Retrospective analysis of neurologic and psychiatric manifestations in 91 children (<18 years old) with a diagnosis of SLE. | Autoimmune | Systemic lupus erythematosus |
| Yancey CL, Doughty RA, Athreya BH. 1981 [191] | Central nervous system involvement in childhood systemic lupus erythematosus. | Retrospective analysis of neurologic and psychiatric manifestations in 37 children with a diagnosis of SLE. | Autoimmune | Systemic lupus erythematosus |
| Zandi MS. 2016 [20] | Autoimmune Encephalitis. | Overview of the most common clinical syndromes of autoimmune encephalitis. | Autoimmune | Limbic encephalitis |
| Nasr JT, Andriola MR, Coyle PK. 2000 [46] | ADEM: literature review and case report of acute psychosis presentation. | Case report of a 14-year-old girl and systematic review of ADEM presenting with acute psychosis. | Autoimmune | Acute disseminated encephalomyelitis |
| Weiss DB, Dyrud J, House RM, Beresford TP. 2005 [192] | Psychiatric manifestations of autoimmune disorders. | Review of psychiatric symptoms in autoimmune disorders. | Autoimmune | |
| O'Rourke L, Murphy KC. 2019 [150] | Recent developments in understanding the relationship between 22q11.2 deletion syndrome and psychosis. | Review including 70 papers focusing on the relationship between 22q11 deletion syndrome and psychosis. | Genetic | 22q11 deletion syndrome |

| Author/Date | Article Title | Article Characteristics | Type of Pathology | Disease |
|---|---|---|---|---|
| Ducharme S, Bajestan S, Dickerson BC, Voon V. 2017 [162] | Psychiatric Presentations of C9orf72 Mutation: What Are the Diagnostic Implications for Clinicians? | Systematic review of the literature, including 43 articles related to psychiatric manifestations of the C9orf72 mutation. | Genetic | C9orf72 mutation |
| Tang SX, Yi JJ, Calkins ME, Whinna DA, Kohler CG, Souders MC, McDonald-McGinn DM, Zackai EH, Emanuel BS, Gur RC, Gur RE. 2014 [149] | Psychiatric disorders in 22q11.2 deletion syndrome are prevalent but undertreated. | Cross-sectional study including 112 patients (ages 8–45) with a diagnosis of 22q11DS to characterize psychiatric manifestations. | Genetic | 22q11 deletion syndrome |
| Al-Owain M, Colak D, Albakheet A, Al-Younes B, Al-Humaidi Z, Al-Sayed M, Al-Hindi H, Al-Sugair A, Al-Muhaideb A, Rahbeeni Z, Al-Sehli A, Al-Fadhli F, Ozand PT, Taylor RW, Kaya N. 2013 [145] | Clinical and biochemical features associated with BCS1L mutation. | Clinical presentation and laboratory results for 9 patients with a BCS1L mutation. | Genetic | BSC1L mutation |
| Anglin RE, Garside SL, Tarnopolsky MA, Mazurek MF, Rosebush PI. 2012 [148] | The psychiatric manifestations of mitochondrial disorders: a case and review of the literature. | Systematic review of the literature, including 50 case reports of patients with mitochondrial disorders who initially presented with psychiatric symptoms. | Genetic | Mitochondrial disorders |
| Bourgeois JA, Coffey SM, Rivera SM, Hessl D, Gane LW, Tassone F, Greco C, Finucane B, Nelson L, Berry-Kravis E, Grigsby J, Hagerman PJ, Hagerman RJ. 2009 [143] | A review of fragile X premutation disorders: expanding the psychiatric perspective. | Review of clinical, genetic, molecular, and neuroimaging manifestations of fragile X premutation disorders. | Genetic | Fragile X premutation disorder |
| Soni S, Whittington J, Holland AJ, Webb T, Maina EN, Boer H, Clarke D. 2008 [158] | The phenomenology and diagnosis of psychiatric illness in people with Prader–Willi syndrome. | Historical cohort study including 119 patients with PWS to investigate clinical psychiatric features. | Genetic | Prader–Willi syndrome |
| Mulle JG, Gambello MJ, Cook EH, Rutkowski TP, Glassford M. 1993 [146] | 3q29 Recurrent Deletion. | Disease overview (clinical characteristics, diagnosis, management). | Genetic | 3q29 deletion |
| Finucane BM, Lusk L, Arkilo D, Chamberlain S, Devinsky O, Dindot S, Jeste SS, LaSalle JM, Reiter LT, Schanen NC, Spence SJ, Thibert RL, Calvert G, Luchsinger K, Cook EH. 1993 [147] | 15q Duplication Syndrome and Related Disorders. | Disease overview (clinical characteristics, diagnosis, management). | Genetic | 15q duplication syndrome |
| Brodziński S, Nasierowski T. 2019 [139] | Psychosis in Borrelia burgdorferi infection -part I: epidemiology, pathogenesis, diagnosis and treatment of neuroborreliosis. | Clinical overview. | Infectious | Neuroborreliosis |
| Yolken RH, Torrey EF. 2008 [130] | Are some cases of psychosis caused by microbial agents? A review of the evidence. | Review of infectious agents causing psychotic symptoms. | Infectious | Toxoplasmosis Cytomegalovirus |
| Pradhan S, Yadav R, Mishra VN. 2007 [129] | Toxoplasma meningoencephalitis in HIV-seronegative patients: clinical patterns, imaging features and treatment outcome. | Group study with 15 patients presenting with toxoplasma meningoencephalitis. | Infectious | HIV |
| Buhrich N, Cooper DA. 1987 [193] | Requests for psychiatric consultation concerning 22 patients with AIDS and ARC. | Retrospective analysis of psychiatric symptoms in 22 patients with AIDS. | Infection | HIV |
| Faoucher M, Demily C. 2019 [50] | The psychopharmacology of Wilson disease and other metabolic disorders. | Disease overview. 30% may initially present with psychotic symptoms. | Metabolic | Wilson's disease |
| Sitarska D, Ługowska A. 2019 [58] | Laboratory diagnosis of the Niemann-Pick type C disease: an inherited neurodegenerative disorder of cholesterol metabolism. | Review of clinical manifestations and laboratory results. | Metabolic | Niemann–Pick disease |
| Rego T, Farrand S, Goh AMY, Eratne D, Kelso W, Mangelsdorf S, Velakoulis D, Walterfang M. 2019 [54] | Psychiatric and Cognitive Symptoms Associated with Niemann-Pick Type C Disease: Neurobiology and Management. | Review of clinical manifestations of NPC. Initial psychotic symptoms range from 40 to 55%. | Metabolic | Niemann–Pick disease |
| Sekijima Y. 2018. [90] | Hereditary Transthyretin Amyloidosis. | Disease overview (clinical characteristics, diagnosis, management). | Metabolic | Hereditary transthyretin amyloidosis |

| Author/Date | Article Title | Article Characteristics | Type of Pathology | Disease |
|---|---|---|---|---|
| Gomez-Ospina N. 2017 [84] | Arylsulfatase A Deficiency. | Disease overview (clinical characteristics, diagnosis, management). | Metabolic | Arylsulfatase A deficiency |
| Biswas S, Paul N, Das SK. 2017 [70] | Nonmotor Manifestations of Wilson's Disease. | Disease overview (clinical characteristics, treatment, imaging). | Metabolic | Wilson's disease |
| Hendriksz CJ, Anheim M, Bauer P, Bonnot O, Chakrapani A, Corvol JC, de Koning TJ, Degtyareva A, Dionisi-Vici C, Doss S, Duning T, Giunti P, Iodice R, Johnston T, Kelly D, Klünemann HH, Lorenzl S, Padovani A, Pocovi M, Synofzik M, Terblanche A, Then Bergh F, Topçu M, Tranchant C, Walterfang M, Velten C, Kolb SA. 2017 [52] | The hidden Niemann-Pick type C patient: clinical niches for a rare inherited metabolic disease. | Review of the literature. Psychotic symptoms at initial presentation are reported in 55% of cases. | Metabolic | Niemann–Pick disease |
| Shulman LM, David NJ, Weiner WJ. 1995 [194] | Psychosis as the initial manifestation of adult-onset Niemann-Pick disease type C. | Review of adult-onset NPC clinical presentations and case report of a 38-year-old man. | Metabolic | Niemann–Pick disease |
| Bonnot O, Herrera PM, Tordjman S, Walterfang M. 2015 [57] | Secondary psychosis induced by metabolic disorders. | Systematic review of psychiatric symptoms and cognitive impairments in neurometabolic diseases, including 63 publications. | Metabolic | Disorders of homocysteine metabolism Urea cycle disorders Porphyria Wilson's disease Niemann-Pick disease Cerebrotendinous xanthomatosis |
| Demily C, Sedel F. 2014 [59] | Psychiatric manifestations of treatable hereditary metabolic disorders in adults. | Review of psychiatric symptoms in hereditary metabolic disorders. | Metabolic | Hereditary metabolic disorders |
| Chawla J, Kvarnberg D. 2014 [109] | Hydrosoluble vitamins. | Clinical presentation overview of hydrosuble vitamin deficiencies. | Metabolic | Wernicke encephalopathy and Korsakoff disease |
| Zimbrean PC, Schilsky ML. 2014 [71] | Psychiatric aspects of Wilson disease: a review. | Systematic review of psychiatric manifestations in Wilson's disease, including 90 articles. | Metabolic | Wilson's disease |
| Huang CC, Chu NS. 1992 [195] | Wilson's disease: clinical analysis of 71 cases and comparison with previous Chinese series. | Comparative study of clinical presentations in 3 series of patients with Wilson's disease. | Metabolic | Wilson's disease |
| Walterfang M, Bonnot O, Mocellin R, Velakoulis D. 2013 [49] | The neuropsychiatry of inborn errors of metabolism. | Review of major metabolic disorders associated with secondary psychiatric illness. | Metabolic | Inborn errors of metabolism |
| Staretz-Chacham O, Choi JH, Wakabayashi K, Lopez G, Sidransky E. 2010 [56] | Psychiatric and behavioral manifestations of lysosomal storage disorders. | Review of psychiatric and behavioral manifestations in lysosomal storage disorders. | Metabolic | Lysosomal storage disorders |
| Roze E, Gervais D, Demeret S, Ogier de Baulny H, Zittoun J, Benoist JF, Said G, Pierrot-Deseilligny C, Bolgert F. 2003 [74] | Neuropsychiatric disturbances in presumed late-onset cobalamin C disease. | Case reports of a 16-year-old girl and her 24-year-old sister. Review of neurologic and psychiatric symptoms in late-onset vitamin B12 disturbances. | Metabolic | Disorders of homocysteine metabolism |
| Thomson AD, Marshall EJ. 2006 [107] | The natural history and pathophysiology of Wernicke's Encephalopathy and Korsakoff's Psychosis. | Review of symptoms related to Wernicke's encephalopathy and Korsakoff's psychosis. | Metabolic | Wernicke encephalopathy and Korsakoff disease |
| Bonnot. 2019 [55] | Systematic review of psychiatric signs in Niemann-Pick type C disease. | Systematic review of psychiatric symptoms in NPC disease, including 40 publications and data from 58 patients. | Metabolic | Niemann–Pick disease |
| Walterfang M, Wood SJ, Velakoulis D, Copolov D, Pantelis C. 2005 [196] | Diseases of white matter and schizophrenia-like psychosis. | Review of diseases affecting white matter tracks associated with psychotic symptoms. | Metabolic | Niemann–Pick disease Arylsulfatase A deficiency Cerebrotendinous xanthomatosis |
| Rosebush PI, MacQueen GM, Clarke JT, Callahan JW, Strasberg PM, Mazurek MF. 1995 [96] | Late-onset Tay-Sachs disease presenting as catatonic schizophrenia: diagnostic and treatment issues. | Case report of a 17-year-old boy and review of psychiatric manifestations and treatment of psychotic symptoms in late-onset Tay-Sachs disease. | Metabolic | Tay-Sachs disease |

| Author/Date | Article Title | Article Characteristics | Type of Pathology | Disease |
|---|---|---|---|---|
| MacQueen GM, Rosebush PI, Mazurek MF. 1998 [95] | Neuropsychiatric aspects of the adult variant of Tay-Sachs disease. | Review of neurologic and psychiatric manifestations in late-onset Tay-Sachs disease, including 64 cases. | Metabolic | Tay-Sachs disease |
| Toro C, Shirvan L, Tifft C. 1999 [97] | HEXA Disorders. | Disease overview (clinical characteristics, diagnosis, management). | Metabolic | Tay-Sachs disease |
| Albers JW, Fink JK. 2004 [197] | Porphyric neuropathy. | Review of neurologic and psychiatric symptoms in porphyria. | Metabolic | Porphyria |
| Qadiri MR, Church SE, McColl KE, Moore MR, Youngs GR. 1986 [198] | Chester porphyria: a clinical study of a new form of acute porphyria. | Retrospective analysis of porphyria clinical characteristics in 41 patients from the same family. | Metabolic | Porphyria |
| Chandrakumar A, Bhardwaj A, 't Jong GW. 2018 [112] | Review of thiamine deficiency disorders: Wernicke encephalopathy and Korsakoff psychosis. | Disease overview (epidemiology, etiopathogeneseis, neuropathology, genetics, clinical presentation, and diagnosis). | Neurologic | Wernicke encephalopathy and Korsakoff disease |
| Ramos ARS, Garrett C. 2017 [99] | Huntington's Disease: Premotor Phase. | Review of the evidence regarding the symptoms in the premotor state of Huntington's disease. | Neurologic | Huntington's disease |
| Sum-Ping O, Guilleminault C. 2016 [116] | Kleine-Levin Syndrome. | Disease overview (epidemiology, clinical presentation, etiology, evaluation, and management). | Neurologic | Kleine–Levin syndrome |
| Cooper JJ, Ovsiew F. 2013 [199] | The relationship between schizophrenia and frontotemporal dementia. | Review of clinical presentations of schizophrenia and frontotemporal dementia. | Neurologic | Frontotemporal dementia |
| Velakoulis D, Walterfang M, Mocellin R, Pantelis C, McLean C. 2009 [103] | Frontotemporaldementia presenting as schizophrenia-like psychosis in young people: clinicopathological series and review of cases. | Case series including 17 patients with FTD and a systematic review including 751 cases from 199 publications. | Neurologic | Frontotemporal dementia |
| Kishi Y, Konishi S, Koizumi S, Kudo Y, Kurosawa H, Kathol RG. 2004 [119] | Schizophrenia and narcolepsy: a review with a case report. | Review of psychotic manifestations in narcolepsy and case report of a 25-year-old woman. | Neurologic | Narcolepsy |
| Douglass AB. 2003 [120] | Narcolepsy: differential diagnosis or etiology in some cases of bipolar disorder and schizophrenia? | Review of psychiatric symptoms in narcolepsy. | Neurologic | Narcolepsy |
| Freudenreich O, Schulz SC, Goff DC. 2009 [127] | Initial medical work-up of first-episode psychosis: a conceptual review. | Conceptual review focusing on laboratory tests and imaging performances to exclude medical causes of psychosis. | Overview | |
| Giannitelli M, Consoli A, Raffin M, Jardri R, Levinson DF, Cohen D, Laurent-Levinson C. 2018 [13] | An overview of medical risk factors for childhood psychosis: Implications for research and treatment. | Systematic review of somatic disorders that can present with psychotic symptoms in children and early adolescents, including 66 publications and clinical data from a cohort of 160 patients who received schizophrenia spectrum diagnoses. | Overview | |
| Griswold KS, Del Regno PA, Berger RC. 2015 [200] | Recognition and Differential Diagnosis of Psychosis in Primary Care. | Overview of medical conditions that can present with acute psychosis. | Overview | |
| Keshavan MS, Kaneko Y. 2013 [14] | Secondary psychoses: an update. | Overview of causes of secondary psychoses and investigations to rule out these causes. | Overview | |
| Falkai P. 1996 [5] | Differential diagnosis in acute psychotic episode. | Review of somatic conditions presenting with acute psychosis. | Overview | |
| Orygen, Early Psychosis Guidelines Writing Group and EPPIC National Support Program. 2016 [1] | Australian Clinical Guidelines for Early Psychosis, 2nd edition update. | Guidelines. | Academic society recommendation (Australia) | |
| Haute Autorité de Santé. 2017 [201] | Guide-Affection de Longue Durée, Schizophrénies. | Guidelines. | Academic society recommendation (France) | |
| McGorry P, Killackey E, Elkins K, Lambert M, Lambert T. 2003 [168] | Summary Australian and New Zealand clinical practice guideline for the treatment of schizophrenia | Guidelines. | Academic society recommendation (Australia and New Zealand) | |

| Author/Date | Article Title | Article Characteristics | Type of Pathology | Disease |
|---|---|---|---|---|
| Canadian Psychiatric Association. 2005 [202] | Clinical practice guidelines. Treatment of schizophrenia. | Guidelines. | Academic society recommendation (Canada) | |
| Lehman AF, Lieberman JA, Dixon LB et al. 2004 [203] | Practice guideline for the treatment of patients with schizophrenia, second edition. | Guidelines. | Academic society recommendation (USA) | |

## Appendix B

| | Pathology | Clinical Signs | Psychiatric Signs | Paraclinical Exams | | |
|---|---|---|---|---|---|---|
| | | | | Laboratory Tests | Imaging | Others |
| Autoimmune | Limbic encephalitis (NMDA) | The prodromal phase of viral appearance Memory disorders Behavioral disorders Temporal or generalized epileptic seizures Orofacial dyskinesias. No localizing signs on neurologic examination | Sudden, noisy onset Personality change Pseudo-catatonic episodes Delusional ideas of persecution Hallucinations (visual and/or auditory) Intolerance to neuroleptics Risk of neuroleptic malignant syndrome | Blood: anti-NMDA-r antibodies CSF: oligoclonal bands, specific antibodies, inflammation | MRI: T2 or FLAIR signal hyperintensity in the temporal region PET: Association of hypo- and hypermetabolisms Anteroposterior gradient with frontal and temporal hypermetabolism and occipital hypometabolism | EEG: Focal or diffuse slow or disorganized activity, epileptic activity, or extreme delta brush |
| | Systemic Lupus Erythematosus | Asthenia Discoid skin rash Photosensitivity Mouth ulcers Arthritis Inflammation of the serous membranes (pleural or pericardial) Renal disorders Neurologic disorders (seizures, psychotic symptoms) Blood disorder | Hallucinations Delusions | Blood: Antinuclear antibodies, anti-DNA antibodies, anti-smith antibodies | MRI: T2 small focal hyperintense lesions in the subcortical and periventricular white matter | |
| | Hashimoto encephalopathy | Acute or insidious symptoms Convulsions Cognitive decline Myoclonus Tremors Fluctuations in the level of consciousness | Psychotic symptoms Depression | Blood: Anti-thyroid antibodies CSF: Anti-thyroid antibodies | MRI: White matter T2 hyperintensities | EEG: Nonspecific abnormalities |
| | Acute disseminated encephalomyelitis | Optic neuritis Ataxia Impairment of consciousness Rapid onset fever Weakness | Irritability Psychosis | CSF: Lymphocytic pleocytosis Elevated level of myelin basic protein | MRI: Multiple, widespread asymmetric T2 hyperintense lesions | EEG: Disturbed sleep pattern Focal or general slowing |
| Metabolic | Niemann–Pick | Dystonia, Dysmetria, Dysarthria, Dysphagia Supranuclear vertical paralysis Convulsions Gelastic cataplexy Liver disorders Developmental retardation Learning difficulties | Paranoid episodes Auditory hallucinations Disorganized thoughts Resistance and intolerance to neuroleptics | | | Cutaneous biopsy: Identification of cholesterol deposits Genetics: Search for specific mutations in the NPC1 and NPC2 genes |
| | Wilson's | Complex cognitive disorders involving executive functions Memory disorders Neurovisual disorders Kayser-Fleisher rings | Mood disorders Personality change Hallucinations Intolerance to neuroleptics | Blood: Copper levels Ceruloplasmin Urines: Copper levels | MRI: Hypersignals in the thalamic and lenticular nuclei Hypodensity of the basal ganglia | EEG: Aspecific defects |
| | Disorders of homocysteine metabolism | Episodes of thrombosis Cognitive decline Dementia Movement disorders Behavioral disorders | Hallucinations | | MRI: Demyelination | Amino acids chromatography |

| | Pathology | Clinical Signs | Psychiatric Signs | Paraclinical Exams | | |
|---|---|---|---|---|---|---|
| | | | | Laboratory Tests | Imaging | Others |
| Metabolic | Acute intermittent porphyria | Intermittent, cyclical pain | Anxiety Impatience Suicide attempts Isolated psychotic symptoms Catatonia | Urine: Increased rates of porphobilinogen | | |
| | Cerebrotendinous xanthomasis | Developmental disorders Chronic diarrhea Seizure Progressive spastic paraparesis Cerebellar ataxia Polyneuropathy Cognitive disorders Tendinous xanthomas | Depression Psychosis Attention deficit hyperactivity disorder | Blood: Cholestanol dosage | MRI: Dendritic hypersignal in regions of the cerebellar nuclei | |
| | Arysulfatase A deficiency | Educational difficulties Progressive spasticity Incontinence Seizure Dementia | Personality change Emotional lability | | MRI: Leukodystrophy | Genetics: Biallelic ARSA pathogens |
| | Hereditary Transthyretin Amyloidosis | Progressive sensorimotor autonomic neuropathy Cardiomyopathy Renal disease Vitreous opacities Amylosis | Psychotic symptoms | | | |
| | Urea Cycle Disorders | Altered level of consciousness Seizures Learning disabilities Developmental delay Hepatomegaly, elevated liver enzymes | Hyperactivity Mood alteration Behavioral changes Psychotic symptoms | Blood: Hyperammonemia | | |
| | Tay Sachs | Speech disorder Muscle weakness Gait disturbance | Mood disorders Psychotic symptoms | Blood: Hexosaminidase levels | | |
| Neurologic | Huntington | Movement disorders Cognitive decline Executive disorder Involuntary choreic movements | Depression Apathy Irritability Psychotic symptoms Sleep disorders | | | Genetic testing |
| | Frontotemporal dementia | Disinhibition Apathy Hyperorality Neurologic disorders | Psychotic symptoms | | | Search for C9ORF72 mutation |
| | Wernicke and Korsakoff | Memory disorders | Hallucinations | Blood: Thiamine concentration Functional enzymatic assay of transketolase activity | MRI: Hyperintensity in the thalamic area, the mammillary bodies, and the periaqueductal area | |
| | Kleine–Levin | Hypersomnia Hyperphagia Hypersexuality | Feelings of derealization Depression Anxiety disorder Suicidal behaviors | | | |
| | Narcolepsy | Excessive daytime sleepiness Cataplexy Sleep attacks | Hallucinations | | | EEG: Nocturnal polysomnography Daytime measurement of sleep latency |
| Infectious | Human Immuno deficiency virus | | Delusions of persecution Ideas of grandeur Hallucinations | Blood: HIV serology | | |
| | Toxoplasmosis | Adenopathy Mononucleosis-like infectious episode Meningoencephalitis | Psychotic symptoms | Blood: IgG and IgM antibodies CSF: Low-key inflammation | MRI: Extended inflammatory lesions abscess | |
| | Cytomegalovirus | HIV infection Encephalitis Enteritis Pneumonia Fever Adenopathy | Auditory hallucinations Delusions Tangential thoughts Blunting of emotions | Blood: IgG and IgM antibodies | | |
| | Syphilis | HIV co-infection | Psychotic symptoms | Direct examination by darkfield microscope immunofluorescence PCR (polymerase chain reaction) test | | |

|  | Pathology | Clinical Signs | Psychiatric Signs | Paraclinical Exams | | |
|---|---|---|---|---|---|---|
|  |  |  |  | Laboratory Tests | Imaging | Others |
| Infectious | Lyme Borreliosis | Radicular pain Paresis Confusion Cerebellar ataxia | Mood disorders Psychotic symptoms | CSF: Elevated cell count Elevated protein Oligoclonal IgG bands Blood: ELISA antibody test |  |  |
| Genetic | 22q11 deletion syndrome | Congenital heart defects Abnormalities of the palate Hypoparathyroidism Immunological disorders Numerous other developmental anomalies | Psychotic symptoms Mood disorders Anxiety disorders Attention deficit hyperactivity disorder |  |  | Genetics: Search for 22q11 mutation |
| Genetic | Prader–Willi syndrome | Hypotonia Hypogonadism Hyperphagia Learning disabilities Small size Tolerance to cutaneous pain | Fluctuating symptoms Anxiety Agitation Delusions of persecution Sleep disorders Emotional involvement |  |  | Genetics: Search for 15q11-q13 mutation |
| Genetic | C9orf72 mutations | Cognitive and behavioral troubles | Delusions Hallucinations Concerns about health |  | MRI: Cortical atrophy |  |

## References

1. *Australian Clinical Guidelines for Early Psychosis-Second Edition Updated-Orygen, Revolution in Mind;* Orygen, The National Centre of Excellence in Youth Mental Health: Melbourne, Australia, 2016.
2. Kirkbride, J.B.; Hameed, Y.; Ankireddypalli, G.; Ioannidis, K.; Crane, C.M.; Nasir, M.; Kabacs, N.; Metastasio, A.; Jenkins, O.; Espandian, A.; et al. The Epidemiology of First-Episode Psychosis in Early Intervention in Psychosis Services: Findings from the Social Epidemiology of Psychoses in East Anglia [SEPEA] Study. *AJP* **2017**, *174*, 143–153. [CrossRef] [PubMed]
3. Albon, E.; Tsourapas, A.; Frew, E.; Davenport, C.; Oyebode, F.; Bayliss, S.; Arvanitis, T.; Meads, C. *Structural Neuroimaging in Psychosis: A Systematic Review and Economic Evaluation;* NIHR Journals Library: Winchester, UK, 2008.
4. Sleurs, D.; Dubertret, C.; Pignon, B.; Tebeka, S.; Le Strat, Y. Psychotic-like Experiences Are Associated with Physical Disorders in General Population: A Cross-Sectional Study from the NESARC II. *J. Psychosom. Res.* **2023**, *165*, 111128. [CrossRef] [PubMed]
5. Falkai, P. Differential Diagnosis in Acute Psychotic Episode. *Int. Clin. Psychopharmacol.* **1996**, *11* (Suppl. S2), 13–17. [CrossRef] [PubMed]
6. Johnstone, E.C.; MacMillan, J.F.; Crow, T.J. The Occurrence of Organic Disease of Possible or Probable Aetiological Significance in a Population of 268 Cases of First Episode Schizophrenia. *Psychol. Med.* **1987**, *17*, 371–379. [CrossRef] [PubMed]
7. Penttilä, M.; Jääskeläinen, E.; Hirvonen, N.; Isohanni, M.; Miettunen, J. Duration of Untreated Psychosis as Predictor of Long-Term Outcome in Schizophrenia: Systematic Review and Meta-Analysis. *Br. J. Psychiatry* **2014**, *205*, 88–94. [CrossRef]
8. Oliver, D.; Davies, C.; Crossland, G.; Lim, S.; Gifford, G.; McGuire, P.; Fusar-Poli, P. Can We Reduce the Duration of Untreated Psychosis? A Systematic Review and Meta-Analysis of Controlled Interventional Studies. *Schizophr. Bull.* **2018**, *44*, 1362–1372. [CrossRef]
9. Bost, C.; Pascual, O.; Honnorat, J. Autoimmune Encephalitis in Psychiatric Institutions: Current Perspectives. *Neuropsychiatr. Dis. Treat.* **2016**, *12*, 2775–2787. [CrossRef]
10. Dalmau, J.; Lancaster, E.; Martinez-Hernandez, E.; Rosenfeld, M.R.; Balice-Gordon, R. Clinical Experience and Laboratory Investigations in Patients with Anti-NMDAR Encephalitis. *Lancet Neurol.* **2011**, *10*, 63–74. [CrossRef]
11. Wang, H.-Y.; Li, T.; Li, X.-L.; Zhang, X.-X.; Yan, Z.-R.; Xu, Y. Anti-N-Methyl-D-Aspartate Receptor Encephalitis Mimics Neuroleptic Malignant Syndrome: Case Report and Literature Review. *Neuropsychiatr. Dis. Treat.* **2019**, *15*, 773–778. [CrossRef]
12. Hutton, B.; Salanti, G.; Caldwell, D.M.; Chaimani, A.; Schmid, C.H.; Cameron, C.; Ioannidis, J.P.A.; Straus, S.; Thorlund, K.; Jansen, J.P.; et al. The PRISMA Extension Statement for Reporting of Systematic Reviews Incorporating Network Meta-Analyses of Health Care Interventions: Checklist and Explanations. *Ann. Intern. Med.* **2015**, *162*, 777. [CrossRef]
13. Giannitelli, M.; Consoli, A.; Raffin, M.; Jardri, R.; Levinson, D.F.; Cohen, D.; Laurent-Levinson, C. An Overview of Medical Risk Factors for Childhood Psychosis: Implications for Research and Treatment. *Schizophr. Res.* **2018**, *192*, 39–49. [CrossRef] [PubMed]
14. Keshavan, M.S.; Kaneko, Y. Secondary Psychoses: An Update. *World Psychiatry* **2013**, *12*, 4–15. [CrossRef] [PubMed]
15. Honnorat, J.; Plazat, L.O. Autoimmune Encephalitis and Psychiatric Disorders. *Rev. Neurol.* **2018**, *174*, 228–236. [CrossRef] [PubMed]
16. Lancaster, E. The Diagnosis and Treatment of Autoimmune Encephalitis. *J. Clin. Neurol.* **2016**, *12*, 1–13. [CrossRef]
17. Gable, M.; Glaser, C. Anti-N-Methyl-d-Aspartate Receptor Encephalitis Appearing as a New-Onset Psychosis: Disease Course in Children and Adolescents Within the California Encephalitis Project. *Pediatr. Neurol.* **2017**, *72*, 25–30. [CrossRef]
18. Hao, Q.; Wang, D.; Guo, L.; Zhang, B. Clinical Characterization of Autoimmune Encephalitis and Psychosis. *Compr. Psychiatry* **2017**, *74*, 9–14. [CrossRef]

19. Kruse, J.L.; Jeffrey, J.K.; Davis, M.C.; Dearlove, J.; IsHak, W.W.; Iii, J.O.B. Anti-N-Methyl-d-Aspartate Receptor Encephalitis: A Targeted Review of Clinical Presentation, Diagnosis, and Approaches to Psychopharmacologic Management. *Ann. Clin. Psychiatry* **2014**, *26*, 10.
20. Zandi, M.S. Autoimmune Encephalitis. *FOC* **2016**, *14*, 432–436. [CrossRef]
21. Ford, B.; McDonald, A.; Srinivasan, S. Anti-NMDA Receptor Encephalitis: A Case Study and Illness Overview. *Drugs Context* **2019**, *8*, 212589. [CrossRef]
22. Kayser, M.S.; Dalmau, J. Anti-NMDA Receptor Encephalitis, Autoimmunity, and Psychosis. *Schizophr. Res.* **2016**, *176*, 36–40. [CrossRef]
23. Lazar-Molnar, E.; Tebo, A.E. Autoimmune NMDA Receptor Encephalitis. *Clin. Chim. Acta* **2015**, *438*, 90–97. [CrossRef] [PubMed]
24. Armangue, T.; Petit-Pedrol, M.; Dalmau, J. Autoimmune Encephalitis in Children. *J. Child Neurol.* **2012**, *27*, 1460–1469. [CrossRef] [PubMed]
25. Al-Diwani, A.; Handel, A.; Townsend, L.; Pollak, T.; Leite, M.I.; Harrison, P.J.; Lennox, B.R.; Okai, D.; Manohar, S.G.; Irani, S.R. The Psychopathology of NMDAR-Antibody Encephalitis in Adults: A Systematic Review and Phenotypic Analysis of Individual Patient Data. *Lancet Psychiatry* **2019**, *6*, 235–246. [CrossRef] [PubMed]
26. Warren, N.; Siskind, D.; O'Gorman, C. Refining the Psychiatric Syndrome of Anti-N-Methyl-d-Aspartate Receptor Encephalitis. *Acta Psychiatr. Scand.* **2018**, *138*, 401–408. [CrossRef]
27. Sarkis, R.A.; Coffey, M.J.; Cooper, J.J.; Hassan, I.; Lennox, B. Anti-N-Methyl-D-Aspartate Receptor Encephalitis: A Review of Psychiatric Phenotypes and Management Considerations: A Report of the American Neuropsychiatric Association Committee on Research. *JNP* **2019**, *31*, 137–142. [CrossRef]
28. Pollak, T.A.; Lennox, B.R.; Müller, S.; Benros, M.E.; Prüss, H.; Tebartz van Elst, L.; Klein, H.; Steiner, J.; Frodl, T.; Bogerts, B.; et al. Autoimmune Psychosis: An International Consensus on an Approach to the Diagnosis and Management of Psychosis of Suspected Autoimmune Origin. *Lancet Psychiatry* **2020**, *7*, 93–108. [CrossRef]
29. Chandra, S.R.; Viswanathan, L.G.; Sindhu, D.M.; Pai, A.R. Subacute Noninfective Inflammatory Encephalopathy: Our Experience and Diagnostic Problems. *Indian J. Psychol. Med.* **2017**, *39*, 183–187. [CrossRef]
30. Brenton, J.N.; Goodkin, H.P. Antibody-Mediated Autoimmune Encephalitis in Childhood. *Pediatr. Neurol.* **2016**, *60*, 13–23. [CrossRef]
31. Graus, F.; Titulaer, M.J.; Balu, R.; Benseler, S.; Bien, C.G.; Cellucci, T.; Cortese, I.; Dale, R.C.; Gelfand, J.M.; Geschwind, M.; et al. A Clinical Approach to Diagnosis of Autoimmune Encephalitis. *Lancet Neurol.* **2016**, *15*, 391–404. [CrossRef]
32. Guasp, M.; Servén, E.; Maudes, E.; Rosa-Justicia, M.; Martinez-Hernandez, E.; Boix-Quintana, E.; Bioque, M.; Casado, V.; Módena-Ouarzi, Y.; Guanyabens, N.; et al. Clinical, Neuroimmunologic, and CSF Investigations in First Episode Psychosis. *Neurology* **2021**, *97*, e61–e75. [CrossRef]
33. Endres, D.; Leypoldt, F.; Bechter, K.; Hasan, A.; Steiner, J.; Domschke, K.; Wandinger, K.-P.; Falkai, P.; Arolt, V.; Stich, O.; et al. Autoimmune Encephalitis as a Differential Diagnosis of Schizophreniform Psychosis: Clinical Symptomatology, Pathophysiology, Diagnostic Approach, and Therapeutic Considerations. *Eur. Arch. Psychiatry Clin. Neurosci.* **2020**, *270*, 803–818. [CrossRef] [PubMed]
34. Steiner, J.; Prüss, H.; Köhler, S.; Frodl, T.; Hasan, A.; Falkai, P. Autoimmune Encephalitis with Psychosis: Warning Signs, Step-by-Step Diagnostics and Treatment. *World J. Biol. Psychiatry* **2018**, *21*, 241–254. [CrossRef] [PubMed]
35. Yazdany, J.; Dall'Era, M. Definition and Classification of Lupus and Lupus-Related Disorders. In *Dubois' Lupus Erythematosus and Related Syndromes*; Wallace, D.J., Hahn, B.H., Eds.; W.B. Saunders: Philadelphia, PA, USA, 2013; pp. 1–7. ISBN 978-1-4377-1893-5.
36. Lisnevskaia, L.; Murphy, G.; Isenberg, D. Systemic Lupus Erythematosus. *Lancet* **2014**, *384*, 1878–1888. [CrossRef]
37. Khajezadeh, M.-A.; Zamani, G.; Moazzami, B.; Nagahi, Z.; Mousavi-Torshizi, M.; Ziaee, V. Neuropsychiatric Involvement in Juvenile-Onset Systemic Lupus Erythematosus. 2018. Available online: https://www.hindawi.com/journals/nri/2018/2548142/ (accessed on 6 April 2020).
38. Liang, M.H.; Corzillius, M.; Bae, S.C.; Lew, R.A.; Fortin, P.R.; Gordon, C.; Isenberg, D.; Alarcón, G.S.; Straaton, K.V.; Denburg, J.; et al. The American College of Rheumatology Nomenclature and Case Definitions for Neuropsychiatric Lupus Syndromes. *Arthritis Rheum.* **1999**, *42*, 599–608. [CrossRef]
39. Hanly, J.G.; Urowitz, M.B.; Siannis, F.; Farewell, V.; Gordon, C.; Bae, S.C.; Isenberg, D.; Dooley, M.A.; Clarke, A.; Bernatsky, S.; et al. Autoantibodies and Neuropsychiatric Events at the Time of Systemic Lupus Erythematosus Diagnosis: Results from an International Inception Cohort Study. *Arthritis Rheum.* **2008**, *58*, 843–853. [CrossRef] [PubMed]
40. Shimizu, Y.; Yasuda, S.; Kako, Y.; Nakagawa, S.; Kanda, M.; Hisada, R.; Ohmura, K.; Shimamura, S.; Shida, H.; Fujieda, Y.; et al. Post-Steroid Neuropsychiatric Manifestations Are Significantly More Frequent in SLE Compared with Other Systemic Autoimmune Diseases and Predict Better Prognosis Compared with de Novo Neuropsychiatric SLE. *Autoimmun. Rev.* **2016**, *15*, 786–794. [CrossRef]
41. Garcia, L.P.W.; Gladman, D.D.; Urowitz, M.; Touma, Z.; Su, J.; Johnson, S.R. New EULAR/ACR 2019 SLE Classification Criteria: Defining Ominosity in SLE. *Ann. Rheum. Dis.* **2021**, *80*, 767. [CrossRef]
42. Chong, J.Y.; Rowland, L.P.; Utiger, R.D. Hashimoto Encephalopathy: Syndrome or Myth? *Arch. Neurol.* **2003**, *60*, 164–171. [CrossRef]
43. Lee, J.; Yu, H.J.; Lee, J. Hashimoto Encephalopathy in Pediatric Patients: Homogeneity in Clinical Presentation and Heterogeneity in Antibody Titers. *Brain Dev.* **2018**, *40*, 42–48. [CrossRef]

44. de Holanda, N.C.P.; de Lima, D.D.; Cavalcanti, T.B.; Lucena, C.S.; Bandeira, F. Hashimoto's Encephalopathy: Systematic Review of the Literature and an Additional Case. *JNP* **2011**, *23*, 384–390. [CrossRef]
45. Krupp, L.B.; Banwell, B.; Tenembaum, S. Consensus Definitions Proposed for Pediatric Multiple Sclerosis and Related Disorders. *Neurology* **2007**, *68*, S7. [CrossRef] [PubMed]
46. Nasr, J.T.; Andriola, M.R.; Coyle, P.K. Adem: Literature Review and Case Report of Acute Psychosis Presentation. *Pediatr. Neurol.* **2000**, *22*, 8–18. [CrossRef] [PubMed]
47. Tahan, A.A.; Arora, S.; Alzeer, A.; Tahan, F.A.; Malabarey, T.; Daif, A. Acute Disseminated Encephalomyelitis: The Importance of Early Magnetic Resonance Imaging. *Eur. J. Neurol.* **1997**, *4*, 52–58. [CrossRef] [PubMed]
48. Tardieu, M.; Banwell, B.; Wolinsky, J.S.; Pohl, D.; Krupp, L.B. Consensus Definitions for Pediatric MS and Other Demyelinating Disorders in Childhood. *Neurology* **2016**, *87*, S8–S11. [CrossRef]
49. Walterfang, M.; Bonnot, O.; Mocellin, R.; Velakoulis, D. The Neuropsychiatry of Inborn Errors of Metabolism. *J. Inherit. Metab. Dis.* **2013**, *36*, 687–702. [CrossRef]
50. Faoucher, M.; Demily, C. Chapter 11—The Psychopharmacology of Wilson Disease and Other Metabolic Disorders. In *Handbook of Clinical Neurology*; Reus, V.I., Lindqvist, D., Eds.; Psychopharmacology of Neurologic Disease; Elsevier: Amsterdam, The Netherlands, 2019; Volume 165, pp. 191–205.
51. Vanier, M.T. Niemann-Pick Disease Type C. *Orphanet J. Rare Dis.* **2010**, *5*, 16. [CrossRef]
52. Hendriksz, C.J.; Anheim, M.; Bauer, P.; Bonnot, O.; Chakrapani, A.; Corvol, J.-C.; de Koning, T.J.; Degtyareva, A.; Dionisi-Vici, C.; Doss, S.; et al. The Hidden Niemann-Pick Type C Patient: Clinical Niches for a Rare Inherited Metabolic Disease. *Curr. Med. Res. Opin.* **2017**, *33*, 877–890. [CrossRef]
53. Patterson, M.C.; Hendriksz, C.J.; Walterfang, M.; Sedel, F.; Vanier, M.T.; Wijburg, F. Recommendations for the Diagnosis and Management of Niemann–Pick Disease Type C: An Update. *Mol. Genet. Metab.* **2012**, *106*, 330–344. [CrossRef]
54. Rego, T.; Farrand, S.; Goh, A.M.Y.; Eratne, D.; Kelso, W.; Mangelsdorf, S.; Velakoulis, D.; Walterfang, M. Psychiatric and Cognitive Symptoms Associated with Niemann-Pick Type C Disease: Neurobiology and Management. *CNS Drugs* **2019**, *33*, 125–142. [CrossRef]
55. Bonnot, O.; Klünemann, H.-H.; Velten, C.; Martin, J.V.T.; Walterfang, M. Systematic Review of Psychiatric Signs in Niemann-Pick Disease Type C. *World J. Biol. Psychiatry* **2019**, *20*, 320–332. [CrossRef]
56. Staretz-Chacham, O.; Choi, J.H.; Wakabayashi, K.; Lopez, G.; Sidransky, E. Psychiatric and Behavioral Manifestations of Lysosomal Storage Disorders. *Am. J. Med. Genet. Part B Neuropsychiatr. Genet.* **2010**, *153B*, 1253–1265. [CrossRef] [PubMed]
57. Bonnot, O.; Herrera, P.M.; Tordjman, S.; Walterfang, M. Secondary Psychosis Induced by Metabolic Disorders. *Front. Neurosci.* **2015**, *9*, 177. [CrossRef] [PubMed]
58. Sitarska, D.; Ługowska, A. Laboratory Diagnosis of the Niemann-Pick Type C Disease: An Inherited Neurodegenerative Disorder of Cholesterol Metabolism. *Metab. Brain Dis.* **2019**, *34*, 1253–1260. [CrossRef]
59. Demily, C.; Sedel, F. Psychiatric Manifestations of Treatable Hereditary Metabolic Disorders in Adults. *Ann. Gen. Psychiatry* **2014**, *13*, 27. [CrossRef] [PubMed]
60. Taly, A.B.; Meenakshi-Sundaram, S.; Sinha, S.; Swamy, H.S.; Arunodaya, G.R. Wilson Disease: Description of 282 Patients Evaluated Over 3 Decades. *Medicine* **2007**, *86*, 112. [CrossRef]
61. Dening, T.R.; Berrios, G.E. Wilson's Disease: Psychiatric Symptoms in 195 Cases. *Arch. Gen. Psychiatry* **1989**, *46*, 1126–1134. [CrossRef]
62. Medalia, A.; Scheinberg, I.H. Psychopathology in Patients with Wilson's Disease. *Am. J. Psychiatry* **1989**, *146*, 662–664. [CrossRef]
63. Akil, M.; Schwartz, J.A.; Dutchak, D.; Yuzbasiyan-Gurkan, V.; Brewer, G.J. The Psychiatric Presentations of Wilson's Disease. *J. Neuropsychiatry Clin. Neurosci.* **1991**, *3*, 377–382. [CrossRef]
64. Dening, T.R. *The Neuropsychiatry of Wilson's Disease*; University of Newcastle upon Tyne: Newcastle upon Tyne, UK, 1989.
65. Akil, M.; Brewer, G.J. Psychiatric and Behavioral Abnormalities in Wilson's Disease. *Adv. Neurol.* **1995**, *65*, 171–178.
66. Srinivas, K.; Sinha, S.; Taly, A.B.; Prashanth, L.K.; Arunodaya, G.R.; Janardhana Reddy, Y.C.; Khanna, S. Dominant Psychiatric Manifestations in Wilson's Disease: A Diagnostic and Therapeutic Challenge! *J. Neurol. Sci.* **2008**, *266*, 104–108. [CrossRef]
67. Sagawa, M.; Takao, M.; Nogawa, S.; Mizuno, M.; Murata, M.; Amano, T.; Koto, A. Wilson's disease associated with olfactory paranoid syndrome and idiopathic thrombocytopenic purpura. *No Shinkei* **2003**, *55*, 899–902.
68. Wichowicz, H.M.; Cubała, W.J.; Sławek, J. Wilson's Disease Associated with Delusional Disorder. *Psychiatry Clin. Neurosci.* **2006**, *60*, 758–760. [CrossRef] [PubMed]
69. Spyridi, S.; Diakogiannis, I.; Michaelides, M.; Sokolaki, S.; Iacovides, A.; Kaprinis, G. Delusional Disorder and Alcohol Abuse in a Patient with Wilson's Disease. *Gen. Hosp. Psychiatry* **2008**, *30*, 585–586. [CrossRef] [PubMed]
70. Biswas, S.; Paul, N.; Das, S.K. Nonmotor Manifestations of Wilson's Disease. In *International Review of Neurobiology*; Chaudhuri, K.R., Titova, N., Eds.; Nonmotor Parkinson's: The Hidden Face; Academic Press: Cambridge, MA, USA, 2017; Volume 134, pp. 1443–1459.
71. Zimbrean, P.C.; Schilsky, M.L. Psychiatric Aspects of Wilson Disease: A Review. *Gen. Hosp. Psychiatry* **2014**, *36*, 53–62. [CrossRef]
72. Gilbody, S.; Lewis, S.; Lightfoot, T. Methylenetetrahydrofolate Reductase (MTHFR) Genetic Polymorphisms and Psychiatric Disorders: A HuGE Review. *Am. J. Epidemiol.* **2007**, *165*, 1–13. [CrossRef]
73. Li, S.C.H.; Stewart, P.M. Homocystinuria and Psychiatric Disorder: A Case Report. *Pathology* **1999**, *31*, 221–224. [CrossRef]

74. Roze, E.; Gervais, D.; Demeret, S.; de Baulny, H.O.; Zittoun, J.; Benoist, J.-F.; Said, G.; Pierrot-Deseilligny, C.; Bolgert, F. Neuropsychiatric Disturbances in Presumed Late-Onset Cobalamin C Disease. *Arch. Neurol.* **2003**, *60*, 1457–1462. [CrossRef]
75. Kühnel, A.; Gross, U.; Doss, M.O. Hereditary Coproporphyria in Germany: Clinical-Biochemical Studies in 53 Patients. *Clin. Biochem.* **2000**, *33*, 465–473. [CrossRef]
76. Crimlisk, H.L. The Little Imitator–Porphyria: A Neuropsychiatric Disorder. *J. Neurol. Neurosurg. Psychiatry* **1997**, *62*, 319–328. [CrossRef]
77. Bonkowsky, H.L.; Schady, W. Neurologic Manifestations of Acute Porphyria. *Semin. Liver Dis.* **1982**, *2*, 108–124. [CrossRef]
78. Kumar, B. Acute Intermittent Porphyria Presenting Solely with Psychosis: A Case Report and Discussion. *Psychosomatics* **2012**, *53*, 494–498. [CrossRef] [PubMed]
79. Jain, G.; Bennett, J.I.; Resch, D.S.; Godwin, J.E. Schizoaffective Disorder with Missed Diagnosis of Acute Porphyria: A Case Report and Overview. *Prim. Care Companion CNS Disord.* **2011**, *13*, 26826. [CrossRef] [PubMed]
80. Salen, G.; Steiner, R.D. Epidemiology, Diagnosis, and Treatment of Cerebrotendinous Xanthomatosis (CTX). *J. Inherit. Metab. Dis.* **2017**, *40*, 771–781. [CrossRef] [PubMed]
81. Nie, S.; Chen, G.; Cao, X.; Zhang, Y. Cerebrotendinous Xanthomatosis: A Comprehensive Review of Pathogenesis, Clinical Manifestations, Diagnosis, and Management. *Orphanet J. Rare Dis.* **2014**, *9*, 179. [CrossRef] [PubMed]
82. Sedel, F.; Baumann, N.; Turpin, J.-C.; Lyon-Caen, O.; Saudubray, J.-M.; Cohen, D. Psychiatric Manifestations Revealing Inborn Errors of Metabolism in Adolescents and Adults. *J. Inherit. Metab. Dis.* **2007**, *30*, 631–641. [CrossRef]
83. Hyde, T.M.; Ziegler, J.C.; Weinberger, D.R. Psychiatric Disturbances in Metachromatic Leukodystrophy: Insights into the Neurobiology of Psychosis. *Arch. Neurol.* **1992**, *49*, 401–406. [CrossRef]
84. Gomez-Ospina, N. Arylsulfatase A Deficiency. In *GeneReviews®*; Adam, M.P., Ardinger, H.H., Pagon, R.A., Wallace, S.E., Bean, L.J., Stephens, K., Amemiya, A., Eds.; University of Washington: Seattle, WA, USA, 1993.
85. Aicardi, J. The Inherited Leukodystrophies: A Clinical Overview. *J. Inherit. Metab. Dis.* **1993**, *16*, 733–743. [CrossRef]
86. Mahmood, A.; Berry, J.; Wenger, D.A.; Escolar, M.; Sobeih, M.; Raymond, G.; Eichler, F.S. Metachromatic Leukodystrophy: A Case of Triplets with the Late Infantile Variant and a Systematic Review of the Literature. *J. Child Neurol.* **2010**, *25*, 572–580. [CrossRef]
87. Baumann, N.; Masson, M.; Carreau, V.; Lefevre, M.; Herschkowitz, N.; Turpin, J.C. Adult Forms of Metachromatic Leukodystrophy: Clinical and Biochemical Approach. *DNE* **1991**, *13*, 211–215. [CrossRef]
88. Benson, M.D.; Uemichi, T. Transthyretin Amyloidosis. *Amyloid* **1996**, *3*, 44–56. [CrossRef]
89. Ando, Y.; Nakamura, M.; Araki, S. Transthyretin-Related Familial Amyloidotic Polyneuropathy. *Arch. Neurol.* **2005**, *62*, 1057–1062. [CrossRef] [PubMed]
90. Sekijima, Y. Hereditary Transthyretin Amyloidosis. In *GeneReviews®*; Adam, M.P., Ardinger, H.H., Pagon, R.A., Wallace, S.E., Bean, L.J., Stephens, K., Amemiya, A., Eds.; University of Washington: Seattle, WA, USA, 1993.
91. Brett, M.; Persey, M.R.; Reilly, M.M.; Revesz, T.; Booth, D.R.; Booth, S.E.; Hawkins, P.N.; Pepys, M.B.; Morgan-Hughes, J.A. Transthyretin Leu12Pro Is Associated with Systemic, Neuropathic and Leptomeningeal Amyloidosis. *Brain* **1999**, *122*, 183–190. [CrossRef] [PubMed]
92. Häberle, J.; Boddaert, N.; Burlina, A.; Chakrapani, A.; Dixon, M.; Huemer, M.; Karall, D.; Martinelli, D.; Crespo, P.S.; Santer, R.; et al. Suggested Guidelines for the Diagnosis and Management of Urea Cycle Disorders. *Orphanet J. Rare Dis.* **2012**, *7*, 32. [CrossRef]
93. Lichter-Konecki, U.; Caldovic, L.; Morizono, H.; Simpson, K. *Ornithine Transcarbamylase Deficiency*; University of Washington: Seattle, WA, USA, 2016.
94. Shapiro, B.E.; Pastores, G.M.; Gianutsos, J.; Luzy, C.; Kolodny, E.H. Miglustat in Late-Onset Tay-Sachs Disease: A 12-Month, Randomized, Controlled Clinical Study with 24 Months of Extended Treatment. *Genet. Med.* **2009**, *11*, 425–433. [CrossRef] [PubMed]
95. MacQueen, G.M.; Rosebush, P.I.; Mazurek, M.F. Neuropsychiatric Aspects of the Adult Variant of Tay-Sachs Disease. *JNP* **1998**, *10*, 10–19. [CrossRef] [PubMed]
96. Rosebush, P.I.; MacQueen, G.M.; Clarke, J.T.R.; Callahan, J.W.; Strasberg, P.M.; Mazurek, M.F. Late-Onset Tay-Sachs Disease Presenting as Catatonic Schizophrenia: Diagnostic and Treatment Issues. *J. Clin. Psychiatry* **1995**, *56*, 347–353. [PubMed]
97. Toro, C.; Shirvan, L.; Tifft, C. HEXA Disorders. In *GeneReviews®*; Adam, M.P., Ardinger, H.H., Pagon, R.A., Wallace, S.E., Bean, L.J., Stephens, K., Amemiya, A., Eds.; University of Washington: Seattle, WA, USA, 1993.
98. Ross, C.A.; Tabrizi, S.J. Huntington's Disease: From Molecular Pathogenesis to Clinical Treatment. *Lancet Neurol.* **2011**, *10*, 83–98. [CrossRef]
99. Ramos, A.R.S.; Garrett, C. Huntington's Disease: Premotor Phase. *NDD* **2017**, *17*, 313–322. [CrossRef]
100. Martinez-Horta, S.; Perez-Perez, J.; van Duijn, E.; Fernandez-Bobadilla, R.; Carceller, M.; Pagonabarraga, J.; Pascual-Sedano, B.; Campolongo, A.; Ruiz-Idiago, J.; Sampedro, F.; et al. Neuropsychiatric Symptoms Are Very Common in Premanifest and Early Stage Huntington's Disease. *Park. Relat. Disord.* **2016**, *25*, 58–64. [CrossRef]
101. Hogarth, P.; Kayson, E.; Kieburtz, K.; Marder, K.; Oakes, D.; Rosas, D.; Shoulson, I.; Wexler, N.S.; Young, A.B.; Zhao, H. Interrater Agreement in the Assessment of Motor Manifestations of Huntington's Disease. *Mov. Disord.* **2005**, *20*, 293–297. [CrossRef]
102. Neary, D.; Snowden, J.; Mann, D. Frontotemporal Dementia. *Lancet Neurol.* **2005**, *4*, 771–780. [CrossRef] [PubMed]

103. Velakoulis, D.; Walterfang, M.; Mocellin, R.; Pantelis, C.; McLean, C. Frontotemporal Dementia Presenting as Schizophrenia-like Psychosis in Young People: Clinicopathological Series and Review of Cases. *Br. J. Psychiatry* **2009**, *194*, 298–305. [CrossRef] [PubMed]
104. Neary, D.; Snowden, J.S.; Gustafson, L.; Passant, U.; Stuss, D.; Black, S.; Freedman, M.; Kertesz, A.; Robert, P.H.; Albert, M.; et al. Frontotemporal Lobar Degeneration. *Neurology* **1998**, *51*, 1546. [CrossRef] [PubMed]
105. McKhann, G.M.; Albert, M.S.; Grossman, M.; Miller, B.; Dickson, D.; Trojanowski, J.Q. Clinical and Pathological Diagnosis of Frontotemporal Dementia: Report of the Work Group on Frontotemporal Dementia and Pick's Disease. *Arch. Neurol.* **2001**, *58*, 1803–1809. [CrossRef]
106. Rascovsky, K.; Hodges, J.R.; Knopman, D.; Mendez, M.F.; Kramer, J.H.; Neuhaus, J.; van Swieten, J.C.; Seelaar, H.; Dopper, E.G.P.; Onyike, C.U.; et al. Sensitivity of Revised Diagnostic Criteria for the Behavioural Variant of Frontotemporal Dementia. *Brain* **2011**, *134*, 2456–2477. [CrossRef] [PubMed]
107. Thomson, A.D.; Marshall, E.J. The Natural History and Pathophysiology of Wernicke's Encephalopathy and Korsakoff's Psychosis. *Alcohol Alcohol.* **2006**, *41*, 151–158. [CrossRef]
108. Thomson, A.D. Mechanisms of Vitamin Deficiency in Chronic Alcohol Misusers and the Development of the Wernicke-Korsakoff Syndrome. *Alcohol Alcohol.* **2000**, *35*, 1–2. [CrossRef]
109. Chawla, J.; Kvarnberg, D. Chapter 59—Hydrosoluble Vitamins. In *Handbook of Clinical Neurology*; Biller, J., Ferro, J.M., Eds.; Neurologic Aspects of Systemic Disease Part II; Elsevier: Amsterdam, The Netherlands, 2014; Volume 120, pp. 891–914.
110. Dhir, S.; Tarasenko, M.; Napoli, E.; Giulivi, C. Neurological, Psychiatric, and Biochemical Aspects of Thiamine Deficiency in Children and Adults. *Front. Psychiatry* **2019**, *10*, 207. [CrossRef]
111. Kopelman, M.D.; Thomson, A.D.; Guerrini, I.; Marshall, E.J. The Korsakoff Syndrome: Clinical Aspects, Psychology and Treatment. *Alcohol Alcohol.* **2009**, *44*, 148–154. [CrossRef]
112. Chandrakumar, A.; Bhardwaj, A.; Jong, G.W. Review of Thiamine Deficiency Disorders: Wernicke Encephalopathy and Korsakoff Psychosis. *J. Basic Clin. Physiol. Pharmacol.* **2018**, *30*, 153–162. [CrossRef]
113. Lavault, S.; Golmard, J.-L.; Groos, E.; Brion, A.; Dauvilliers, Y.; Lecendreux, M.; Franco, P.; Arnulf, I. Kleine–Levin Syndrome in 120 Patients: Differential Diagnosis and Long Episodes. *Ann. Neurol.* **2015**, *77*, 529–540. [CrossRef] [PubMed]
114. AlShareef, S.M.; Smith, R.M.; BaHammam, A.S. Kleine-Levin Syndrome: Clues to Aetiology. *Sleep Breath* **2018**, *22*, 613–623. [CrossRef] [PubMed]
115. Arnulf, I.; Rico, T.J.; Mignot, E. Diagnosis, Disease Course, and Management of Patients with Kleine-Levin Syndrome. *Lancet Neurol.* **2012**, *11*, 918–928. [CrossRef] [PubMed]
116. Sum-Ping, O.; Guilleminault, C. Kleine-Levin Syndrome. *Curr. Treat. Options Neurol.* **2016**, *18*, 24. [CrossRef]
117. Arnulf, I. Kleine-Levin Syndrome. *Sleep Med. Clin.* **2015**, *10*, 151–161. [CrossRef]
118. Sateia, M.J. International Classification of Sleep Disorders-Third Edition. *Chest* **2014**, *146*, 1387–1394. [CrossRef]
119. Kishi, Y.; Konishi, S.; Koizumi, S.; Kudo, Y.; Kurosawa, H.; Kathol, R.G. Schizophrenia and Narcolepsy: A Review with a Case Report. *Psychiatry Clin. Neurosci.* **2004**, *58*, 117–124. [CrossRef]
120. Douglass, A.B. Narcolepsy: Differential Diagnosis or Etiology in Some Cases of Bipolar Disorder and Schizophrenia? *CNS Spectr.* **2003**, *8*, 120–126. [CrossRef]
121. Guelfi, J.D.; Rouillon, F. *Manuel de Psychiatrie*; Elsevier Masson: Issy Les Moulineaux, France, 2017; ISBN 978-2-294-74976-6.
122. Ey, H.; Bernard, P. *Manuel de Psychiatrie (6ème Edition)*; Elsevier Masson: Issy Les Moulineaux, France, 2010.
123. Alciati, A.; Fusi, A.; D'Arminio Monforte, A.; Coen, M.; Ferri, A.; Mellado, C. New-Onset Delusions and Hallucinations in Patients Infected with HIV. *J. Psychiatry Neurosci.* **2001**, *26*, 229–234.
124. Sewell, D.D. Schizophrenia and HIV. *Schizophr. Bull.* **1996**, *22*, 465–473. [CrossRef]
125. Dolder, C.R.; Patterson, T.L.; Jeste, D.V. HIV, Psychosis and Aging: Past, Present and Future. *AIDS* **2004**, *18*, 35. [CrossRef]
126. Shedlack, K.J.; Soldato-Couture, C.; Swanson, C.L. Rapidly Progressive Tardive Dyskinesia in AIDS. *Biol. Psychiatry* **1994**, *35*, 147–148. [CrossRef] [PubMed]
127. Freudenreich, O.; Schulz, S.C.; Goff, D.C. Initial Medical Work-up of First-Episode Psychosis: A Conceptual Review. *Early Interv. Psychiatry* **2009**, *3*, 10–18. [CrossRef]
128. Montoya, J.G.; Rosso, F. Diagnosis and Management of Toxoplasmosis. *Clin. Perinatol.* **2005**, *32*, 705–726. [CrossRef]
129. Pradhan, S.; Yadav, R.; Mishra, V.N. Toxoplasma Meningoencephalitis in HIV-Seronegative Patients: Clinical Patterns, Imaging Features and Treatment Outcome. *Trans. R. Soc. Trop. Med. Hyg.* **2007**, *101*, 25–33. [CrossRef] [PubMed]
130. Yolken, R.H.; Torrey, E.F. Are Some Cases of Psychosis Caused by Microbial Agents? A Review of the Evidence. *Mol. Psychiatry* **2008**, *13*, 470–479. [CrossRef]
131. Villard, O.; Cimon, B.; L'Ollivier, C.; Fricker-Hidalgo, H.; Godineau, N.; Houze, S.; Paris, L.; Pelloux, H.; Villena, I.; Candolfi, E. Serological Diagnosis of Toxoplasma Gondii Infection: Recommendations from the French National Reference Center for Toxoplasmosis. *Diagn. Microbiol. Infect. Dis.* **2016**, *84*, 22–33. [CrossRef]
132. Duchowny, M.; Caplan, L.; Siber, G. Cytomegalovirus Infection of the Adult Nervous System. *Ann. Neurol.* **1979**, *5*, 458–461. [CrossRef]
133. Torrey, E.F. Functional Psychoses and Viral Encephalitis. *Integr. Psychiatry* **1986**, *4*, 224–230.
134. LaFond, R.E.; Lukehart, S.A. Biological Basis for Syphilis. *Clin. Microbiol. Rev.* **2006**, *19*, 29–49. [CrossRef]

135. Singh, A.E.; Romanowski, B. Syphilis: Review with Emphasis on Clinical, Epidemiologic, and Some Biologic Features. *Clin. Microbiol. Rev.* **1999**, *12*, 187–209. [CrossRef] [PubMed]
136. Morshed, M.G. Current Trend on Syphilis Diagnosis: Issues and Challenges. In *Proceedings of the Infectious Diseases and Nanomedicine II*; Adhikari, R., Thapa, S., Eds.; Springer: New Delhi, India, 2014; pp. 51–64.
137. Rizzoli, A.; Hauffe, H.C.; Carpi, G.; Vourc'h, G.I.; Neteler, M.; Rosà, R. Lyme Borreliosis in Europe. *Eurosurveillance* **2011**, *16*, 19906. [CrossRef]
138. Fallon, B.A.; Nields, J.A. Lyme Disease: A Neuropsychiatric Illness. *Am. J. Psychiatry* **1994**, *151*, 13.
139. Brodziński, S.; Nasierowski, T. Psychosis in Borrelia Burgdorferi Infection—Part I: Epidemiology, Pathogenesis, Diagnosis and Treatment of Neuroborreliosis. *Psychiatr. Pol.* **2019**, *53*, 629–640. [CrossRef] [PubMed]
140. Fallon, B.A.; Levin, E.S.; Schweitzer, P.J.; Hardesty, D. Inflammation and Central Nervous System Lyme Disease. *Neurobiol. Dis.* **2010**, *37*, 534–541. [CrossRef] [PubMed]
141. Mygland, Å.; Ljøstad, U.; Fingerle, V.; Rupprecht, T.; Schmutzhard, E.; Steiner, I. EFNS Guidelines on the Diagnosis and Management of European Lyme Neuroborreliosis. *Eur. J. Neurol.* **2010**, *17*, 8-e4. [CrossRef]
142. Propping, P. Genetic Disorders Presenting as "Schizophrenia". Karl Bonhoeffer's Early View of the Psychoses in the Light of Medical Genetics. *Hum. Genet.* **1983**, *65*, 1–10. [CrossRef] [PubMed]
143. Bourgeois, J.; Coffey, S.; Rivera, S.M.; Hessl, D.; Gane, L.W.; Tassone, F.; Greco, C.; Finucane, B.; Nelson, L.; Berry-Kravis, E.; et al. Fragile X Premutation Disorders—Expanding the Psychiatric Perspective. *J. Clin. Psychiatry* **2009**, *70*, 852–862. [CrossRef]
144. Franke, P.; Leboyer, M.; Gänsicke, M.; Weiffenbach, O.; Biancalana, V.; Cornillet-Lefebre, P.; Françoise Croquette, M.; Froster, U.G.; Schwab, S.; Poustka, F.; et al. Genotype–Phenotype Relationship in Female Carriers of the Premutation and Full Mutation of FMR-1. *Psychiatry Res.* **1998**, *80*, 113–127. [CrossRef]
145. Al-Owain, M.; Colak, D.; Albakheet, A.; Al-Younes, B.; Al-Humaidi, Z.; Al-Sayed, M.; Al-Hindi, H.; Al-Sugair, A.; Al-Muhaideb, A.; Rahbeeni, Z.; et al. Clinical and Biochemical Features Associated with BCS1L Mutation. *J. Inherit Metab. Dis.* **2013**, *36*, 813–820. [CrossRef]
146. Mulle, J.G.; Gambello, M.J.; Cook, E.H.; Rutkowski, T.P.; Glassford, M. 3q29 Recurrent Deletion. In *GeneReviews®*; Adam, M.P., Ardinger, H.H., Pagon, R.A., Wallace, S.E., Bean, L.J., Stephens, K., Amemiya, A., Eds.; University of Washington: Seattle, WA, USA, 1993.
147. Finucane, B.M.; Lusk, L.; Arkilo, D.; Chamberlain, S.; Devinsky, O.; Dindot, S.; Jeste, S.S.; LaSalle, J.M.; Reiter, L.T.; Schanen, N.C.; et al. 15q Duplication Syndrome and Related Disorders. In *GeneReviews®*; Adam, M.P., Ardinger, H.H., Pagon, R.A., Wallace, S.E., Bean, L.J., Stephens, K., Amemiya, A., Eds.; University of Washington: Seattle, WA, USA, 1993.
148. Anglin, R.; Garside, S.; Tarnopolsky, M.; Mazurek, M.; Rosebush, P. The Psychiatric Manifestations of Mitochondrial Disorders: A Case and Review of the Literature. *J. Clin. Psychiatry* **2012**, *73*, 506–512. [CrossRef] [PubMed]
149. Tang, S.X.; Yi, J.J.; Calkins, M.E.; Whinna, D.A.; Kohler, C.G.; Souders, M.C.; McDonald-McGinn, D.M.; Zackai, E.H.; Emanuel, B.S.; Gur, R.C.; et al. Psychiatric Disorders in 22q11.2 Deletion Syndrome Are Prevalent but Undertreated. *Psychol. Med.* **2014**, *44*, 1267–1277. [CrossRef] [PubMed]
150. O'Rourke, L.; Murphy, K.C. Recent Developments in Understanding the Relationship between 22q11.2 Deletion Syndrome and Psychosis. *Curr. Opin. Psychiatry* **2019**, *32*, 67–72. [CrossRef] [PubMed]
151. Green, T.; Gothelf, D.; Glaser, B.; Debbane, M.; Frisch, A.; Kotler, M.; Weizman, A.; Eliez, S. Psychiatric Disorders and Intellectual Functioning Throughout Development in Velocardiofacial (22q11.2 Deletion) Syndrome. *J. Am. Acad. Child Adolesc. Psychiatry* **2009**, *48*, 1060–1068. [CrossRef] [PubMed]
152. Bassett, A.S.; Chow, E.W.C.; AbdelMalik, P.; Gheorghiu, M.; Husted, J.; Weksberg, R. The Schizophrenia Phenotype in 22q11 Deletion Syndrome. *AJP* **2003**, *160*, 1580–1586. [CrossRef] [PubMed]
153. Schreiner, M.J.; Lazaro, M.T.; Jalbrzikowski, M.; Bearden, C.E. Converging Levels of Analysis on a Genomic Hotspot for Psychosis: Insights from 22q11.2 Deletion Syndrome. *Neuropharmacology* **2013**, *68*, 157–173. [CrossRef]
154. Whittington, J.; Holland, T. *Prader-Willi Syndrome: Development and Manifestations*; Cambridge University Press: Cambridge, UK, 2004; ISBN 978-1-139-45245-8.
155. Clarke, D.J. Prader-Willi Syndrome and Psychoses. *Br. J. Psychiatry* **1993**, *163*, 680–684. [CrossRef]
156. Bouras, N.; Verhoeven, W.M.A.; Curfs, L.M.G.; Tuinier, S. Prader–Willi Syndrome and Cycloid Psychoses. *J. Intellect. Disabil. Res.* **1998**, *42*, 455–462. [CrossRef]
157. Bouras, N.; Beardsmore, A.; Dorman, T.; Cooper, S.-A.; Webb, T. Affective Psychosis and Prader–Willi Syndrome. *J. Intellect. Disabil. Res.* **1998**, *42*, 463–471. [CrossRef]
158. Soni, S.; Whittington, J.; Holland, A.J.; Webb, T.; Maina, E.N.; Boer, H.; Clarke, D. The Phenomenology and Diagnosis of Psychiatric Illness in People with Prader-Willi Syndrome. *Psychol. Med.* **2008**, *38*, 1505–1514. [CrossRef]
159. Rohrer, J.D.; Isaacs, A.M.; Mizielinska, S.; Mead, S.; Lashley, T.; Wray, S.; Sidle, K.; Fratta, P.; Orrell, R.W.; Hardy, J.; et al. C9orf72 Expansions in Frontotemporal Dementia and Amyotrophic Lateral Sclerosis. *Lancet Neurol.* **2015**, *14*, 291–301. [CrossRef] [PubMed]
160. Snowden, J.S.; Rollinson, S.; Thompson, J.C.; Harris, J.M.; Stopford, C.L.; Richardson, A.M.T.; Jones, M.; Gerhard, A.; Davidson, Y.S.; Robinson, A.; et al. Distinct Clinical and Pathological Characteristics of Frontotemporal Dementia Associated with C9ORF72 Mutations. *Brain* **2012**, *135*, 693–708. [CrossRef]

161. Dobson-Stone, C.; Hallupp, M.; Bartley, L.; Shepherd, C.E.; Halliday, G.M.; Schofield, P.R.; Hodges, J.R.; Kwok, J.B.J. C9ORF72 Repeat Expansion in Clinical and Neuropathologic Frontotemporal Dementia Cohorts. *Neurology* **2012**, *79*, 995. [CrossRef] [PubMed]
162. Ducharme, S.; Bajestan, S.; Dickerson, B.C.; Voon, V. Psychiatric Presentations of C9orf72 Mutation: What Are the Diagnostic Implications for Clinicians? *JNP* **2017**, *29*, 195–205. [CrossRef] [PubMed]
163. Pruessner, M.; Cullen, A.E.; Aas, M.; Walker, E.F. The Neural Diathesis-Stress Model of Schizophrenia Revisited: An Update on Recent Findings Considering Illness Stage and Neurobiological and Methodological Complexities. *Neurosci. Biobehav. Rev.* **2017**, *73*, 191–218. [CrossRef] [PubMed]
164. Howes, O.D.; McCutcheon, R. Inflammation and the Neural Diathesis-Stress Hypothesis of Schizophrenia: A Reconceptualization. *Transl. Psychiatry* **2017**, *7*, e1024. [CrossRef]
165. Howick, J.; Glasziou, P.; Aronson, J.K. The Evolution of Evidence Hierarchies: What Can Bradford Hill's 'Guidelines for Causation' Contribute? *J. R. Soc. Med.* **2009**, *102*, 186–194. [CrossRef]
166. Manu, P.; Correll, C.U.; Wampers, M.; Mitchell, A.J.; Probst, M.; Vancampfort, D.; Hert, M.D. Markers of Inflammation in Schizophrenia: Association vs. Causation. *World Psychiatry* **2014**, *13*, 189–192. [CrossRef]
167. Congrès de Psychiatrie et de Neurologie de Langue Française; Krebs, M.-O. *Signes Précoces de Schizophrénie des Prodromes à la Notion de Prévention*; Dunod: Paris, France, 2015; ISBN 978-2-10-073964-6.
168. McGorry, P.; Killackey, E.; Elkins, K.; Lambert, M.; Lambert, T. RANZCP Clinical Practice Guideline Team for the Treatment of Schizophrenia. Summary Australian and New Zealand Clinical Practice Guideline for the Treatment of Schizophrenia 2003. *Australas. Psychiatry* **2003**, *11*, 136–147. [CrossRef]
169. Greenberg, B.M. The Neurologic Manifestations of Systemic Lupus Erythematosus. *Neurologist* **2009**, *15*, 115. [CrossRef]
170. Debbabi, W.; Essid, A.; Chiboub, M.; Kharrat, I.; Samet, S. Encéphalopathie corticosensible associée à une thyroïdite auto-immune. *Ann. D'endocrinologie* **2017**, *78*, 346. [CrossRef]
171. Branson, B.M.; Handsfield, H.H.; Lampe, M.A.; Janssen, R.S.; Taylor, A.W.; Lyss, S.B.; Clark, J.E. Revised Recommendations for HIV Testing of Adults, Adolescents, and Pregnant Women in Health-Care Settings. *Morb. Mortal. Wkly. Rep. Recomm. Rep.* **2006**, *55*, 1–17.
172. Horowitz, A.; Shifman, S.; Rivlin, N.; Pisanté, A.; Darvasi, A. A Survey of the 22q11 Microdeletion in a Large Cohort of Schizophrenia Patients. *Schizophr. Res.* **2005**, *73*, 263–267. [CrossRef]
173. Bertsias, G.; Ioannidis, J.P.A.; Boletis, J.; Bombardieri, S.; Cervera, R.; Dostal, C.; Font, J.; Gilboe, I.M.; Houssiau, F.; Huizinga, T.; et al. EULAR Recommendations for the Management of Systemic Lupus Erythematosus. Report of a Task Force of the EULAR Standing Committee for International Clinical Studies Including Therapeutics. *Ann. Rheum. Dis.* **2008**, *67*, 195–205. [CrossRef]
174. González-Valcárcel, J.; Rosenfeld, M.R.; Dalmau, J. Differential Diagnosis of Encephalitis Due to Anti-NMDA Receptor Antibodies. *Neurología* **2010**, *25*, 409–413. [CrossRef] [PubMed]
175. León-Caballero, J.; Pacchiarotti, I.; Murru, A.; Valentí, M.; Colom, F.; Benach, B.; Pérez, V.; Dalmau, J.; Vieta, E. Bipolar Disorder and Antibodies against the N-Methyl-d-Aspartate Receptor: A Gate to the Involvement of Autoimmunity in the Pathophysiology of Bipolar Illness. *Neurosci. Biobehav. Rev.* **2015**, *55*, 403–412. [CrossRef]
176. Falkenberg, I.; Benetti, S.; Raffin, M.; Wuyts, P.; Pettersson-Yeo, W.; Dazzan, P.; Morgan, K.D.; Murray, R.M.; Marques, T.R.; David, A.S.; et al. Clinical Utility of Magnetic Resonance Imaging in First-Episode Psychosis. *Br. J. Psychiatry* **2017**, *211*, 231–237. [CrossRef]
177. Lancaster, E. Continuum: The Paraneoplastic Disorders. *Contin. Minneap. Minn.* **2015**, *21*, 452–475. [CrossRef]
178. Fénelon, G. Les hallucinations en neurologie. *Prat. Neurol. FMC* **2014**, *5*, 277–286. [CrossRef]
179. Gresa-Arribas, N.; Titulaer, M.J.; Torrents, A.; Aguilar, E.; McCracken, L.; Leypoldt, F.; Gleichman, A.J.; Balice-Gordon, R.; Rosenfeld, M.R.; Lynch, D.; et al. Antibody Titres at Diagnosis and during Follow-up of Anti-NMDA Receptor Encephalitis: A Retrospective Study. *Lancet Neurol.* **2014**, *13*, 167–177. [CrossRef]
180. Bechter, K.; Deisenhammer, F. Chapter 17—Psychiatric Syndromes Other than Dementia. In *Handbook of Clinical Neurology*; Deisenhammer, F., Teunissen, C.E., Tumani, H., Eds.; Cerebrospinal Fluid in Neurologic Disorders; Elsevier: Amsterdam, The Netherlands, 2017; Volume 146, pp. 285–296.
181. Wang, D.; Hao, Q.; He, L.; He, L.; Wang, Q. LGI1 Antibody Encephalitis—Detailed Clinical, Laboratory and Radiological Description of 13 Cases in China. *Compr. Psychiatry* **2018**, *81*, 18–21. [CrossRef] [PubMed]
182. Hermans, T.; Santens, P.; Matton, C.; Oostra, K.; Heylens, G.; Herremans, S.; Lemmens, G.M.D. Anti-NMDA Receptor Encephalitis: Still Unknown and Underdiagnosed by Physicians and Especially by Psychiatrists? *Acta Clin. Belg.* **2018**, *73*, 364–367. [CrossRef] [PubMed]
183. Voice, J.; Ponterio, J.M.; Lakhi, N. Psychosis Secondary to an Incidental Teratoma: A "Heads-up" for Psychiatrists and Gynecologists. *Arch. Womens Ment. Health* **2017**, *20*, 703–707. [CrossRef] [PubMed]
184. Mantere, O.; Saarela, M.; Kieseppä, T.; Raij, T.; Mäntylä, T.; Lindgren, M.; Rikandi, E.; Stoecker, W.; Teegen, B.; Suvisaari, J. Anti-Neuronal Anti-Bodies in Patients with Early Psychosis. *Schizophr. Res.* **2018**, *192*, 404–407. [CrossRef] [PubMed]
185. Xiao, X.; Gui, S.; Bai, P.; Bai, Y.; Shan, D.; Hu, Y.; Bui-Nguyen, T.M.; Zhou, R. Anti-NMDA-Receptor Encephalitis during Pregnancy: A Case Report and Literature Review. *J. Obstet. Gynaecol. Res.* **2017**, *43*, 768–774. [CrossRef] [PubMed]
186. Singh, R.K.; Bhoi, S.K.; Kalita, J.; Misra, U.K. Cerebral Venous Sinus Thrombosis Presenting Feature of Systemic Lupus Erythematosus. *J. Stroke Cerebrovasc. Dis.* **2017**, *26*, 518–522. [CrossRef] [PubMed]

187. Schou, M.; Sæther, S.G.; Borowski, K.; Teegen, B.; Kondziella, D.; Stoecker, W.; Vaaler, A.; Reitan, S.K. Prevalence of Serum Anti-Neuronal Autoantibodies in Patients Admitted to Acute Psychiatric Care. *Psychol. Med.* **2016**, *46*, 3303–3313. [CrossRef]
188. Pollak, T.A.; McCormack, R.; Peakman, M.; Nicholson, T.R.; David, A.S. Prevalence of Anti-N-Methyl-D-Aspartate (NMDA) Receptor [Corrected] Antibodies in Patients with Schizophrenia and Related Psychoses: A Systematic Review and Meta-Analysis. *Psychol. Med.* **2014**, *44*, 2475–2487. [CrossRef]
189. Bertsias, G.K.; Ioannidis, J.P.A.; Aringer, M.; Bollen, E.; Bombardieri, S.; Bruce, I.N.; Cervera, R.; Dalakas, M.; Doria, A.; Hanly, J.G.; et al. EULAR Recommendations for the Management of Systemic Lupus Erythematosus with Neuropsychiatric Manifestations: Report of a Task Force of the EULAR Standing Committee for Clinical Affairs. *Ann. Rheum. Dis.* **2010**, *69*, 2074–2082. [CrossRef]
190. Steinlin, M.I.; Blaser, S.I.; Gilday, D.L.; Eddy, A.A.; Logan, W.J.; Laxer, R.M.; Silverman, E.D. Neurologic Manifestations of Pediatric Systemic Lupus Erythematosus. *Pediatr. Neurol.* **1995**, *13*, 191–197. [CrossRef]
191. Yancey, C.L.; Doughty, R.A.; Athreya, B.H. Central Nervous System Involvement in Childhood Systemic Lupus Erythematosus. *Arthritis Rheum* **1981**, *24*, 1389–1395. [CrossRef] [PubMed]
192. Weiss, D.B.; Dyrud, J.; House, R.M.; Beresford, T.P. Psychiatric Manifestations of Autoimmune Disorders. *Curr. Treat. Options Neurol.* **2005**, *7*, 413–417. [CrossRef] [PubMed]
193. Buhrich, N.; Cooper, D.A. Requests for Psychiatric Consultation Concerning 22 Patients with AIDS and ARC. *Aust. N. Z. J. Psychiatry* **1987**, *21*, 346–353. [CrossRef]
194. Shulman, L.M.; David, N.J.; Weiner, W.J. Psychosis as the Initial Manifestation of Adult-Onset Niemann-Pick Disease Type C. *Neurology* **1995**, *45*, 1739–1743. [CrossRef]
195. Huang, C.C.; Chu, N.S. Wilson's Disease: Clinical Analysis of 71 Cases and Comparison with Previous Chinese Series. *J. Formos. Med. Assoc.* **1992**, *91*, 502–507.
196. Walterfang, M.; Wood, S.J.; Velakoulis, D.; Copolov, D.; Pantelis, C. Diseases of White Matter and Schizophrenia-like Psychosis. *Aust. N. Z. J. Psychiatry* **2005**, *39*, 746–756. [CrossRef]
197. Albers, J.W.; Fink, J.K. Porphyric Neuropathy. *Muscle Nerve* **2004**, *30*, 410–422. [CrossRef]
198. Qadiri, M.R.; Church, S.E.; McColl, K.E.; Moore, M.R.; Youngs, G.R. Chester Porphyria: A Clinical Study of a New Form of Acute Porphyria. *Br. Med. J. Clin. Res. Ed.* **1986**, *292*, 455–459. [CrossRef]
199. Cooper, J.J.; Ovsiew, F. The Relationship between Schizophrenia and Frontotemporal Dementia. *J. Geriatr. Psychiatry Neurol.* **2013**, *26*, 131–137. [CrossRef]
200. Griswold, K.S.; Del Regno, P.A.; Berger, R.C. Recognition and Differential Diagnosis of Psychosis in Primary Care. *Am. Fam. Physician* **2015**, *91*, 856–863.
201. ALD n° 23—Schizophrénies. Available online: https://www.has-sante.fr/jcms/c_565630/fr/ald-n-23-schizophrenies (accessed on 17 August 2023).
202. Canadian Psychiatric Association Clinical Practice Guidelines. Treatment of Schizophrenia. *Can. J. Psychiatry* **2005**, *50*, 7S–57S.
203. Lehman, A.F.; Lieberman, J.A.; Dixon, L.B.; McGlashan, T.H.; Miller, A.L.; Perkins, D.O.; Kreyenbuhl, J.; American Psychiatric Association; Steering Committee on Practice Guidelines. Practice Guideline for the Treatment of Patients with Schizophrenia, Second Edition. *Am. J. Psychiatry* **2004**, *161*, 1–56. [PubMed]

**Disclaimer/Publisher's Note:** The statements, opinions and data contained in all publications are solely those of the individual author(s) and contributor(s) and not of MDPI and/or the editor(s). MDPI and/or the editor(s) disclaim responsibility for any injury to people or property resulting from any ideas, methods, instructions or products referred to in the content.

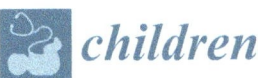 

*Perspective*

# Sympathy-Empathy and the Radicalization of Young People

Nathalie Lavenne-Collot [1,2,3], Nolwenn Dissaux [1,2], Nicolas Campelo [4,5], Charlotte Villalon [1], Guillaume Bronsard [1,2,6,7], Michel Botbol [2,8] and David Cohen [4,9,*]

[1] Service de Psychiatrie de l'Enfant et de l'Adolescent, Centre Hospitalier Universitaire de Brest, 29200 Brest, France
[2] Faculté de Médecine, Université de Bretagne Occidentale, 29200 Brest, France
[3] Laboratoire du Traitement de l'Information Médicale, Inserm U1101, 29200 Brest, France
[4] Service de Psychiatrie de l'Enfant et de l'Adolescent, Assistance Publique-Hôpitaux de Paris, Hôpital Pitié-Salpêtrière, 75006 Paris, France
[5] Laboratoire de Psychologie Clinique, Psychopathologie, Psychanalyse (EA 4056), Institut de Psychologie, Université Paris Descartes, Sorbonne Paris Cité, 92100 Boulogne-Billancourt, France
[6] Département de Sciences Humaines et Sociales, Laboratoire Soins Primaires, Santé Publique, Registre des Cancers de Bretagne Occidentale (EA 7479), 29200 Brest, France
[7] Laboratoire de Santé Publique (EA3279), Aix Marseille Université, 13005 Marseille, France
[8] Professeur Émérite de Psychiatrie de l'Enfant et de l'Adolescent, Université de Bretagne Occidentale, 29000 Brest, France
[9] CNRS, UMR 7222, Institut des Systèmes Intelligents et de Robotiques, Sorbonne Université, 75006 Paris, France
* Correspondence: david.cohen@aphp.fr

**Abstract:** Background: The sympathy-empathy (SE) system is commonly considered a key faculty implied in prosocial behaviors, and SE deficits (also called callous-unemotional traits, CUTs) are associated with nonprosocial and even violent behaviors. Thus, the first intuitive considerations considered a lack of SE among young people who undergo radicalization. Yet, their identification with a cause, their underlying feelings of injustice and grievance, and the other ways in which they may help communities, suggest that they may actually have a lot of empathy, even an excess of it. As a consequence, the links between SE and radicalization remain to be specified. This critical review aims to discuss whether and how SE is associated with developmental trajectories that lead young people to radicalization. Method: We first recall the most recent findings about SE development, based on an interdisciplinary perspective informed by social neuroscience. Then, we review sociological and psychological studies that address radicalization. We will critically examine the intersections between SE and radicalization, including neuroscientific bases and anthropologic modulation of SE by social factors involved in radicalization. Results: This critical review indicates that the SE model should clearly distinguish between sympathy and empathy within the SE system. Using this model, we identified three possible trajectories in young radicalized individuals. In individuals with SE deficit, the legitimization of violence is enough to engage in radicalization. Concerning individuals with normal SE, we hypothesize two trajectories. First, based on SE inhibition/desensitization, individuals can temporarily join youths who lack empathy. Second, based on an SE dissociation, combining emotional sympathy increases for the in-group and cognitive empathy decreases toward the out-group. Conclusions: While confirming that a lack of empathy can favor radicalization, the counterintuitive hypothesis of a favorable SE development trajectory also needs to be considered to better specify the cognitive and affective aspects of this complex phenomenon.

**Keywords:** radicalization; empathy; callous unemotional traits; adolescence; violent extremism

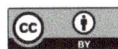

## 1. Introduction

Radicalization is a complex phenomenon representing a significant threat worldwide. Young people, from the age of 12/13, have also been concerned, thus manifesting specific adolescent issues that have not been studied as much as other forms of juvenile violence [1]. While the growing threat of Right-Wing Extremism in some countries is associated with a tendency to recruit older rather than younger people, Islamic radicalization of young people remains an ongoing threat and a social challenge.

In addition, the radicalization epidemic that occurred in European countries from 2014/2015 among young people who converted to Islam without Muslim backgrounds has raised unsolved issues: Why does someone radicalize against his own people? What type of empathy do radicalized people feel for someone toward whom they direct their radicalized violence, given that the development of the sympathy-empathy (SE) system is particularly activated during adolescence and young adulthood [2,3]?

The SE system is commonly involved in prosocial behavior, and SE deficits are associated with many conditions involving antisocial and violent behavior. An SE deficit is notably one of the hallmarks of psychopaths [4] and a subgroup of adolescents with severe conduct disorders and callous unemotional traits (CUTs) [5]. Terrorists do indeed kill civilians in large numbers, suggesting an obvious lack of empathy. However, the recent implications of 'ordinary adolescents' without any psychiatric disorder put this hypothesis into perspective. Moreover, their identification with a cause, the underlying feelings of injustice and grievance that motivate their radicalization, and the other ways in which they may help communities, suggest that they may instead demonstrate preserved empathetic abilities. Indeed, several case studies and surveys have shown that at least some young people actively involved in radicalized violent behaviors, especially suicide bombing, have been strongly committed to volunteering and philanthropic engagement, thus suggesting empathetic capacities that might be higher than those of the usual offenders [6–8]. Moreover, the apparent contradiction between preserved empathy and violent behaviors has already been noticed among adults in other circumstances (e.g., Syndrome E [9]).

In an attempt to overcome this apparent contradiction and compensate for the lack of in-depth data about the role of the SE system in radicalization, this literature review aims to explore whether and how SEs are involved in the radicalization among youth from the first stage of enrollment to possible violent action. In doing so, we will propose that the above-mentioned contradiction may well have to do with SE itself, especially with the modulation of SE by several factors that may be involved in the radicalization of young individuals. Moreover, while the SE model has relevance regardless of age, it is particularly important to consider this with young people as they are progressing through important stages of development and socialization, and this enhances the potential for protective measures to have some concrete effect.

In Section 1, after an introduction to the SE system, we will examine its role in the sensitivity to the face-to-face encounters in group or virtual social media propaganda discourse; we will then consider both the influence of emotional contagion in increasing group identification and the factors involved in the SE-based motivational aspects of radical commitment. These findings will ground the question at the center of this paper detailed in Section 2: the consistency between empathy and radical views and between beliefs and behaviors and the type of empathy that may be involved in this consistency. We will distinguish, in addition to radicalized youth showing a deficit of empathy classically described in young offenders, other radicalized young people who might present a dissociated profile combining a higher affective component (including emotional) contrasting with a weaker cognitive component of empathy.

After a brief intermediary summary, Section 5 will examine how this dissociated profile may be triggered by the environmental context in which radicalization occurs; e.g., in certain contexts, the opposition between in-group and out-group relations may contribute to a dehumanization of the out-group, and this dehumanization may favor violent radicalized behaviors toward the out-group's members.

The last section (Section 4) will lead to one of the main contributions of this this work: the hypothesis of a so-called "double dissociation model of sympathy/empathy in youth radicalization". This model of adolescent radicalization is summarized in Figure 1 from a micro-macro perspective. The first dissociation occurs at the individual level (micro) and is characterized by high affective SE contrasting with diminished cognitive empathy. The second occurs at the intergroup level (macro), thus combining high in-group empathy and low out-group empathy both inversely related according to a parochial empathy effect; i.e., an increase in one leads to a decrease in the other. The implications of these hypotheses will be discussed as well as the need for specific empirical research to confirm them.

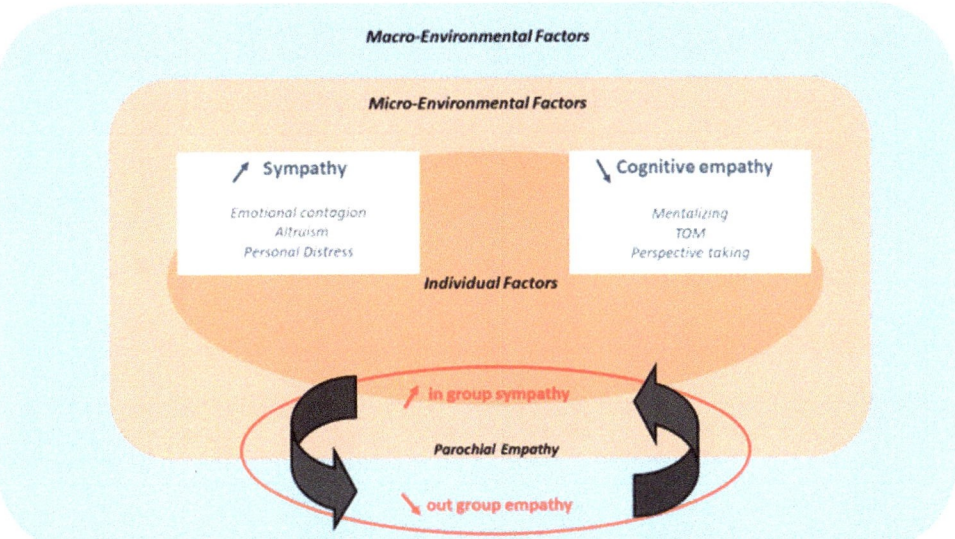

**Figure 1.** The double dissociation model of sympathy/empathy in youth radicalization. The model shows how sympathy/empathy may change during radicalization with a dissociative mode combining increased sympathy (emotional sharing and affective contagion) and decreased empathy (the cognitive ability to feel what the other feels) according to the sympathy/empathy status at the baseline and specific trajectories summarized.

## 2. Relationship between the Sympathy/Empathy System and Radicalization in Young People

### 2.1. The Sympathy/Empathy System

Empathy has a broad understanding in folk psychology and is influenced by information-processing biases, perspective tacking, theory of mind, and reasoning. Empathy is composed of at least a spontaneous transfer of emotion and a concern for others' well-being and has several possible behavioral outcomes, such as altruism, compassion, kindness, liking, and trust [10,11]. Therefore, empathy is a multidimensional construct (with emotional, cognitive and motivational facets) reflecting an ability to feel and understand another person's lived experience and associated mental state while mentally adopting that person's perspective [12]. Empathy encompasses the automatic embodiment of internally feeling what another person is experiencing. Empathy implies emotional processing, a cognitive theory of mind, and self-regulation and relies on the interaction of interacting neural regions within topographically and functionally distinct networks [13]. From an evolutionary perspective, an empathetic response is composed of several layers that build upon each other and remain functionally integrated and related to different levels of empathy. At the core of the empathetic response lies emotional contagion (or sympathy), the middle layer includes empathetic concern, and the outer layer contains perspective-taking and targeted helping [14]. More importantly, this theorization supports a developmental perspective of empathy: while some empathic abilities are present from early infancy, others depend on higher cognitive functions that emerge later in development due to brain progressive maturation under the influence of environmental factors [15].

Empathy is involved in many aspects of emotional processing, notably through the mechanism of emotional sharing (also called emotional contagion or affective resonance or sympathy) [12]. The basic tenet of these models is that observing an action in another individual directly activates the matching neural substrates in the observer through which the action can be understood and leads the observer to vicariously experience similar feelings [16]. This state-matching reaction has been related to simulation theory relying on the mirror neuron system (MNS), which is the first primitive resonance mechanism involved in empathy processes since early infancy [17]. Individual differences in empathy, notably among subjects who score higher on a measure of empathy, activate the subjects' MNS more strongly when the subjects hear about the actions of others [18].

Indeed, emotional contagion refers to sympathy. However, empathy requires the ability to distinguish between simultaneous representations of both the other's and one's own current experiences or feelings [19]. Maintaining a self/other distinction (SOD) is a fundamental prerequisite also supported by neuroimagery data showing that empathy does not involve a complete self-other merging [20]. Notably, SOD permits one to shift from emotional contagion to empathy by distinguishing that the primary source of one's feeling is the perception of someone else's experience. Another important difference relies on an own-body-transformation (OBT) that helps one decenter from oneself into the other's body and mind within a shift from an ego-centered (sympathy) to heterocentered (empathy) perspective [21]. Previous research has demonstrated the existence of separate brain networks recruited from egocentric and allocentric perspectives [22] and decoupling mechanisms between self- and other-centered processes [23]. If perspective-taking also involves executive functions (e.g., inhibition [24]), SOD must be conceived as an independent mechanism that relies on others' brain networks and is related to self-consciousness and awareness in its different dimensions [25]. The best evidence of the essential place of self-awareness in empathy comes from Bischof, who found time synchronicity in the onset of mirror recognition and empathic behaviors for peers during early development [26].

Thus, although empathy is a complex and multifaceted concept [27], it is legitimate to distinguish, as modern neuroscience does, sympathy (affective sharing/emotional contagion) from empathy (a concept that requires being in the other's shoes).

*2.2. Sympathy/Empathy and Sensitivity to Propaganda*

Youth radicalization occurs through both face-to-face group encounters and internet and virtual contacts and is more likely to result when these two processes happen simultaneously [28–30]. Despite their important role in affecting recipients' beliefs, attitudes, and intentions, little is known about individual dispositional factors involved in sensitivity to propaganda whether online or offline [31]. We propose to explore here to what extent empathic abilities may be involved at this early stage of radicalization.

First, SE is involved in the way one reacts to media viewing. SE has been associated with (i) increased physiological activation when one views movie clips containing graphic scenes of horror [32]; (ii) coping strategies [33]; (iii) adoption of altruistic behaviors [34]; and (iv) perception of a higher level of danger severity and risk for oneself when one views victimization stories [35]. One of the most powerful communication tools used by terrorist groups is narratives [36]. The crucial role of narratives in radicalizing adolescents is supported by numerous authors who have highlighted the fundamental place of narratives in building an attractive epic or in mythological storytelling [28,37–40]. The powerful effect of narrative propaganda relies on eliciting affective reactions in the reader [41], and empathy is involved in many aspects of emotional processing, notably through the mechanism of emotional sharing (also called emotional contagion or affective resonance or sympathy) [12].

The main themes and emotions elicited in a propaganda narrative are scenes of victimization (for instance, animal experimentation) that may arouse high empathetic abilities (such as empathetic concern and even compassion) and emotional responses (especially disgust, anger, sadness and guilt) [42,43]. Interestingly, most of these emotions have adaptive and survival values and thus elicit rapid nonconscious responses [44]. More importantly, emotional contagion involves many components: unconscious and automatic mimicry [45] and a conglomerate of somatosensory sensations that facilitate physiological and motor feedback inducing emotion in the receiver. For instance, observing and feeling disgust activate the same sites on the anterior insula and visceral sensations, such as nausea [46]. Disgust is particularly relevant since it is related to violations of internalized moral duties [47], frequently associated with the adoption of obsessive and compulsive behaviors [48] and with dehumanization [49], which occupies a prominent position in radicalization (see below). The limbic system plays an important role in this stage because amygdala activity has been shown to be higher in adolescents than in adults who view social threat-related stimuli [50]; therefore, this first emotional response may be increased.

Several arguments support the idea that emotional contagion or sympathy also has a central place far beyond recruitment [51]. Social psychology emphasizes the central role of emotional contagion in group cohesion [52]. Notably, sharing emotions is an important factor in the differentiation of friends from foes because of an in-group favoritism involved in emotion recognition [53,54]. Moreover, activation of the premotor cortex of the MNS when one observes an action performed by someone else is not neutral for the observer's desires: this activation may increase the attractiveness of the goal pursued by the action. Such mimetic desire involves an influence of the MNS on the brain valuation system (BVS), thereby increasing the value of the goal targeted by the observed [55]. This phenomenon may be an effective way of acquiring new values and behaviors through a mechanism of non-verbal contagion [56].

Second, case reports of young people engaged in radicalization sometimes connect engagement to the repetitive viewing of propaganda movies [37,39]. Importantly, SE involves not only these first bottom-up primitive resonance mechanisms but also higher top-down abilities needed to moderate its effects [12]. Previous research notably showed that repetitive exposure to painful situations might lead to an inhibition of the representation of pain in the observer when painful procedures are inflicted [57]. Interestingly, such sympathy inhibition mechanisms may provide young people engaging in radicalization with the feeling of reaching a superhuman status [39,40,58].

Third, the persuasive effect of narratives relies on narrative transportation, i.e., the ability to be totally immersed in a story [59]. In particular, identification with protagonists of narratives mediates this effect: as readers mentally simulate the events that happen to a character, readers may come to understand what it is like to experience the described events [60]. As empathy perspective-taking is related to mental imagery and transformation aimed at the ability to feel like someone else, empathy perspective-taking should be involved in both narrative transportation and identification. Some studies indeed found a positive correlation between empathy and identification with the characteristics of a story [61]. Interestingly, positive associations were also found between empathy and "fan identity" in media viewing [62], whereas identification with a charismatic leader is supposed to be an important determinant in young radical commitment [63,64].

Recently, in an EEG study, Yoder et al. presented 238 adult participant video clips containing ISIS propaganda (either heroic or social martyr narratives) and collected behavioral measures of appeal, narrative transportation, sympathy/empathy and attraction to terrorism [31]. The findings confirmed that sympathy/empathy plays an important role in psychological predispositions to attraction by terrorism since individuals with higher dispositional empathy reported greater narrative transportation. Moreover, higher empathetic subjects preferred heroic narratives, thereby indicating that at least a subgroup of subjects with high empathy would be the intentional targets of narratives emphasizing individual benefits, notably personal glory and empowerment through sacrifice and righteous violence; this indication is stunning with regard to motivations commonly related to empathy.

### 2.3. Empathy/Sympathy and Radical Group Identification

In the previously mentioned EEG study exploring neural processes impacted by propaganda videos, heroic narratives were associated with electrophysiological patterns accompanying autobiographical remembering [31]. Autobiographical memory deals with identity [65], which is a central issue in adolescents' motivation for radical commitment, according to uncertainty-identity theory [66,67]. Some clinical observations support this self-other identification in radicalized young people; for instance, an adolescent became engaged after viewing a propaganda video showing violence against women who looked like her own mother [63], or reactivating suffering linked to personal family history [64].

Since several authors do not distinguish between empathy (self-other distinction) and sympathy (self-other identification) [27], especially in the field of social psychology, it is rather perspective-taking that is conceived as activating the self-concept and leading perspective-takers to attribute a greater proportion of their self-traits to the other according to the self-other overlap hypothesis [68,69]. In the context of radicalization, some authors have emphasized this identity fusion by using a series of increasingly overlapping circles, one of which represented the self and the others a given group [70,71]. Moreover, we argue that several factors would favor a total loss of SOD (or complete self/other merging) in adolescents as compared to older subjects for the following reasons:

(1) Developmental immaturity of the SE system with regard to the development of top-down regulation abilities. Several studies suggest that adolescents' neural response patterns may differ from adults' patterns in situations that evoke cognitive or emotional empathy [72]. The development of neural circuits underlying empathy from childhood (7 years) to adulthood (40 years) through fMRI starts with emotional empathy that appears earlier than cognitive empathy, but this development also shows a gradual shift from a visceral response to pain as a potential threat to a more detached and regulated appraisal of the stimulus [73]. Neuroimagery studies have shown the following: stronger automatic responses in adolescents who witness another in a painful situation [74]; a negative relationship between empathetic accuracy and brain activation (this relationship is compatible with adolescents becoming immersed in their own emotions while sharing the emotional experience of the target) [75]; and compensatory hyperactivation of emotionally related brain areas to compensate for adolescents' lower emotional empathy ability [76].

(2) SOD is weaker in adolescents due to fragility in self-consciousness and awareness [25,77]. In addition, individual vulnerabilities may also increase this trend. As the development of self-consciousness is closely linked with self-emotional development, SOD has been shown to be disturbed in some psychopathologies such as borderline personality disorder [78].

(3) Collusion between adolescence and radicalization. Emotions and issues elicited by radicalization echo normal adolescent issues (such as guilt, shame, sexuality, and the need for rupture and change), just as the offering of radicalization resonates with adolescents' usual coping mechanisms (such as projective identification, polarized attribution of values, intellectualization, and ascetism) [58,79], thus increasing self-other merging.

(4) Adaptation of propaganda to target. We must acknowledge that recruiters have shown acute abilities in the cognitive aspects of empathy; these abilities are supported by recruiters' ability to propose a wide range of propaganda messages [31] and then to subsequently adapt the message to each specific target [37]. This is not neutral for these young people; the perception of being the target of a perspective-taker have been shown to lead to an important self-other merging [80] as well as a soothing feeling of being understood [81]. This relief of no longer being alone to face uncertainty seems to play an important role in the early stages of the radicalization of young people [79].

Among adolescents, this process may favor bonding with one favorite person, often a charismatic leader [63]. Among young women who became especially affected by recent radicalization [28], this process may promote love fusion with a "charming prince" as frequent "sleeping beauty" storytelling suggests [37,82]. This privileged link then extends to the other members of the terrorist group; research has indeed robustly demonstrated that perspective-taking reduces stereotyping [83–85], with stereotype reduction extending to the whole target group [63,69,86]. This self-other overlap leads to acting stereotypically by adopting the behaviors of the target group [87], thus favoring a loss of personal identity, as highlighted among young radicalized people [88,89].

Taken together, these considerations support that the S/E system may be strongly involved in the process leading to radical group membership. In particular, these findings support the hypothesis that at least some of the young people who engage in radicalization would not be characterized by a lack of empathy per se; normal or even enhanced dispositional empathic capacities, and the interplay of internal and external factors, may, on the contrary, favor a sympathetic relationship with group members, thereby leading to self-identification and an altered sense of identity (or group contagion).

*2.4. Motivational Aspects of SE and Radical Commitment*

2.4.1. Altruism

Another possible implication of empathy in radicalization relies on the importance of the motivational facets of empathy. Empathy includes moral values that involve caring for others' well-being. This intuition is based on empathetic concern, which is the empathy subcomponent that reflects an other-oriented motivation that merges very early in development, i.e., earlier than the full acquisition of theory of mind and verbal abilities [90]. This intuition is the motivational part of what is called altruism.

Youth who engage in radicalization are often driven by humanitarian concerns rather than by violent radicalism [40,91,92]. Moreover, biographies of such youth often reveal pro-altruistic characteristics, such as the realization of humanitarian camps or vocations of medical and social careers, especially among girls [37]. These pro-altruistic characteristics do not always protect these youth from becoming violent extremists; i.e., these characteristics have often been identified and used by ISIS recruiters to select and convert potential violent extremists, particularly among adolescents and young adults [30]. Those who become involved can then give up everything, including family, friends, and usual activities, even when doing so is costly; i.e., becoming involved in violent extremism can lead to martyrdom, or what has been described as an altruistic suicidal behavior [8,93]. These findings show how, according to SE theory, high-level empathy profiles can favor violent actions rather than inhibit them [94].

Moreover, if empathy is commonly associated with unconditionally helping those in need, there is some evidence indicating that several interpersonal factors can interfere; these factors include how similar the target is to the observer [95] or how likable the target is. For example, empathy-related responses to pain in others are significantly reduced when one observes an unfair person receiving pain and when the observation co-occurs with increased activation in reward-related areas; the reduction in empathy-related responses to pain in others is correlated with an expressed desire for revenge [96]. This study underlines that empathy is shaped not only (at least in men) by the evaluation of other people's social behavior but also by the promotion of the physical punishment of unfair opponents; this finding echoes evidence for altruistic punishment. A priori stigmatization of the target may also interfere with empathy, especially if the target is blamed: participants are more sensitive to the pain of targets infected with AIDS as a result of blood transfusion and less sensitive to pain caused by intravenous drug use. Importantly, the more the participants blamed these targets, the less pain the participants attributed to the targets [97].

These findings are all the more important if we consider that people who do not belong to the terrorist group are blamed and perceived as worthless and responsible for the threat [98]. In addition, empathy is also modulated by other factors in intergroup relations; these factors will be further specified.

### 2.4.2. Group Belongingness

Group belongingness is central in adolescence when identity is at stake. In the context of radicalization, youth build new affiliation links in a surrogate family: they exchange names and identities with new sisters and brothers with whom they can find significance [99]. Importantly, brain regions [100] and neurochemical pathways (e.g., oxytocin, see [101]) involved in empathetic concern are similar to those implicated in parental and care-giving behavior selected through evolutionary perspectives across many species, supporting a major role of empathy in group belongingness [102], including in radicalization [103].

### 2.4.3. Self-Regulatory Emotional Control

The failure to apply sufficient self-regulatory emotional control over the shared state leads to the experience of emotional contagion and, in the case of negative emotion, to personal distress (PD) [104]. PD is an aversive emotional reaction to the vicarious experience of another's emotion; this experience results from perceiving another's distress and is similar to the target's state [105]. Importantly, the motivational behavioral response resulting from PD differs from empathetic concern since PD is a self-oriented motivated response [106] that has also been shown to be unrelated to prosocial behaviors [107] in adolescents [108].

Some factors may even foster PD upon empathetic concern, such as (i) psychological state of the observer (especially depression) [104] (depression is frequent among radicalized young people); (ii) exposure to physical rather than psychological pain [109]; and (iii) psychological inflexibility in adolescents' prejudices [110]. Conversely, the adoption of radical views has been shown to reduce PD [111]; therefore, PD may have an important role as an acute coping mechanism possibly involved in the radical belief system.

PD may also mediate the relation between empathy and obedience. The famous Milgram paradigm is a paradigmatic form of dilemma eliciting empathy where people obey an instruction that involves harming another person [112]. Interestingly, using this obedience paradigm in 'virtual' life with virtual reality technology, Cheetham showed an atypical pattern of brain activity distinct from those commonly associated with affect sharing and compatible with PD [113]. These findings provide interesting insight into the way killing people may be perceived as the lesser of two evils when people are under threat (for example, compared to when pain is potentially inflicted on a person's in-group relatives). The obedience paradigm supports the idea that inflicting pain on others may be seen as less important when it is committed under the pressure of an authority figure; this issue is easily transposable to radicalization, given that radicalization is generally influenced by a more or less legitimate religious authority [103].

### 2.4.4. Perceived Injustice or Unfairness

Another determinant motivation for young radical commitment is unfairness [114,115]. Indeed, perceived injustice is an important determinant of radicalization in adolescence [98]. A triggering event that deals with injustice may become a determining factor in acting out [116]. These findings support that radicalized youth may react with stronger resentment when facing justice issues; such a reaction depends highly on the concept of justice sensitivity [117]. While some authors thought justice sensitivity to be linked with emotional components [118], some more recent studies indicate that it is more related to cognitive components of empathy [119]. Experiencing unjust events (directed against oneself or one's community) can intensify justice sensitivity [120]. Interviews with young people who engage in radicalization often contain distressing events, such as emotional deficiencies, trauma, and abandonment [1,121,122]. Interestingly, the severity of past adversity, including adverse life events and childhood trauma [123], can lead to an increase in prosocial and altruistic behavior mediated by empathy [124]. Taken together, these findings suggest that empathy, including justice sensitivity, may be higher in radicalized young people. In addition, social neuroscience studies have shown that when participants are exposed to moral decision-making, cognitive empathy modulates functional connectivity across several domain-general systems, particularly in regions of the prefrontal cortex involved in goal representations in the service of moral decision-making [125]. These findings support that among those with higher empathy, perceiving injustice may provide a strong motivation to act to avoid injustice or restore justice. Generally, this research emphasizes the centrality of the motivational aspects of empathy in radicalization.

## 3. Consistency between Empathy and Radical Beliefs and Behaviors and the Type of Empathy Possibly Involved in Radicalization

### 3.1. Is Empathy Consistent with Radical Views, Beliefs and Behaviors?

Religious fundamentalism represents a distinctive attitude of certainty in the ultimate truth of one's religious faith [126]. The relationship between religious fundamentalism and radicalization in youth is complex. Although some authors have downplayed the role of religious fundamentalism in radicalization [127], several scholars have noted the major role of religious fundamentalism in providing an identity figure [58,128]. However, in regard to strict fundamentalism, radicalization in youth is generally associated with radical views, beliefs and behaviors and can occur outside religion [129].

Although motivational aspects involved in radical views have been largely studied, little is known about the specificities of the cognitive processes and style of radicalized people. Several authors have suggested that cognitive inflexibility, defined as the inability to switch between modes of thinking and changing rules of categories, may predict extremist attitudes [130]. From cognitive functioning [131] to moral reasoning [132], the ability to entertain different perspectives is a crucial mechanism related to empathy. Notably, at least empathy's cognitive aspects, such as perspective-taking and theory of mind, require the individual to hold in mind multiple perceived realities and active considerations of beliefs and views that differ from one's own [133]. For these reasons, it might be natural to assume that these abilities may be decreased under fundamentalism and, more generally, negatively associated with radical thinking.

Importantly, the onset of a heterocentered perspective follows different stages of complexity during development [134]. The operational capacity of such a perspective is acquired between the ages of seven and ten, which is a critical period in the child's development; during this period, the capacity of understanding, interpreting and accepting the plurality of viewpoints emerges [24]. This ability can be altered by neurodevelopmental disorders [135] and environmental factors, e.g., parents' attention to their child's mental states nurtures symbolic abilities [136]. Some authors noticed specificities in the family environment of youth who engage in radicalization, such as absence of countervailing opinions, lack of corrective answers to the subject's radical position [137] and permissive arenas with little response to radical opinion [138]. When radicalization is underway, the isolation of the subject increases this trend even more [103].

Fundamentalism is also generally associated with violence, authoritarianism and aggression and has been negatively associated with empathy [139]. However, personality characteristics driving religious and nonreligious fundamentalism show a divergent relationship between fundamentalism and empathy, as religious fundamentalists scored higher for empathy than nonreligious ones [140]. In addition, empathy networks involve two brain networks that are anatomically dissociable and functionally antagonistic, namely, the task-positive network (TPN) also called the analytic network, and the default mode network (DMN), also referred to as the social brain. These two networks allow different types of thinking related to different belief considerations [141]. The thought process of people cycles between the two networks. In the religious fundamentalist's mind, the DMN appears to dominate, while in the nonreligious fundamentalist's mind, the TPN appears to rule [140]. As a consequence, empathic concern can be linked to hostility in individuals who focus on potential threats to protect what they regard as precious or sacred. Interestingly, the neural basis of sacred value showed activation in the left inferior frontal gyrus, a region associated with rule retrieval, opposite to utilitarian cost–benefit reasoning [142], and this brain region is also the core structure of emotional empathy involved in the MNS [143]. Collectively, these findings suggest that affective empathy may be higher in some radicalized people defined as "devoted actors" (as opposed to rational actors), who are particularly prone to making costly and extreme sacrifices in the defense of sacred values [70].

*3.2. Disentangling Affective and Cognitive Empathy*

Relationships between empathy and radicalization are complex, especially because most studies used multifaceted sympathy/empathy scales that do not enable disentangling the specific links that each component might have with radicalization.

Regarding the cognitive components of empathy, most research has focused on religious beliefs. Several authors have claimed that there is a positive association between mentalizing and belief in God, while considering that the capacity to perceive minds is not limited to human targets [144] and evidence of TOM network activation during prayer [145]. However, other authors found contradictory results [146]. Interestingly, these conflicting results may be related not to the degree but rather to different styles of belief: higher TOM may facilitate symbolic religious belief [147], while at the other extreme, TOM may be negatively related to a tendency to an "overliteral" understanding of language [148]. This overliteral understanding appears to be frequent among religiously radicalized youths [39], as has been previously observed in a population of alexithymic adolescents and young adults [149].

More generally, the literature mostly identifies a positive association between religiosity and empathy [150], cognitive flexibility and openness [151] and prosocial behaviors [152]. The theological account of the relationship between empathy and religion derives from the theory that religion generally promotes helping behavior and openness. Interestingly, some authors directly compared mentalizing measures to empathetic concern and found that the latter was a more robust and substantive correlate of religious belief [153].

Very recent research went further to clarify reciprocal relationships between empathy and religious beliefs. To determine whether holding religious beliefs promotes cognitive flexibility and openness or biases the development of such beliefs, Cristofori et al. studied neurological patients with brain lesions involving the main regions of TOM (notably the VmPFC) [111]. The authors tested two alternative hypotheses: whether empathy promotes religious belief or whether religious belief promotes greater prosocial tendencies. They concluded that, contrary to what was commonly admitted, empathy does not influence the development of religious beliefs, whereas religious cognition (relying on TOM) regulates empathetic responses to others. Interestingly, in this study, the image of God was the mediator between religious cognition and empathy. This echoes previous experiments that showed that among adolescents, an image of God as the "God of mercy" was associated with higher levels of empathy, while an image of God as the "God of justice" was associated with lower levels of empathy. Interestingly, in the same study, the image of God was associated with self-concept and self-esteem [154].

Importantly, if religious cognition modulates empathic abilities, there is serious concern about the potential deleterious effects of sustained radical thinking when shared religious beliefs no longer influence empathetic tendencies. This issue may be particularly important for young people who, between 2015 and 2018, fled France to join the war zones in Syria, as shown by the experts' clinical observations of those returning from Syria in the qualitative study mentioned above [39].

## 4. Intermediary Summary

Let us summarize some key points: (i) empathy is a multifaceted construct, with affective and cognitive components both relying on different brain networks [13]; (ii) possible dissociation between cognitive and affective empathy has been shown in these networks in the context of lesion models [155] and psychopathology [156,157]; (iii) weaker TOM was associated with a greater God image thought that was associated with higher empathic concern [111]; (iv) lower perspective-taking abilities were associated with higher affective empathy among religious fundamentalists [140]; and (v) motivational components may modify the SE system [10,158].

Taken together, these findings support that in addition to radicalized youth possibly showing a deficit of empathy, other youth might present a dissociated profile combining a higher affective (including emotional) component of empathy and weaker cognitive components of empathy driven by motivational components. This can result in a strong adhesion of the emotional system to radical beliefs without adequate cognitive evaluation and criticism.

## 5. Radicalization and Empathy in an Intergroup Context
### 5.1. In-Group vs. Out-Group

The ontogenetic development of empathy shows that empathy constitutes an advanced skill that has been selected to enable thriving within a group context since group living offers several reproductive and long-term survival advantages compared to the advantages of going solo [103]. This suggests a double-edged feature of empathy when considering intergroup context: on the one hand, empathy enables strong cooperation, in-group efficiency and prosperity; on the other hand, when doing so, empathy implies that outsiders are excluded or harmed.

Numerous authors have supported the importance of in-group versus out-group polarization among macroenvironmental factors involved in radicalization (e.g., [98]). According to Social Identity Theory [159], people are inclined to perceive their group as better than most other groups and to develop an 'us and them' perspective as a consequence of this social categorization, leading to antagonism between groups. This categorization also maximizes intergroup differences; this maximization is not without consequences as far as empathy is concerned. Studies of empathy in an intergroup context indeed have shown that group membership can compromise all levels of empathic response (i.e., affective, cognitive, and motivational) and helping behavior [160]. Indeed, despite the common opinion that affective resonance is automatic, group membership can affect its induction in the observer. For instance, in a transcranial magnetic stimulation study, no vicarious mapping of the pain of individuals culturally marked as outgroup members on the basis of their skin color was found [161]. This reduction in emotional sharing in response to outgroup members also extends to emotional pain [162]. Importantly, in these studies, higher levels of racial prejudice were associated with a greater absence of empathetic response to outgroup members. In the same way, cognitive empathy is also modulated by group membership and can lead to biases that affect decision-making [163].

In-group favoritism also exists in group contexts other than ethnicity, for instance, in the context of a sports team [164], but also when group differences are generated artificially by using the minimal group paradigm according to minimal group theory [165]. Notably, Van Bavel showed that an arbitrary temporary novel group can override the effects of predominant group membership by inhibiting automatic racial biases in the context of mixed race teams [166]. As far as religious allegiance is concerned, empathetic response has been shown to be larger when participants viewed a painful event occurring to a hand labeled with their own religion than to a hand labeled with a different religion, and this classifier was generalized successfully to validation experiments in which the in-group condition was based on an arbitrary group assignment [167]. Interestingly, in this study, the neural empathetic response was modulated by minimally differentiating information (e.g., a simple text label indicating another's religious belief).

A very important aspect of intergroup empathy bias is that such bias appears to depend highly on the social motivation of the perceiver. Indeed, various studies have shown that self-categorization along an in-group/out-group distinction is flexible and that recategorization with an arbitrarily defined group may be sufficient to overcome automatic response biases [168]. This is of special importance in the context of radicalization since young people recategorize their group of membership by establishing new kinship relations as an effect of propaganda [103].

Interestingly, social group membership is highly flexible and context-dependent, and not all outgroups elicit the same intergroup empathy bias. Cikara et al. highlighted two critical factors: functional relationships between groups (shared, competing, or independent goals) and relative group status [169]. These findings are of special relevance since the same conditions have been identified among macroenvironmental factors involved in group polarization in radicalization [89,129,170,171].

Previous research has shown that minimal group manipulation can enhance intergroup biases when groups are in competition. Notably, similar group membership between a helper and a target (whether the group is real or artificially determined) reinforced the role of empathy and helping thought. Simply categorizing participants into irrelevant social groups appears to be sufficient to facilitate an in-group bias in empathy for physical pain [172].

Importantly, intergroup empathy bias has been shown to be associated with enhanced hostility and pleasure in response to the out-group target's misfortune (schadenfreude) [173]. In a neuroimaging study involving passionate fans of two baseball teams, in-group team failures were associated with increased activity in neural areas associated with the subjective experience of pain [174]. In contrast, out-group team failures were associated with increased self-reported pleasure and activity in neural areas associated with reward processing. Furthermore, the more positive value (pleasure) participants attached to the rival team's failures, the more willing they were to assault a rival team fan. These results support the idea that outcomes of social group competition can directly affect primary reward-processing neural systems, with implications for intergroup harm [175].

Moreover, dissymmetry of status and resources even without overt competition can affect the intergroup empathy response [176]. These findings may be of special importance in the context of radicalization since, as shown by various authors working specifically with this population, dissymmetry of status and resources (real or symbolic) is an important macroenvironmental factor in hostility toward the out-group [40,98,170].

*5.2. Empathy and Dehumanization*

In regard to violent radicalization, dehumanization of the out-group is also of special importance. Surprisingly, several findings indicate that empathy processes may contribute to dehumanization against the out-group. Dehumanization is enabled by the formation of stereotypes, and research in social cognition firmly establishes that people differentiate each other not simply along an in-group vs. out-group boundary but also according to the extent to which they (dis)-like and (dis)-respect a target. In particular, the stereotype content model organizes beliefs about social groups along two fundamental dimensions: perceived warmth and competence [177].

Although numerous studies support the fact that empathy and specifically perspective-taking components can help form social bonds by decreasing prejudice and stereotyping [69,84,86], other findings indicate that perspective-taking can be a double-edged sword that also leads to exacerbated intergroup relations [178,179]. Indeed, assuming the perspective of a stereotype-consistent target may increase stereotyping when the target individual is highly stereotypic [180] and in the case of the perspective-taker's need for cognitive closure [181]. Moreover, perspective-takers have been shown to be more likely than nonperspective-takers to adopt the negative stereotypical traits and behaviors of the person he or she is perspective-taking with [87].

Importantly, empathy can not only increase stereotyping but also be shaped by the stereotypes that result from it. Fiske examined social groups that elicit dehumanized emotions, such as disgust, and demonstrated that these individuals' judgment is processed in a region anatomically distinct from that which is used in the case of social groups that elicit exclusively social emotions (such as pity, envy, and pride) [49]. These findings suggest that extreme out-groups do not elicit these complex social emotions in the perceiver and that the in-groups judge the out-groups as not experiencing complex emotions in the same way in which the in-group does [182]. These findings are compatible with infrahumanization theory [183], which states that people see some groups as less human than others and suggests that empathy may paradoxically contribute to this less human perception or dehumanization [184].

## 6. Discussion

To understand how empathy as a general concept (with its emotional, cognitive and social levels and its motivational and environmental influences) contributes to radicalization among adolescents and young adults, it is crucial to consider two contradictions.

*6.1. The Contradiction of Empathy*

First, several arguments seriously reduce the hegemonic strength of the commonly admitted empathy-altruism theory. Critically, this depends on the separateness of the self from the other. Without a distinct self and other and without distinct motivations to help the self or the other, it is impossible to detach altruism from egoism [185]. However, studying both sympathy and empathy provides interesting insight into how seemingly similar behaviors can be underpinned by different or even opposite phenomenological realities, especially in martyrdom cases [186]: while some pursue a more narcissistic motivation to die "in apotheosis" [187], others are driven by identity fusion and willingness to fight and die for the in-group [76].

Second, both sympathy and empathy, like social cognition in general, always depend on the context in which they occur [188]. Significantly, this implies that SE failures toward out-groups do not seem to depend on a person's characteristics and that even the most deeply sympathetic person can mute his or her sympathy response to a perceived enemy under certain circumstances. This is especially true in situations such as radicalization, which involves several possible targets of the SE system (in-group members versus out-group members that can become potential victims).

Finally, the best predictor of meaningful intergroup attitudes and behaviors might not be the general capacity for sympathy but rather "parochial empathy" [189] or "intergroup empathy bias" [174], i.e., how empathy is distributed and especially the difference in sympathy felt for the in-group versus the out-group. In other words, the more sympathy one feels for one's own group, the more likely one may be to endorse, support, or commit violence against the out-group and may lose the ability to feel what an out-group individual may feel (lack of empathy). This hypothesis has been confirmed by Bruneau, who found in three different intergroup contexts that out-group empathy inhibited intergroup harm and promoted intergroup helping, whereas in-group sympathy had the opposite effect. In all samples, in-group and out-group sympathy/empathy had independent, significant, and opposite effects on intergroup outcomes, thus controlling trait empathic concern [189].

Thus, at the end of this review, we hypothesize a double dissociation model of empathy in radicalization:

The first dissociation occurs at the individual level and is characterized by high affective SE contrasting with diminished cognitive empathy. This dissociation can lead to a strong identification with the radical group and adherence to a radical belief system due to the absence of adequate emotional regulation and cognitive criticism mechanisms.

The second occurs at the intergroup level, thus combining high in-group empathy and low out-group empathy, both inversely related according to a parochial empathy effect; i.e., an increase in one leads to a decrease in the other.

This double dissociation model is summarized in Figure 1 from a micro-macro perspective, as proposed in Campelo et al.'s model of adolescent radicalization [1]. Importantly, this model has both theoretical and very concrete applications; i.e., this model can explain why programs aimed at increasing empathy to prevent radicalization may have mixed results or even paradoxical effects [190]. In particular, Feddes et al. found unwanted harmful effects, as participants showed increased narcissistic traits (an identified risk factor for radicalization) after the implementation of this type of program among adolescents [191]. Consequently, although it still needs to be confirmed systematically, this model may be a first step toward practical implications of the SE system on countering violent extremism intervention programs.

*6.2. The Contradiction of Radicalization among Adolescents*

The issue of preserved or altered SE systems seems to be quite paradigmatic of a more general apparent contradiction concerning the complex relationships between radicalization and young people. Indeed, the same contradictory results are found in the literature regarding the prevalence of mental disorders among radicalized adolescents and young adults: while several authors emphasize their rarity and the lack of any consistent psychiatric or psychological profile, other studies consider that the situation is less contrasted and show an overrepresentation of mental disorders in the radicalized young [39,192,193]. This contradiction is probably due to the imprecise definition of radicalization: which motive do we refer to when we talk about radicalization? Is there a radical claim? Is there an intention? Does radicalization mean acting out? This is a crucial issue because while radicalization may be a "new symptom" related to the complex issues of adolescence in some cases [79], serious acts may also be the prerogative of another youth typology that differs from the first one.

Significantly, forensic reports of youth involved in serious terrorist acts also find characteristic unemotional traits with real sympathy deficits in which ideology is used as violence. Some authors even underlined the observation that the radicalized individuals who committed radicalized murders were all engaged in severe delinquent behaviors when they were adolescents [121], especially in France [194], thus raising the possibility that these individuals should be considered as a particular subgroup needing to be specifically studied to shed some more clinical light on their psychopathological profile. However, a comparison between minors convicted in France for 'criminal association to commit terrorism' and teenagers convicted for nonterrorist delinquency shows that adolescents engaged in radicalization and terrorism do not have a significant prevalence of psychiatric disorders, suicidal tendencies or lack of SE. In addition, radicalized adolescents show better intellectual skills, insight capacities, coping strategies and less history of nonterrorist delinquent acts prior radicalization [195].

Those who join the ranks of terrorists to become warriors may constitute a third subgroup on the empathy continuum. If an SE deficit is not primitive in some radicalized individuals, it may perhaps emerge as the radicalization unfolds through a desensitization mechanism or a temporary dissociation. Some insight into this temporary dissociation in the SE system can be gained by exploring recent works about Syndrome E [196]. In particular, some authors have stressed the importance of distinguishing between the rule system and the brain valuation system which do not rely on the same brain networks. Obsessive compliance with rituals and procedures, such as those observed in radicalization, may play a major role in the rule system overriding the BVS [197]. In other cases, BVS may also be completely deviated by cognitive distortions amplified by transmission and social contagion in the belief, for example, that killing heretics can get one into heaven [56]. To favor violent engagement, recruiters have indeed well understood the power of dehumanizing out-group members to help recruits move to violent radicalization. Adolescents may be more concerned with this rule system overriding the BVS, considering the immaturity of their decision-making system [198]. This hypothesis however remains to be confirmed.

Moreover, the SE system is not a reliable source of information in moral decision-making as this system is unconsciously and rapidly modulated by various social signals and situational/motivational factors [10]. In the case of adolescent radicalization, we individuate at least three different contributions related to three possible trajectories of young radicalized individuals according to their SE status at baseline. In Figure 2, we describe the SE trajectories related to these three subgroups.

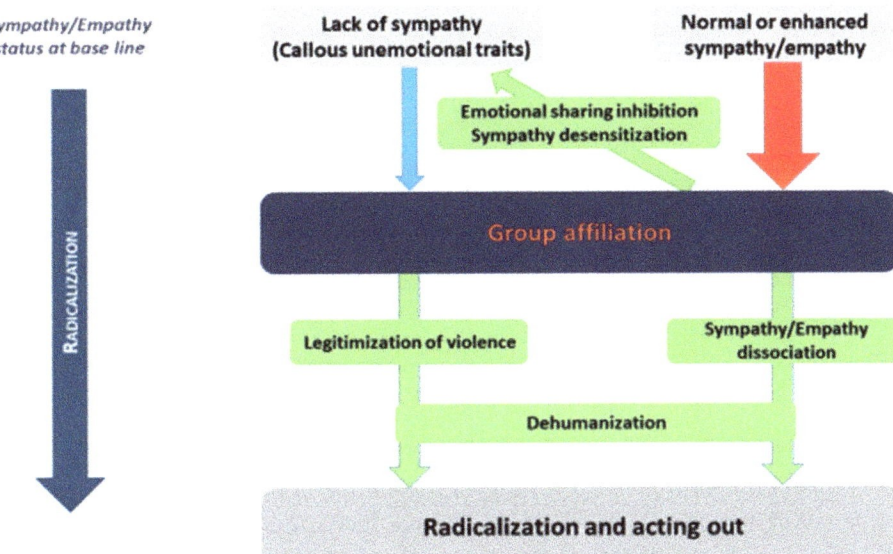

**Figure 2.** The sympathy/empathy trajectories and changes during radicalization according to the youth empathy status at the baseline. The model shows 3 trajectories in green. Among individuals with a lack of sympathy (callous unemotional traits, left), legitimization of violence is enough to engage in radicalization and violence. Concerning individuals with normal or enhanced sympathy/empathy, we hypothesize two trajectories. First, based on sympathy inhibition/desensitization, the individual joins youth who lack empathy. The second trajectory is based on a sympathy/empathy dissociation (that combines ↗ sympathy for the in-group and ↘ cognitive empathy toward the out-group) favoring violence against the out-group.

The first group includes individuals with SE deficits or CUTs. In this group, legitimization of violence would be sufficient to move toward radicalization and possibly violent acts.

For individuals with normal SE, we hypothesize two trajectories: First, based on SE sympathy inhibition/desensitization, the individual joins youths who lack empathy. Second, based on an SE dissociation combining an increase in emotional sympathy for the in-group and a decrease in cognitive empathy for the out-group, the individual favors violence toward the out-group.

This hypothesis requires further work to be demonstrated notably by assessing empathetic functioning of young individuals at different levels of the radicalization process and among different sub-groups. Especially, comparison could be made between empathic profile of non-terrorist habitual offenders, terrorist offenders, and actual terrorist perpetrators. This assessment may go further Bronsard's study [195] by using a multidimensional scale, such as the Interpersonal Reactivity Index (IRI), which would allow for separate assessment of cognitive and affective components of empathy. More specifically, the search for correlations between, one the one hand, the different components of empathy and, on the other hand, the loss of SOD (such as that assessed by Sheikh et al. [70]) might confirm that increased affective contrasting with decreased cognitive empathic abilities may be involved in identity fusion with terrorists groups.

Furthermore, given the previously demonstrated relationships between empathetic profiles and personality traits [199–201] as well as psychopathological alterations [202], correlational analyses may be usefully conducted to examine whether some psychopathological categories highlighted in the literature about radicalization might reflect some dominance of one SE profile over the other. This may be particularly useful in some extreme cases, such as that studied by Merari [7] who compared psychological profiles of suicide bombers with terrorists imprisoned for unrelated offences. They found in the first group more avoidant-dependent personality disorders (60% vs. 17%), fewer psychopathic tendencies (0% vs. 25%) as well as fewer impulsive and unstable tendencies (27% vs. 67%).

Finally, without claiming to find a strict concordance between both neurocognitive and psychopathological profiles, we may assume that, following the three SE trajectories shown in Figure 2: (i) youth with low cognitive and affective developmental empathy may be predominant among youth with psychopathic traits (engaging in chronic antisocial behavior); (ii) youth with high affective empathy and low cognitive empathy in youth with borderline/paranoid functioning (with high inhibition of sympathy referring) (iii) youth with increased sympathy for in-group and reduced cognitive empathy for out-group may be predominant in youth with severe narcissistic vulnerability with dependency traits.

## 7. Conclusions

The conclusion of this review supports the hypothesis that young radicalized people may have specificities in the development of SE abilities leading to an atypical SE profile that differs from that of young people with other nonprosocial behaviors.

We claim that, far from being rooted in a total deficit in SE, radicalization may be related to a paradox combining normal and even enhanced empathy promoted by the accentuation of social identification with the in-group as opposed to poor empathy for the out-group. More importantly, preserved and even enhanced in-group empathic abilities among these individuals may play a crucial role in the violence directed at an out-group. Moreover, a hypothetical dissociation between higher affective versus lower cognitive empathic abilities may favor an overload of the emotional system with no compensation of either top-down regulation mechanisms or cognitive criticism. A transitory dissociation of empathy leading to radical acting out may occur, but such a dissociation remains scarce in youth. It should nevertheless be underlined that this profile may apply only to some of the adolescents who engage in radicalization and should not lead to the trivialization of this issue or to exclusion of the fact that some of them may indeed present a frank empathy deficit.

Finally, SE development suggests differences among evolutionary trajectories that may lead to radicalization. This is an essential prerequisite for a better specification of the clinical and neuropsychological underpinnings of radicalization, not only to detect but also to develop, at both the individual and collective levels, the appropriate responses.

**Author Contributions:** All authors have read and agreed to the published version of the manuscript.

**Funding:** This research received no external funding.

**Institutional Review Board Statement:** Not applicable.

**Informed Consent Statement:** Not applicable.

**Data Availability Statement:** Not applicable.

**Acknowledgments:** The authors thank Alain Berthoz for his careful review and advice on this work.

**Conflicts of Interest:** The authors declare no conflict of interest.

## References

1. Campelo, N.; Oppetit, A.; Neau, F.; Cohen, D.; Bronsard, G. Who are the European youths willing to engage in radicalisation? A multidisciplinary review of their psychological and social profiles. *Eur. Psychiatry J. Assoc. Eur. Psychiatr.* **2018**, *52*, 1–14. [CrossRef] [PubMed]
2. Allemand, M.; Steiger, A.E.; Fend, H.A. Empathy development in adolescence predicts social competencies in adulthood. *J. Pers.* **2015**, *83*, 229–241. [CrossRef] [PubMed]
3. Van der Graaff, J.; Carlo, G.; Crocetti, E.; Koot, H.M.; Branje, S. Prosocial Behavior in Adolescence: Gender Differences in Development and Links with Empathy. *J. Youth. Adolesc.* **2018**, *47*, 1086–1099. [CrossRef] [PubMed]
4. Van Dongen, J.D.M. The Empathic Brain of Psychopaths: From Social Science to Neuroscience in Empathy. *Front. Psychol.* **2020**, *11*, 695. [CrossRef]

5. Milone, A.; Cerniglia, L.; Cristofani, C.; Inguaggiato, E.; Levantini, V.; Masi, G.; Paciello, M.; Simone, F.; Muratori, P. Empathy in Youths with Conduct Disorder and Callous-Unemotional Traits. *Neural. Plast.* **2019**, *2019*, 9638973. [CrossRef]
6. Bruneau, E. The Marionettes's Threads: How the Tugs of Empathy and Dehumanization Can Lead to Intergroup Conflict. In *The Brains That Pull the Triggers*; Fried, I., Berthoz, A., Mirdal, M., Eds.; Odile Jacob: Paris, France; New York, NY, USA, 2021; pp. 336–351.
7. Merari, A.; Diamant, I.; Bibi, A.; Broshi, Y.; Zakin, G. Personality Characteristics of "Self Martyrs"/"Suicide Bombers" and Organizers of Suicide Attacks. *Terror. Polit. Violence* **2009**, *22*, 87–101. [CrossRef]
8. Pedahzur, A.; Perliger, A.; Weinberg, L. Altruism and Fatalism: The Characteristics of Palestinian Suicide Terrorists. *Deviant. Behav.* **2003**, *24*, 405–423. [CrossRef]
9. Fried, I. Syndrome E. *Lancet* **1997**, *350*, 1845–1847. [CrossRef]
10. Decety, J. Why Empathy Is Not a Reliable Source of Information in Moral Decision Making. *Curr. Dir. Psychol. Sci.* **2021**, *30*, 425–430. [CrossRef]
11. Botbol, M.; Garret-Gloanec, N.; Besse, A. L'empathie: Au Carrefour des Sciences et de la Clinique. Doin: Montrogue, France, 2014; p. 332.
12. Decety, J.; Jackson, P.L. The functional architecture of human empathy. *Behav. Cogn. Neurosci. Rev.* **2004**, *3*, 71–100. [CrossRef]
13. Decety, J. The neural pathways, development and functions of empathy. *Curr. Opin. Behav. Sci.* **2015**, *3*, 1–6. [CrossRef]
14. De Waal, F.B.M. The "Russian doll" model of empathy and imitation. In *On Being Moved: From Mirror Neurons to Empathy*; John Benjamins Publishing: Amsterdam, The Netherlands, 2007; pp. 49–69.
15. Tooley, U.A.; Bassett, D.S.; Mackey, A.P. Environmental influences on the pace of brain development. *Nat. Rev. Neurosci.* **2021**, *22*, 372–384. [CrossRef] [PubMed]
16. Preston, S. A perception-action model for empathy. *Empathy Ment. Illn.* **2007**, *1*, 428–447.
17. Gallese, V. The roots of empathy: The shared manifold hypothesis and the neural basis of intersubjectivity. *Psychopathology* **2003**, *36*, 171–180. [CrossRef] [PubMed]
18. Gazzola, V.; Aziz-Zadeh, L.; Keysers, C. Empathy and the somatotopic auditory mirror system in humans. *Curr. Biol.* **2006**, *16*, 1824–1829. [CrossRef]
19. Lamm, C.; Bukowski, H.; Silani, G. From shared to distinct self-other representations in empathy: Evidence from neurotypical function and socio-cognitive disorders. *Philos. Trans. R. Soc. B Biol. Sci.* **2016**, *371*, 20150083. [CrossRef]
20. Jackson, P.; Brunet, E.; Meltzoff, A.; Decety, J. Empathy examined through the neural mechanisms involved in imagining how I feel versus how you feel pain. *Neuropsychologia* **2006**, *44*, 752–761. [CrossRef]
21. Berthoz, A.; Thirioux, B. A Spatial and Perspective Change Theory of the Difference Between Sympathy and Empathy. *Paragrana* **2010**, *19*, 32–61. [CrossRef]
22. Lambrey, S.; Doeller, C.; Berthoz, A.; Burgess, N. Imagining being somewhere else: Neural basis of changing perspective in space. *Cereb. Cortex* **2012**, *22*, 166–174. [CrossRef]
23. Thirioux, B.; Mercier, M.R.; Blanke, O.; Berthoz, A. The cognitive and neural time course of empathy and sympathy: An electrical neuroimaging study on self-other interaction. *Neuroscience* **2014**, *267*, 286–306. [CrossRef]
24. Berthoz, A. Physiologie du changement de point de vue. *L'Empathie. Odile Jacob* **2004**, 251–275. [CrossRef]
25. Steinbeis, N. The role of self-other distinction in understanding others' mental and emotional states: Neurocognitive mechanisms in children and adults. *Philos. Trans. R. Soc. B Biol. Sci.* **2016**, *371*, 20150074. [CrossRef]
26. Bischof-Köhler, D. Self object and interpersonal emotions. Identification of own mirror image, empathy and prosocial behavior in the 2nd year of life. *Z Psychol. Z Angew Psychol.* **1994**, *202*, 349–377.
27. Håkansson Eklund, J.; Summer Meranius, M. Toward a consensus on the nature of empathy: A review of reviews. *Patient. Educ. Couns.* **2021**, *104*, 300–307. [CrossRef] [PubMed]
28. Oppetit, A.; Campelo, N.; Bouzar, L.; Pellerin, H.; Hefez, S.; Bronsard, G.; Bouzar, D.; Cohen, D. Do Radicalized Minors Have Different Social and Psychological Profiles From Radicalized Adults? *Front. Psychiatry* **2019**, *10*, 644. [CrossRef] [PubMed]
29. Hassan, G.; Brouillette-Alarie, S.; Séraphin, A.; Frau-Meigs, D.; Lavoie, L.; Fetiu, A.; Varela, W.; Borokhovski, E.; Venkatesh, V.; Rousseau, S.; et al. Exposure to Extremist Online Content Could Lead to Violent Radicalization: A Systematic Review of Empirical Evidence. *Int. J. Dev. Sci.* **2018**, *12*, 1–18. [CrossRef]
30. Sikkens, E.; van San, M.; Sieckelinck, S.; Boeije, H.; de Winter, M. Participant Recruitment through Social Media: Lessons Learned from a Qualitative Radicalization Study Using Facebook. *Field. Methods* **2017**, *29*, 130–139. [CrossRef]
31. Yoder, K.J.; Ruby, K.; Pape, R.; Decety, J. EEG distinguishes heroic narratives in ISIS online video propaganda. *Sci. Rep.* **2020**, *10*, 19593. [CrossRef]
32. Tamborini, R.; Stiff, J.; Heidel, C. Reacting to Graphic Horror: A Model of Empathy and Emotional Behavior. *Commun. Res.* **1990**, *17*, 616–640. [CrossRef]
33. Hoffner, C.A.; Levine, K.J. Enjoyment of Mediated Fright and Violence: A Meta-Analysis. In *Mass Media Effects Research: Advances Through Meta-Analysis*; Lawrence Erlbaum Associates Publishers: Mahwah, NJ, USA, 2007; pp. 215–244.
34. Bagozzi, R.P.; Moore, D.J. Public Service Advertisements: Emotions and Empathy Guide Prosocial Behavior. *J. Mark.* **1994**, *58*, 56–70. [CrossRef]
35. Zillmann, D. Mechanisms of emotional involvement with drama. *Poetics* **1995**, *23*, 33–51. [CrossRef]

36. Holbrook, D.; Taylor, M. Terrorism as Process Narratives: A Study of Pre-Arrest Media Usage and the Emergence of Pathways to Engagement. *Terror. Polit. Violence* **2019**, *31*, 1307–1326. [CrossRef]
37. Bouzar, D.; Martin, M. Pour quels motifs les jeunes s'engagent-ils dans le djihad? *Neuropsychiatr. Enfance. Adolesc.* **2016**, *64*, 353–359. [CrossRef]
38. Pemberton, A.; Aarten, P.G.M. Narrative in the Study of Victimological Processes in Terrorism and Political Violence: An Initial Exploration. *Stud. Confl. Terror.* **2018**, *41*, 541–556. [CrossRef]
39. Botbol, M.; Campelo, N.; Lacour-Gonay, C.; Roche-Rabreau, D.; Teboul, R.; Chambry, J.; Michel, D. Psychiatrie et Radicalisation—Rapport du groupe de travail de la Fédération Française de Psychiatrie. 2020. Available online: https://fedepsychiatrie.fr/wp-content/uploads/2020/08/FFP-Rapport-Psychiatrie-et-Radicalisation-Janvier-2020-V3.pdf (accessed on 15 September 2022).
40. Khosrokhavar, F. Radicalisation. Éditions de la Maison des Sciences de L'homme: Paris, France, 2017.
41. Mar, R.A.; Oatley, K.; Djikic, M.; Mullin, J. Emotion and narrative fiction: Interactive influences before, during, and after reading. *Cogn. Emot.* **2011**, *25*, 818–833. [CrossRef]
42. Braddock, K. The utility of narratives for promoting radicalization: The case of the Animal Liberation Front. *Dyn. Asymmetric. Confl.* **2014**, *8*, 38–59. [CrossRef]
43. Mahood, S.; Rane, H. Islamist narratives in ISIS recruitment propaganda. *J. Int. Commun.* **2017**, *23*, 15–35. [CrossRef]
44. Lazarus, R. *Emotion and Adaptation*; Oxford University Press: New York, NY, USA, 1991.
45. Holland, A.C.; O'Connell, G.; Dziobek, I. Facial mimicry, empathy, and emotion recognition: A meta-analysis of correlations. *Cogn. Emot.* **2021**, *35*, 150–168. [CrossRef]
46. Wicker, B.; Keysers, C.; Plailly, J.; Royet, J.P.; Gallese, V.; Rizzolatti, G. Both of us disgusted in My insula: The common neural basis of seeing and feeling disgust. *Neuron* **2003**, *40*, 655–664. [CrossRef]
47. Oaten, M.; Stevenson, R.J.; Williams, M.A.; Rich, A.N.; Butko, M.; Case, T.I. Moral Violations and the Experience of Disgust and Anger. *Front. Behav. Neurosci.* **2018**, *12*, 179. [CrossRef]
48. Bhikram, T.; Abi-Jaoude, E.; Sandor, P. OCD: Obsessive-compulsive disgust? The role of disgust in obsessive-compulsive disorder. *J. Psychiatry Neurosci. JPN* **2017**, *42*, 300–306. [CrossRef] [PubMed]
49. Harris, L.T.; Fiske, S.T. Social groups that elicit disgust are differentially processed in mPFC. *Soc. Cogn. Affect. Neurosci.* **2007**, *2*, 45–51. [CrossRef] [PubMed]
50. Hare, T.A.; Tottenham, N.; Galvan, A.; Voss, H.U.; Glover, G.H.; Casey, B.J. Biological substrates of emotional reactivity and regulation in adolescence during an emotional go-nogo task. *Biol. Psychiatry* **2008**, *63*, 927–934. [CrossRef] [PubMed]
51. Van Stekelenburg, J. Radicalization and Violent Emotions. *PS Polit. Sci. Polit.* **2017**, *50*, 936–939. [CrossRef]
52. Barsade, S. The Ripple Effect: Emotional Contagion and Its Influence on Group Behavior. *Adm. Sci. Q.* **2002**, *47*, 644–675. [CrossRef]
53. Lazerus, T.; Ingbretsen, Z.A.; Stolier, R.M.; Freeman, J.B.; Cikara, M. Positivity bias in judging ingroup members' emotional expressions. *Emotion* **2016**, *16*, 1117–1125. [CrossRef]
54. Weisbuch, M.; Ambady, N. Affective divergence: Automatic responses to others' emotions depend on group membership. *J. Pers. Soc. Psychol.* **2008**, *95*, 1063–1079. [CrossRef] [PubMed]
55. Lebreton, M.; Kawa, S.; Forgeot d'Arc, B.; Daunizeau, J.; Pessiglione, M. Your goal is mine: Unraveling mimetic desires in the human brain. *J. Neurosci. Off. J. Soc. Neurosci.* **2012**, *32*, 7146–7157. [CrossRef]
56. Pessiglione, M. The brain Valuation System That Pulls the trigger. In *The Brains That Pull the Triggers*; Fried, I., Berthoz, A., Mirdal, M., Eds.; Odile Jacob: Paris, France; New York, NY, USA, 2020; pp. 313–330.
57. Cheng, Y.; Lin, C.P.; Liu, H.L.; Hsu, Y.Y.; Lim, K.E.; Hung, D.; Decety, J. Expertise Modulates the Perception of Pain in Others. *Curr. Biol.* **2007**, *17*, 1708–1713. [CrossRef]
58. Benslama, F. The subjective impact of the jihadist offer. *Interdiscip. J. Relig. Transform. Contemp. Soc.* **2016**, *2*, 75–85. [CrossRef]
59. Busselle, R.; Bilandzic, H. Fictionality and Perceived Realism in Experiencing Stories: A Model of Narrative Comprehension and Engagement. *Commun. Theory* **2008**, *18*, 255–280. [CrossRef]
60. Graaf, A.; Hoeken, H.; Sanders, J.; Beentjes, J. Identification as a Mechanism of Narrative Persuasion. *Commun Res.* **2011**, *29*, 39. [CrossRef]
61. Argo, J.J.; Zhu, R.; Dahl, D.W. Article JD served as editor and BS served as associate editor for this. Fact or Fiction: An Investigation of Empathy Differences in Response to Emotional Melodramatic Entertainment. *J. Consum. Res.* **2008**, *34*, 614–623. [CrossRef]
62. Taylor, L. Investigating Fans of Fictional Texts: Fan Identity Salience, Empathy, and Transportation. *Psychol. Pop. Media Cult.* **2014**, *1*, 4. [CrossRef]
63. Schuurman, B.; Horgan, J. Rationales for terrorist violence in homegrown jihadist groups: A case study from The Netherlands. *Aggress. Violent Behav.* **2016**, *27*, 55–63. [CrossRef]
64. Bazex, H.; Mensat, J.Y. Qui sont les djihadistes français? Analyse de 12 cas pour contribuer à l'élaboration de profils et à l'évaluation du risque de passage à l'acte. *Ann. Méd.-Psychol. Rev. Psychiatr.* **2016**, *174*, 257–265. [CrossRef]
65. Prebble, S.C.; Addis, D.R.; Tippett, L.J. Autobiographical memory and sense of self. *Psychol. Bull.* **2013**, *139*, 815–840. [CrossRef]
66. Hogg, M.A.; Kruglanski, A.; van den Bos, K. Uncertainty and the Roots of Extremism. *J. Soc. Issues* **2013**, *69*, 407–418. [CrossRef]
67. Ludot, M.; Radjack, R.; Moro, M.R. Radicalisation djihadiste et psychiatrie de l'adolescent. *Neuropsychiatry Enfance. Adolesc.* **2016**, *64*, 522–528. [CrossRef]

68. Davis, M.H.; Conklin, L.; Smith, A.; Luce, C. Effect of perspective taking on the cognitive representation of persons: A merging of self and other. *J. Pers. Soc. Psychol.* **1996**, *70*, 713–726. [CrossRef]
69. Galinsky, A.D.; Moskowitz, G.B. Perspective-taking: Decreasing stereotype expression, stereotype accessibility, and in-group favoritism. *J. Pers. Soc. Psychol.* **2000**, *78*, 708–724. [CrossRef] [PubMed]
70. Sheikh, H.; Gómez, Á.; Atran, S. Empirical evidence for the devoted actor model. *Curr. Anthropol.* **2016**, *57*, S13. [CrossRef]
71. Swann, W.B.; Jetten, J.; Gómez, Á.; Whitehouse, H.; Bastian, B. When group membership gets personal: A theory of identity fusion. *Psychol. Rev.* **2012**, *119*, 441–456. [CrossRef] [PubMed]
72. Khanjani, Z.; Mosanezhad jeddi, E.; Hekmati, I.; Khalilzade, S.; Etemadinia, M.; Andalib, M. Comparison of Cognitive Empathy, Emotional Empathy, and Social Functioning in Different Age Groups. *Aust. Psychol.* **2015**, *50*, 80–85. [CrossRef]
73. Decety, J.; Michalska, K. Neurodevelopmental changes in the circuits underlying empathy and sympathy from childhood to adulthood. *Dev. Sci.* **2010**, *13*, 886–899. [CrossRef]
74. Mella, N.; Studer, J.; Gilet, A.L.; Labouvie-Vief, G. Empathy for Pain from Adolescence through Adulthood: An Event-Related Brain Potential Study. *Front. Psychol.* **2012**, *3*, 501. [CrossRef]
75. Kral, T.R.A.; Solis, E.; Mumford, J.A.; Schuyler, B.S.; Flook, L.; Rifken, K.; Patsenko, E.G.; Davidson, R.J. Neural correlates of empathic accuracy in adolescence. *Soc. Cogn. Affect. Neurosci.* **2017**, *12*, 1701–1710. [CrossRef]
76. Kim, E.J.; Son, J.W.; Park, S.K.; Chung, S.; Ghim, H.R.; Lee, S.; Shin, C.; Kim, S.; Ju, G. Cognitive and Emotional Empathy in Young Adolescents: An fMRI Study. Soa–Chongsonyon Chongsin Uihak. *J. Child. Adolesc. Psychiatry* **2020**, *31*, 121–130.
77. Sebastian, C.; Burnett, S.; Blakemore, S.J. Development of the self-concept during adolescence. *Trends Cogn. Sci.* **2008**, *12*, 441–446. [CrossRef]
78. Baptista, A.; Cohen, D.; Jacquet, P.O.; Chambon, V. The Cognitive, Ecological, and Developmental Origins of Self-Disturbance in Borderline Personality Disorder. *Front. Psychiatry* **2021**, *12*, 707091. [CrossRef]
79. Rolling, J.; Corduan, G. La radicalisation, un nouveau symptôme adolescent? *Neuropsychiatry Enfance. Adolesc.* **2017**, *66*. [CrossRef]
80. Goldstein, N.J.; Vezich, I.S.; Shapiro, J.R. Perceived perspective taking: When others walk in our shoes. *J. Pers. Soc. Psychol.* **2014**, *106*, 941–960. [CrossRef] [PubMed]
81. Rogers, C.R. Empathic: An unappreciated way of being. *Couns. Psychol.* **1975**, *5*, 2–10. [CrossRef]
82. Karagiannis, E. European Converts to Islam: Mechanisms of Radicalization. *Polit. Relig. Ideol.* **2012**, *13*, 99–113. [CrossRef]
83. Galinsky, A.; Ku, G.; Wang, C.S. Perspective-Taking and Self-Other Overlap: Fostering Social Bonds and Facilitating Social Coordination. *Group Process. Intergroup Relat.* **2005**, *8*, 109–124. [CrossRef]
84. Vescio, T.K.; Sechrist, G.B.; Paolucci, M.P. Perspective taking and prejudice reduction: The mediational role of empathy arousal and situational attributions. *Eur. J. Soc. Psychol.* **2003**, *33*, 455–472. [CrossRef]
85. Finlay, K.; Stephan, W. Improving Intergroup Relations: The Effects of Empathy on Racial Attitudes. *J. Appl. Soc. Psychol.* **2006**, *30*, 1720–1737. [CrossRef]
86. Batson, C.; Polycarpou, M.; Harmon-Jones, E.; Imhoff, H.; Mitchener, E.; Bednar, L.; Klein, T.; Highberger, L. Empathy and Attitudes: Can Feeling for a Member of a Stigmatized Group Improve Feelings Toward the Group? *J. Pers. Soc. Psychol.* **1997**, *72*, 105–118. [CrossRef]
87. Galinsky, A.D.; Wang, C.S.; Ku, G. Perspective-takers behave more stereotypically. *J. Pers. Soc. Psychol.* **2008**, *95*, 404–419. [CrossRef]
88. Smith, L.G.E.; Blackwood, L.; Thomas, E.F. The Need to Refocus on the Group as the Site of Radicalization. *Perspect. Psychol. Sci.* **2020**, *15*, 327–352. [CrossRef]
89. Ferguson, N.; McAuley, J.W. Dedicated to the cause: Identity development and violent extremism. *Eur. Psychol.* **2021**, *26*, 6–14. [CrossRef]
90. Davidov, M.; Zahn-Waxler, C.; Roth-Hanania, R.; Knafo, A. Concern for Others in the First Year of Life: Theory, Evidence, and Avenues for Research. *Child Dev. Perspect.* **2013**, *7*, 126–131. [CrossRef]
91. Khosrokhavar, F. Les trajectoires des jeunes jihadistes français. *Etudes* **2015**, *6*, 33–44.
92. Campelo, N.; Bouzar, L.; Oppetit, A.; Pellerin, H.; Hefez, S.; Bronsard, G.; Cohen, D.; Bouzar, D. Joining the Islamic State from France between 2014 and 2016: An observational follow-up study. *Palgrave Commun.* **2018**, *4*, 1–10. [CrossRef]
93. Paraschakis, A.; Michopoulos, I.; Douzenis, A. Profile of Islamic suicide bombers: A literature review. *Eur. Psychiatry* **2016**, *33*, 754.
94. Batson, C.D.; Batson, J.G.; Slingsby, J.K.; Harrell, K.L.; Peekna, H.M.; Todd, R.M. Empathic joy and the empathy-altruism hypothesis. *J. Pers. Soc. Psychol.* **1991**, *61*, 413–426. [CrossRef]
95. Batson, C.D.; Sager, K.; Garst, E.; Kang, M.; Rubchinsky, K.; Dawson, K. Is empathy-induced helping due to self–other merging? *J. Pers. Soc. Psychol.* **1997**, *73*, 495–509. [CrossRef]
96. Singer, T.; Seymour, B.; O'Doherty, J.P.; Stephan, K.E.; Dolan, R.J.; Frith, C.D. Empathic neural responses are modulated by the perceived fairness of others. *Nature* **2006**, *439*, 466–469. [CrossRef]
97. Decety, J.; Echols, S.; Correll, J. The blame game: The effect of responsibility and social stigma on empathy for pain. *J. Cogn. Neurosci.* **2010**, *22*, 985–997. [CrossRef] [PubMed]
98. Doosje, B.; Loseman, A.; van den Bos, K. Determinants of Radicalization of Islamic Youth in the Netherlands: Personal Uncertainty, Perceived Injustice, and Perceived Group Threat. *J. Soc. Issues* **2013**, *69*, 586–604. [CrossRef]
99. Kruglanski, A.W.; Gelfand, M.J.; Bélanger, J.J.; Sheveland, A.; Hetiarachchi, M.; Gunaratna, R. The psychology of radicalization and deradicalization: How significance quest impacts violent extremism. *Polit. Psychol.* **2014**, *35*, 69–93. [CrossRef]

100. FeldmanHall, O.; Dalgleish, T.; Evans, D.; Mobbs, D. Empathic concern drives costly altruism. *NeuroImage* **2015**, *105*, 347–356. [CrossRef]
101. Barchi-Ferreira, A.; Osório, F. Associations between oxytocin and empathy in humans: A systematic literature review. *Psychoneuroendocrinology* **2021**, *129*, 105268. [CrossRef]
102. Decety, J.; Svetlova, M. Putting together phylogenetic and ontogenetic perspectives on empathy. *Dev. Cogn. Neurosci.* **2012**, *2*, 1–24. [CrossRef] [PubMed]
103. Decety, J.; Pape, R.; Workman, C.I. A multilevel social neuroscience perspective on radicalization and terrorism. *Soc. Neurosci.* **2018**, *13*, 511–529. [CrossRef] [PubMed]
104. Decety, J.; Lamm, C. Empathy versus personal distress: Recent evidence from social neuroscience. In *The Social Neuroscience of Empathy*; MIT Press: Cambridge, MA, USA, 2009.
105. Singer, T.; Lamm, C. The social neuroscience of empathy. *Ann. Acad. Sci.* **2009**, *1156*, 81–96. [CrossRef]
106. Batson, C.D.; Fultz, J.; Schoenrade, P.A. Distress and empathy: Two qualitatively distinct vicarious emotions with different motivational consequences. *J. Pers.* **1987**, *55*, 19–39. [CrossRef]
107. Eisenberg, N.; Fabes, R.A.; Miller, P.A.; Fultz, J.; Shell, R.; Mathy, R.M.; Reno, R.R. Relation of sympathy and personal distress to prosocial behavior: A multimethod study. *J. Pers. Soc. Psychol.* **1989**, *57*, 55–66. [CrossRef] [PubMed]
108. Eisenberg, N.; Fabes, R.A.; Schaller, M.; Miller, P.A. Sympathy and personal distress: Development, gender differences, and interrelations of indexes. *New Dir. Child Dev.* **1989**, *44*, 107–126. [CrossRef]
109. Fabi, S.; Weber, L.; Leuthold, H. Empathic concern and personal distress depend on situational but not dispositional factors. *PLoS ONE* **2019**, *14*, e0225102. [CrossRef]
110. Valdivia-Salas, S.; Martín-Albo, J.; Cruz, A.; Villanueva-Blasco, V.J.; Jiménez, T.I. Psychological Flexibility with Prejudices Increases Empathy and Decreases Distress Among Adolescents: A Spanish Validation of the Acceptance and Action Questionnaire–Stigma. *Front. Psychol.* **2021**, *11*, 3911. [CrossRef]
111. Cristofori, I.; Zhong, W.; Cohen-Zimerman, S.; Bulbulia, J.; Gordon, B.; Krueger, F.; Grafman, J. Brain networks involved in the influence of religion on empathy in male Vietnam War veterans. *Sci. Rep.* **2021**, *11*, 11047. [CrossRef] [PubMed]
112. Milgram, S. Behavioral Study of obedience. *J. Abnorm. Soc. Psychol.* **1963**, *67*, 371–378. [CrossRef]
113. Cheetham, M.; Pedroni, A.F.; Antley, A.; Slater, M.; Jäncke, L. Virtual milgram: Empathic concern or personal distress? Evidence from functional MRI and dispositional measures. *Front. Hum. Neurosci.* **2009**, *3*, 29. [CrossRef] [PubMed]
114. Van den Bos, K. Unfairness and Radicalization. *Annu. Rev. Psychol.* **2020**, *71*, 563–588. [CrossRef]
115. Charkawi, W.; Dunn, K.; Bliuc, A.M. The influences of social identity and perceptions of injustice on support to violent extremism. *Behav. Sci. Terror. Polit. Aggress.* **2021**, *13*, 177–196. [CrossRef]
116. Leuzinger-Bohleber, M. From Free Speech to IS—Pathological Regression of Some Traumatized Adolescents from a Migrant Background in Germany. *Int. J. Appl. Psychoanal. Stud.* **2016**, *13*, 213–223. [CrossRef]
117. Schmitt, M.; Baumert, A.; Gollwitzer, M.; Maes, J. The Justice Sensitivity Inventory: Factorial Validity, Location in the Personality Facet Space, Demographic Pattern, and Normative Data. *Soc. Justice Res.* **2010**, *23*, 211–238. [CrossRef]
118. Baumert, A.; Schmitt, M. Justice Sensitivity. In *Handbook of Social Justice and Research*; Springer: Berlin/Heidelberg, Germany, 2016.
119. Decety, J.; Yoder, K.J. Empathy and motivation for justice: Cognitive empathy and concern, but not emotional empathy, predict sensitivity to injustice for others. *Soc. Neurosci.* **2016**, *11*, 1–14. [CrossRef] [PubMed]
120. Wijn, R.; Bos, K. Toward a better understanding of the justice judgment process: The influence of fair and unfair events on state justice sensitivity. *Eur. J. Soc. Psychol.* **2010**, *40*, 1294–1301. [CrossRef]
121. Simi, P.; Sporer, K.; Bubolz, B.F. Narratives of Childhood Adversity and Adolescent Misconduct as Precursors to Violent Extremism: A Life-Course Criminological Approach. *J. Res. Crime Delinq.* **2016**, *53*, 536–563. [CrossRef]
122. Koehler, D. Violent extremism, mental health and substance abuse among adolescents: Towards a trauma psychological perspective on violent radicalization and deradicalization. *J. Forensic Psychiatry Psychol.* **2020**, *31*, 455–472. [CrossRef]
123. Greenberg, D.M.; Baron-Cohen, S.; Rosenberg, N.; Fonagy, P.; Rentfrow, P.J. Elevated empathy in adults following childhood trauma. *PLoS ONE* **2018**, *13*, e0203886. [CrossRef] [PubMed]
124. Lim, D.; DeSteno, D. Suffering and compassion: The links among adverse life experiences, empathy, compassion, and prosocial behavior. *Emotion* **2016**, *16*, 175–182. [CrossRef] [PubMed]
125. Yoder, K.J.; Decety, J. The Good, the Bad, and the Just: Justice Sensitivity Predicts Neural Response during Moral Evaluation of Actions Performed by Others. *J. Neurosci.* **2014**, *34*, 4161–4166. [CrossRef]
126. Altemeyer, B.; Hunsberger, B.E. Authoritarianism, religious fundamentalism, quest, and prejudice. *Int. J. Psychol. Relig.* **1992**, *2*, 113–133. [CrossRef]
127. Roy, O. *Le Djihad et la mort*; Seuil: Paris, France, 2016.
128. Verkuyten, M. Religious Fundamentalism and Radicalization Among Muslim Minority Youth in Europe. *Eur. Psychol.* **2018**, *23*, 21–31. [CrossRef]
129. McCauley, C.; Moskalenko, S. Mechanisms of Political Radicalization: Pathways Toward Terrorism. *Terror. Polit. Violence* **2008**, *20*, 415–433. [CrossRef]
130. Zmigrod, L.; Rentfrow, P.; Robbins, T. Cognitive Inflexibility Predicts Extremist Attitudes. *Front. Psychol.* **2019**, *10*, 989. [CrossRef]
131. Piaget, J. The moral judgment of the child. Harcourt, Brace: Oxford, UK, 1932.
132. Kohlberg, L. Moral stages and moralization. A cognitive developmental approach. *J. Study Educ. Dev.* **1982**, *5*, 33–51. [CrossRef]

133. Kloo, D.; Perner, J.; Aichhorn, M.; Schmidhuber, N. Perspective taking and cognitive flexibility in the Dimensional Change Card Sorting (DCCS) task. *Cogn. Dev.* **2010**, *25*, 208–217. [CrossRef]
134. Hirai, M.; Muramatsu, Y.; Nakamura, M. Role of the Embodied Cognition Process in Perspective-Taking Ability during Childhood. *Child Dev.* **2020**, *91*, 214–235. [CrossRef] [PubMed]
135. Gauthier, S.; Anzalone, S.M.; Cohen, D.; Zaoui, M.; Chetouani, M.; Villa, F.; Berthoz, A.; Xavier, J. Behavioral Own-Body-Transformations in Children and Adolescents With Typical Development, Autism Spectrum Disorder, and Developmental Coordination Disorder. *Front. Psychol.* **2018**, *9*, 676. [CrossRef]
136. Meins, E.; Fernyhough, C.; Arnott, B.; Leekam, S.R.; de Rosnay, M. Mind-mindedness and theory of mind: Mediating roles of language and perspectival symbolic play. *Child Dev.* **2013**, *84*, 1777–1790. [CrossRef] [PubMed]
137. Sikkens, E.; van San, M.; Sieckelinck, S.; de Winter, M. Parents' Perspectives on Radicalization: A Qualitative Study. *J. Child Fam. Stud.* **2018**, *27*, 2276–2284. [CrossRef] [PubMed]
138. San, M.; Sieckelinck, S.; Winter, M. Ideals adrift: An educational approach to radicalization. *Ethics Educ.* **2013**, *8*, 276–289. [CrossRef]
139. Bradley, C. The Interconnections Between Religious Fundamentalism, Spirituality and the Four Dimensions of Empathy. *Sociol. Fac. Publ.* **2009**, *51*.
140. Friedman, J.P.; Jack, A.I. What Makes You So Sure? Dogmatism, Fundamentalism, Analytic Thinking, Perspective Taking and Moral Concern in the Religious and Nonreligious. *J. Relig. Health.* **2018**, *57*, 157–190. [CrossRef]
141. Jack, A.I.; Friedman, J.P.; Boyatzis, R.E.; Taylor, S.N. Why Do You Believe in God? Relationships between Religious Belief, Analytic Thinking, Mentalizing and Moral Concern. *PLoS ONE* **2016**, *11*, e0149989.
142. Pretus, C.; Hamid, N.; Sheikh, H.; Ginges, J.; Tobeña, A.; Davis, R.; Villarroya, O.; Atran, S. Neural and Behavioral Correlates of Sacred Values and Vulnerability to Violent Extremism. *Front. Psychol.* **2018**. [CrossRef]
143. Li, Y.; Li, W.; Zhang, T.; Zhang, J.; Jin, Z.; Li, L. Probing the role of the right inferior frontal gyrus during Pain-Related empathy processing: Evidence from fMRI and TMS. *Hum. Brain Mapp.* **2020**, *42*, 1518–1531. [CrossRef]
144. Gervais, W.M. Perceiving Minds and Gods: How Mind Perception Enables, Constrains, and Is Triggered by Belief in Gods. *Perspect. Psychol. Sci. J. Assoc. Psychol. Sci.* **2013**, *8*, 380–394. [CrossRef] [PubMed]
145. Schjoedt, U.; Stødkilde-Jørgensen, H.; Geertz, A.W.; Roepstorff, A. Highly religious participants recruit areas of social cognition in personal prayer. *Soc. Cogn. Affect. Neurosci.* **2009**, *4*, 199–207. [CrossRef] [PubMed]
146. Vonk, J.; Pitzen, J. Believing in other minds: Accurate mentalizing does not predict religiosity. *Personal. Individ. Differ.* **2017**, *115*, 70–76. [CrossRef]
147. Lillard, A.S.; Kavanaugh, R.D. The contribution of symbolic skills to the development of an explicit theory of mind. *Child Dev.* **2014**, *85*, 1535–1551. [CrossRef] [PubMed]
148. Happé, F.G.E. An advanced test of theory of mind: Understanding of story characters' thoughts and feelings by able autistic, mentally handicapped, and normal children and adults. *J. Autism Dev. Disord.* **1994**, *24*, 129–154. [CrossRef] [PubMed]
149. Speranza, M.; Corcos, M.; Guilbaud, O.; Loas, G.; Jeammet, P. Alexithymia, Personality, and Psychopathology. *Am. J. Psychiatry* **2005**, *162*, 1029–1030. [CrossRef]
150. Watson, P.; Hood, R.; Morris, R. Dimensions of Religiosity and Empathy. *J. Psychol. Christ.* **1985**, *4*, 73–85.
151. Saroglou, V. Religion and the five factors of personality: A meta-analytic review. *Pers. Individ. Differ.* **2002**, *32*, 15–25. [CrossRef]
152. Batson, C.; Gray, R.A. Religious orientation and helping behavior: Responding to one's own or the victim's needs? *J. Personal. Soc. Psychol.* **1981**, *40*, 511–520. [CrossRef]
153. Łowicki, P.; Zajenkowski, M.; Cappellen, P.V. It's the heart that matters: The relationships among cognitive mentalizing ability, emotional empathy, and religiosity. *Personal. Individ. Differ.* **2020**, *161*, 109976. [CrossRef]
154. Francis, L.J.; Croft, J.S.; Pyke, A. Religious diversity, empathy, and God images: Perspectives from the psychology of religion shaping a study among adolescents in the UK. In *Religion, Education and Society*; Routledge: London, UK, 2014.
155. Shamay-Tsoory, S.; Aharon-Peretz, J.; Perry, D. Two Systems for Empathy: A Double Dissociation Between Emotional and Cognitive Empathy in Inferior Frontal Gyrus Versus Ventromedial Prefrontal Lesions. *Brain J. Neurol.* **2008**, *132*, 617–627. [CrossRef]
156. Pino, M.C.; De Berardis, D.; Mariano, M.; Vellante, F.; Serroni, N.; Valchera, A.; Valenti, M.; Mazza, M. Two systems for empathy in obsessive-compulsive disorder: Mentalizing and experience sharing. *Rev. Bras. Psiquiatr.* **2016**, *38*, 307–313. [CrossRef] [PubMed]
157. Kerr-Gaffney, J.; Harrison, A.; Tchanturia, K. Cognitive and Affective Empathy in Eating Disorders: A Systematic Review and Meta-Analysis. *Front. Psychiatry* **2019**, *10*, 102. [CrossRef]
158. Hein, G.; Singer, T. I feel how you feel but not always: The empathic brain and its modulation. *Curr. Opin. Neurobiol.* **2008**, *18*, 153–158. [CrossRef]
159. Tajfel, H.; Turner, J.C. An integrative theory of inter-group conflict. In *The Social Psychology of Inter-Group Relations*; Brooks/Cole: Monterey, CA, USA, 1979.
160. Fourie, M.; Subramoney, S.; Gobodo-Madikizela, P. A Less Attractive Feature of Empathy: Intergroup Empathy Bias. In *Empathy: An Evidencebased Interdisciplinary Perspective*; INTECH: London, UK, 2017.
161. Avenanti, A.; Sirigu, A.; Aglioti, S.M. Racial bias reduces empathic sensorimotor resonance with other-race pain. *Curr. Biol.* **2010**, *20*, 1018–1022. [CrossRef] [PubMed]

162. Gutsell, J.; Inzlicht, M. Intergroup differences in the sharing of emotive states: Neural evidence of an empathy gap. *Soc. Cogn. Affect. Neurosci.* **2011**, *7*, 596–603. [CrossRef]
163. Olenski, A.R.; Zimerman, A.; Coussens, S.; Jena, A.B. Behavioral Heuristics in Coronary-Artery Bypass Graft Surgery. *N. Engl. J. Med.* **2020**, *382*, 778–779. [CrossRef]
164. Hein, G.; Silani, G.; Preuschoff, K.; Batson, C.D.; Singer, T. Neural responses to ingroup and outgroup members' suffering predict individual differences in costly helping. *Neuron* **2010**, *68*, 149–160. [CrossRef]
165. Tajfel, H.; Billig, M.G.; Bundy, R.P.; Flament, C. Social categorization and intergroup behaviour. *Eur. J. Soc. Psychol.* **1971**, *1*, 149–178. [CrossRef]
166. Van Bavel, J.J.; Packer, D.J.; Cunningham, W.A. The Neural Substrates of In-Group Bias: A Functional Magnetic Resonance Imaging Investigation. *Psychol. Sci.* **2008**, *19*, 1131–1139. [CrossRef]
167. Vaughn, D.; Savjani, R.; Cohen, M.; Eagleman, D. Empathic Neural Responses Predict Group Allegiance. *Front. Hum. Neurosci.* **2018**, *12*, 302. [CrossRef] [PubMed]
168. Amodio, D.M. The neuroscience of prejudice and stereotyping. *Nat. Rev. Neurosci.* **2014**, *15*, 670–682. [CrossRef]
169. Cikara, M.; Van Bavel, J. The Neuroscience of Intergroup Relations: An Integrative Review. *Perspect. Psychol. Sci.* **2014**, *9*, 245–274. [CrossRef]
170. Doosje, B.; Moghaddam, F.M.; Kruglanski, A.W.; de Wolf, A.; Mann, L.; Feddes, A.R. Terrorism, radicalization and de-radicalization. *Curr. Opin. Psychol.* **2016**, *11*, 79–84. [CrossRef]
171. Moghaddam, F.M. The staircase to terrorism: A psychological exploration. *Am. Psychol.* **2005**, *60*, 161–169. [CrossRef]
172. Montalan, B.; Lelard, T.; Godefroy, O.; Mouras, H. Behavioral Investigation of the Influence of Social Categorization on Empathy for Pain: A Minimal Group Paradigm Study. *Front. Psychol.* **2012**, *3*, 389. [CrossRef]
173. Cikara, M.; Fiske, S.T. Their pain, our pleasure: Stereotype content and schadenfreude. *Ann. Acad. Sci.* **2013**, *1299*, 52–59. [CrossRef]
174. Cikara, M.; Botvinick, M.M.; Fiske, S.T. Us Versus Them: Social Identity Shapes Neural Responses to Intergroup Competition and Harm. *Psychol. Sci.* **2011**, *22*, 306–313. [CrossRef]
175. Cikara, M.; Jenkins, A.C.; Dufour, N.; Saxe, R. Reduced self-referential neural response during intergroup competition predicts competitor harm. *NeuroImage* **2014**, *96*, 36–43. [CrossRef] [PubMed]
176. Trawalter, S.; Hoffman, K.M.; Waytz, A. Racial bias in perceptions of others' pain. *PLoS ONE* **2012**, *7*, e48546. [CrossRef]
177. Fiske, S.; Cuddy, A.J.C.; Glick, P. Universal dimensions of social cognition: Warmth and competence. *Trends Cogn. Sci.* **2007**, *11*, 77–83. [CrossRef] [PubMed]
178. Vorauer, J.D.; Sucharyna, T.A. Potential negative effects of perspective-taking efforts in the context of close relationships: Increased bias and reduced satisfaction. *J. Pers. Soc. Psychol.* **2013**, *104*, 70–86. [CrossRef]
179. Vorauer, J.D.; Martens, V.; Sasaki, S.J. When trying to understand detracts from trying to behave: Effects of perspective taking in intergroup interaction. *J. Pers. Soc. Psychol.* **2009**, *96*, 811–827. [CrossRef] [PubMed]
180. Skorinko, J.L.; Sinclair, S.A. Perspective taking can increase stereotyping: The role of apparent stereotype confirmation. *J. Exp. Soc. Psychol.* **2013**, *49*, 10–18. [CrossRef]
181. Sun, S.; Zuo, B.; Wu, Y.; Wen, F. Does perspective taking increase or decrease stereotyping? The role of need for cognitive closure. *Pers. Individ. Differ.* **2016**, *94*, 21–25. [CrossRef]
182. Harris, L.T.; Fiske, S.T. Dehumanizing the lowest of the low: Neuroimaging responses to extreme out-groups. *Psychol. Sci.* **2006**, *17*, 847–853. [CrossRef]
183. Leyens, J.P.; Rodríguez, A.; Rodriguez-Torres, R.; Gaunt, R.; Paladino, M.; Vaes, J.; Demoulin, S. Psychological Essentialism and the Differential Attribution of Uniquely Human Emotions to Ingroups and Outgroups. *Eur. J. Soc. Psychol.* **2001**, *31*, 395–411. [CrossRef]
184. Fiske, S. How Ordinary People Become Violent: Dehumanizing Out-Groups. In *The Brains That Pull the Triggers*; Fried, I., Berthoz, A., Mirdal, M., Eds.; Odile Jacob: Paris, France; New York, NY, USA, 2021; pp. 146–159.
185. Cialdini, R.B.; Schaller, M.; Houlihan, D.; Arps, K.; Fultz, J.; Beaman, A.L. Empathy-based helping: Is it selflessly or selfishly motivated? *J. Pers. Soc. Psychol.* **1987**, *52*, 749–758. [CrossRef]
186. Perry, S.; Hasisi, B. Rational Choice Rewards and the Jihadist Suicide Bomber. *Terror Polit Violence.* **2015**, *27*, 53–80. [CrossRef]
187. Zagury Zagury, D. Du deuil de soi à l'idéal en apothéose. In *Idéal et Cruauté*; Editions lignes: Paris, France, 2015.
188. Todorov, A.; Harris, L.T.; Fiske, S. Toward socially inspired social neuroscience. *Brain Res.* **2006**, *1079*, 76–85. [CrossRef]
189. Bruneau, E.; Cikara, M.; Saxe, R. Parochial Empathy Predicts Reduced Altruism and the Endorsement of Passive Harm. *Soc. Psychol. Pers. Sci.* **2017**, *8*, 934–942. [CrossRef]
190. Bruneau, E.; Saxe, R. The Power of Being Heard: The Benefits of "Perspective-Giving" in the Context of Intergroup Conflict. *J. Exp. Soc. Psychol.* **2012**, *48*, 855–866. [CrossRef]
191. Feddes, A.; Mann, L.; Doosje, B. Increasing self-esteem and empathy to prevent violent radicalization: A longitudinal quantitative evaluation of a resilience training focused on adolescents with a dual identity. *J. Appl. Soc. Psychol.* **2015**, *45*, 400–411. [CrossRef]
192. Misiak, B.; Samochowiec, J.; Bhui, K.; Schouler-Ocak, M.; Demunter, H.; Kuey, L.; Raballo, A.; Gorwood, P.; Frydecka, D.; Dom, G. A systematic review on the relationship between mental health, radicalization and mass violence. *Eur. Psychiatry* **2019**, *56*, 51–59. [CrossRef] [PubMed]

193. Coid, J.; Bhui, K.; Macmanus, D.; Kallis, C.; Bebbington, P.; Ullrich, S. Extremism, religion and psychiatric morbidity in a population-based sample of young men. *Br. J. Psychiatry* **2016**, *209*. [CrossRef] [PubMed]
194. Botbol, M. Clinical Approach to Difficult Adolescents: Implication for Syndrome E. In *The Brains That Pull the Triggers*; Fried, I., Berthoz, A., Mirdal, M., Eds.; Odile Jacob: Paris, France; New York, NY, USA, 2021; pp. 277–292.
195. Bronsard, G.; Cohen, D.; Diallo, I.; Pellerin, H.; Varnoux, A.; Podlipski, M.A.; Gerardin, P.; Boyer, L.; Campelo, N. Adolescents Engaged in Radicalisation and Terrorism: A Dimensional and Categorical Assessment. *Front. Psychiatry* **2022**, *12*, 774063. [CrossRef]
196. Berthoz, A.; Thirioux, B. Empathy, Sympathy, Empathy Breakdown and Dehumanization: New Phenomenological and Neurobiological H. In *The Brains That Pull The Triggers*; Fried, I., Berthoz, A., Mirdal, M., Eds.; Odile Jacob: Paris, France; New York, NY, USA, 2021; pp. 168–180.
197. Koechlin, E. Neural Cognitive Foundations of Rule Compliance in Humans. In *The Brains That Pull The Triggers*; Fried, I., Berthoz, A., Mirdal, M., Eds.; Odile Jacob: Paris, France; New York, NY, USA, 2021; pp. 257–276.
198. Ernst, M.; Pine, D.S.; Hardin, M. Triadic model of the neurobiology of motivated behavior in adolescence. *Psychol. Med.* **2006**, *36*, 299–312. [CrossRef]
199. Wai, M.; Tiliopoulos, N. The affective and cognitive empathic nature of the dark triad of personality. *Pers. Individ. Differ.* **2012**, *52*, 794–799. [CrossRef]
200. Paulhus, D.L.; Williams, K.M. The Dark Triad of personality: Narcissism, Machiavellianism, and psychopathy. *J. Res. Pers.* **2002**, *36*, 556–563. [CrossRef]
201. Czarna, A.Z.; Wróbel, M.; Dufner, M.; Zeigler-Hill, V. Narcissism and Emotional Contagion: Do Narcissists "Catch" the Emotions of Others? *Soc. Psychol. Pers. Sci.* **2015**, *6*, 318–324. [CrossRef]
202. Dinsdale, N.; Crespi, B.J. The borderline empathy paradox: Evidence and conceptual models for empathic enhancements in borderline personality disorder. *J. Pers. Disord.* **2013**, *27*, 172–195. [CrossRef] [PubMed]

MDPI
St. Alban-Anlage 66
4052 Basel
Switzerland
www.mdpi.com

*Children* Editorial Office
E-mail: children@mdpi.com
www.mdpi.com/journal/children

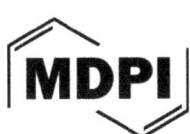

Disclaimer/Publisher's Note: The statements, opinions and data contained in all publications are solely those of the individual author(s) and contributor(s) and not of MDPI and/or the editor(s). MDPI and/or the editor(s) disclaim responsibility for any injury to people or property resulting from any ideas, methods, instructions or products referred to in the content.